Cytokines in the Treatment of Infectious Diseases

Options for the Modulation of Host Defense

edited by

B.-J. KULLBERG and J.W.M. VAN DER MEER

University Hospital Nijmegen,
Department of Medicine,
Division of General Internal Medicine,
Nijmegen, The Netherlands

Reprinted from *Biotherapy*, Volume 7, Nos. 3–4 (1994)

Kluwer Academic Publishers
Dordrecht / Boston / London

A C.I.P. Catalogue record for this book is available from the Library of Congress

ISBN 0-7923-3267-9

Published by Kluwer Academic Publishers,
P.O. Box 17, 3300 AA Dordrecht, The Netherlands.

Kluwer Academic Publishers incorporates
the publishing programmes of
D. Reidel, Martinus Nijhoff, Dr W. Junk and MTP Press.

Sold and distributed in the U.S.A. and Canada
by Kluwer Academic Publishers,
101 Philip Drive, Norwell, MA 02061, U.S.A.

In all other countries, sold and distributed
by Kluwer Academic Publishers Group,
P.O. Box 322, 3300 AH Dordrecht, The Netherlands.

Cover illustration: Electromicrograph of a cerebral postcapillary venule of a mouse infected with *Plasmodium berhei*. Endothelial cell having phagocytozed intravascular material – a step in the pathogenesis of cerebral malaria. Courtesy of W.M.C. Eling, Ph.D., Catholic University Nijmegen, the Netherlands.

Printed on acid-free paper

Printed in the Netherlands

Contents

Introduction 149

1. Cytokines in the treatment of virus infections 151
N.B. Finter

2. Interleukin-1 and related pro-inflammatory cytokines in the treatment of bacterial infections in neutropenic and non-neutropenic animals 161
J.W.M. van der Meer, M.T.E. Vogels & B.-J. Kullberg

3. Cytokines and the host defense against *Listeria monocytogens* and *Salmonella typhimurium* 169
J.A.M. Langermans & R. van Furth

4. Cytokines and legionellosis 179
T.F. Byrd

5. The role of cytokines in mycobacterial infection 187
J.H. Champsi, L.E. Bermudez & L.S. Young

6. Cytokines in the treatment of fungal infections 195
B.-J. Kullberg & J.W. van 't Wout

7. Cytokines in malaria, pathology and protection 211
W.M.C. Eling & P.G. Kremsner

8. Cytokines in the treatment of leishmaniasis: From studies of immunopathology to patient therapy 223
J.L. Ho, R. Badaro, D. Hatzigeorgiou, S.G. Reed & W.D. Johnson, Jr.

9. The role of cytokines in toxoplasmosis 237
C.A. Hunter, C.S. Subauste & J.S. Remington

10. Cytokines in the treatment of primary immunodeficiency 249
B.A. Kruskal & R.A.B. Ezekowitz

11. Cytokines as potential vaccine adjuvants 261
A. Nohria & R.H. Rubin

Biotherapy 7: 149–150, 1994.

Introduction: Cytokines in the biotherapy of infectious diseases

Bart-Jan Kullberg & Jos W.M. van der Meer
Department of Medicine, University Hospital Nijmegen, The Netherlands

The use of antimicrobial agents and vaccines has been very successful in reducing the morbidity and mortality associated with many infectious diseases. However, especially for the growing number of patients with compromised host defense mechanisms, infections remain a serious and increasing problem. The normal relationship between host and microorganism appears to be finely balanced, since the microorganisms can easily take advantage of any disequilibrium, such as alteration of the bacterial flora or impairment of the host defense system. It is therefore desirable to focus on the modulation of host defense mechanisms in addition to antimicrobial therapy, in order to restore the equilibrium between the host and the invading agents in these patients. Only recently a new range of agents has become available that are capable of stimulating and regulating host defense systems. Interleukins, interferons, and hematopoietic growth factors are now being produced by biotechnology industry and are being evaluated for clinical use in this area.

The success of interferon-γ in patients with chronic granulomatous disease (CGD) provides an example of biotherapy that already has become standard practice to restore host defense mechanisms and thereby prevent infection. CGD is a rare congenital disease in which the ability of phagocytes to mount a respiratory burst and to kill ingested microorganisms is impaired. The contribution of Kruskal and Ezekowitz in this issue addresses the application of interferon-γ, interleukin-2 and hematopoietic growth factors in CGD and a variety of other primary immunodeficiencies.

During the past decade, much work has been devoted to establish the role of interferon-γ in macrophage activation. Activation of macrophages by lymphokines that are produced mainly by $CD4^+$ T-lymphocytes is essential for the host defense against intracellular pathogens. There is abundant evidence that interferon-γ is the main lymphokine involved, and especially infection with *Toxoplasma gondii* is an elegant model demonstrating the importance of activation of macrophages. As a consequence of the AIDS epidemic, toxoplasmosis has emerged as one of the most important opportunistic infections, and new strategies for the management of this disease are needed. The contribution of Hunter *et al.* reviews the possibilities for biotherapy with cytokines in toxoplasmosis.

Leishmania is another species that has served as a model to study the regulation of killing mechanisms of macrophages. The profile of cytokines released in mice infected with *L. major* determines whether protective immunity or exacerbation occurs. *Leishmania*-resistant strains of mice produced IFN-γ but not IL-4, whereas susceptible strains produced IL-4 and IL-10 but not IFN-γ mRNA. The knowledge of the immunopathology of *Leishmania* infection now opens the door to an alternative therapy, as is discussed by Ho *et al.* in this issue. The treatment of visceral leishmaniasis (kala azar) had not changed for 70 years, pentavalent antimony being the drug of choice. However, the response rate is only 70–80%, and toxicity is significant. A number of studies with interferon-γ in patients with visceral leishmaniasis has now been performed, and even in those who had not responded to pentavalent antimony the clinical outcome is encouraging.

As is discussed in the contribution of Langermans and Van Furth, the view that the host defense against intracellular bacteria is exclusively mediated by macrophages that phagocytose and kill these bacteria is no longer valid. *Listeria monocytogenes*, and probably also *Salmonella* species, are able to escape form macrophages and to invade hepatocytes. Activation of hepatocytes by interferon-γ and tumor necrosis factor-α is therefore essential in host defense to these infections, together with invading granulocytes that lyse infected hepatocytes.

Legionella pneumophila, the agent responsible for Legionnaires' disease, is probably the most important new opportunistic pathogen identified as a major cause of infection in immunocompromized hosts. The central role of T-cell mediated cellular immunity in host defense to this pathogen and the effect of interferon-γ is discussed by Byrd in this issue. The availability of iron is required for growth of *L. pneumophila*, and it is shown that interferon-γ-activated macrophages inhibit progression of the disease through limitation of iron.

Not only newly described bacteria are important pathogens in the immunocompromized host. Mycobacterial infections are still a major cause for morbidity and mortality. The presentation and outcome of leprosy, tuberculosis, and infection with *Mycobacterium avium-complex* are largely dependent on the host's immune status, and tumor necrosis factor is required at the site of infection for the formation of granulomas and to restrain the infection. As is reviewed in the contribution of Champsi *et al.*, a large variety of agents – interferon-γ, tumor necrosis factor, interleukin-2, granulocyte-macrophage colony stimulating factor – may improve the course of mycobacterial infection. Other cytokines like transforming growth factor-ß, interleukin-6, and interleukin 10 counteract the effects of immunostimulating cytokines, resulting in immunosuppression and progression of infection. Eling and Kremsner review the cells and cytokines involved in the pathogenesis of cerebral malaria, and the application of IFN-γ, TNF-α, interleukin-1 and IL-1-receptor antagonist as treatment modalities to attenuate or prevent the disease.

In granulocytopenic cancer patients, Gram-negative infections have long been the most important life-threatening pathogens. The therapy of Gram-negative bacterial infections in these patients has reached a cure rate of around 80%. It is expected that the development of new antibiotics will not significantly alter these results. The development of immunotherapy aimed at either the infectious agent itself or the systemic mediators of sepsis may improve the outcome of Gram-negative infection. Whereas the contribution of Gram-negative infections to the mortality of granulocytopenic patients has declined, the incidence of other pathogens has risen dramatically. Fungal infections, especially those caused by *Candida* and *Aspergillus* species, are now responsible for the majority of fatal infections in neutropenic cancer patients. Cure of these infections is almost entirely dependent on the recovery from granulocytopenia, indicating that host defense mechanisms are extremely important in the clearance of fungal pathogens. The modulation of host resistance to both Gram-negative bacterial and fungal infections in granulocytopenic hosts will be discussed in detail in this issue of Biotherapy.

As our understanding of the immunopathology and molecular biology underlying these diseases increases, it will become possible to select specific candidate cytokines for therapy and prevention of a variety of infectious diseases. Clinical trials will have to be designed to assess the value of these biological response modifiers in addition to conventional antimicrobial therapy and to indicate the appropriate applications of these new drugs.

Address for correspondence: Division of General Internal Medicine, Department of Medicine, University Hospital Nijmegen, P.O. Box 9101, 6500 HB Nijmegen, The Netherlands

Biotherapy 7: 151–159, 1994.

Cytokines in the treatment of virus infections

N. B. Finter
9 Burntwood Road, Sevenoaks, Kent TN13 1PS, UK

Key words: Interferons, IFN-α subtypes, chronic virus infections, hepatitis viruses, papillomaviruses

Abstract

The interferon (IFN) system consists of both the formation of the various IFN proteins, and the diverse cellular responses which these induce: these result from the intracellular changes which follow their binding to a specific cell surface receptor.

There is only a single human gamma, omega and beta IFN; in contrast, there are 13 closely related chemical species ("subtypes") of human alpha IFN, which are nevertheless chemically and biologically distinct.

IFN preparations made from mass cultured human cells or by using recombinant DNA techniques are now readily available for clinical use. IFN have a major role in the defence of the body against virus infections. In acute virus infections, preformed exogenous IFN cannot be given soon enough to be of value. However, IFN-α and IFN-β have proved of considerable value in some chronic virus infections, particularly chronic virus hepatitis and chronic papillomavirus infections. The doses routinely used are associated with both acute and chronic toxic side effects. Also, some patients form specific neutralising antibodies against the particular IFN preparation injected, which may abrogate all the benefits of the treatment. Nevertheless, IFN are now established as agents for use in routine medical practice.

Abbreviations: TNF: Tumour necrosis factor, IL-6: Interleukin-6, eIF2: The protein initiation factor

Introduction

Although other cytokines such as TNF and IL-6 may directly or indirectly affect the growth of viruses, only the human interferons (HuIFN) are currently used for treating patients with certain virus infections [1,2]. These are therefore the subject of this review, which will give the background to the IFN, and discuss in general terms the infections in which they have been used, and the rationale for these uses.

The interferon system

Conceptually, the IFN system consists of two parts, the formation of IFN by cells exposed to various stimuli, especially a virus infection; and the diverse cellular responses resulting from the IFN formed. *In vivo*, these are closely co-ordinated, and form an important homeostatic mechanism.

From a prototype IFN some 600–800 million years ago [3], many different IFN proteins have evolved. They are classified as Type I and Type II, with the human Type I IFN comprising three families, IFN-α, IFN-β, and IFN-ω. In turn, the HuIFN-α family consists of many chemically distinct but related chemical species or "subtypes", the products of 13 closely spaced genes on chromosome 9 [4]. Because of various post-translational modifications, the number of antiviral proteins in IFN preparations made from human cells is even larger [G Allen, personal communication]. All these subtypes share some 116 amino acids out of the total of 165 or 166 in the polypeptide chain, but some differ obviously from the others in terms of antigenicity or biological activities [5,6], and many, and perhaps all, have a unique spectrum of biological properties [7].

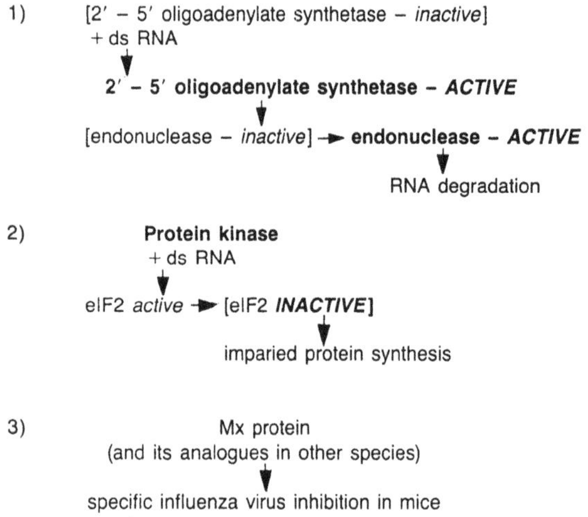

Fig. 1. Antiviral proteins synthesised in cells treated with interferon

The HuIFN-β and HuIFN-ω families each contain a single protein. IFN-β, originally made from fibroblasts and termed accordingly, shares about 35% of its amino acids with the HuIFN-α, and has many of the same properties, but it is antigenically distinct. HuIFN-ω is chemically closely related to the IFN-α, but has an additional 6 amino acids and different antigenic and biological properties. It is present in IFN-α preparations made from human cells, but has not as yet been separately used in patients.

Gamma interferon (HuIFN-γ) is the only Type II interferon. It has antiviral properties *in vitro* like the Type I IFN, but has not proved clinically useful even in virus infections in which Type I IFN have beneficial effects, or it has no apparent advantages, and so will not be further considered here.

An IFN binds to one of the specific IFN receptors on the cell surface. This triggers a complex chain of intracellular biochemical events [8], which result after several hours in the formation of many proteins [9] that mediate its biological effects. Among these are two enzymes with broad-spectrum activity against many viruses: one, 2'-5' oligoadenylate synthetase (2–5A), activates the formation of an endonuclease [10] which breaks down newly synthesised virus RNA; the other, a protein kinase activated by double-stranded RNA, indirectly interferes with protein synthesis [10] - see Fig. 1. A third protein, MxA, inhibits the growth only of influenza and a few other viruses [11].

IFN have many other biological actions, and some may contribute to the overall antiviral effects *in vivo*. There is usually increased expression of histocompatibility antigens (HLA) on the cell surface, with in general Class II HLA stimulated mainly by IFN-γ, and Class I HLA by IFN-α. [12]. Increased expression of HLA is thought to play an important part in the beneficial effects of IFN-α in chronic hepatitis B virus (HBV) infections, and perhaps also in other chronic virus infections.

IFN also affect the immune system in other ways, stimulating or, more usually, depressing its functions depending on the dose and the time of its administration relative to the immune event. The reduced delayed type hypersensitivity in children with an acute virus infection, first noted clinically many years ago, almost certainly reflects IFN formed during the infection.

Cells exposed to small amounts of IFN subsequently form IFN faster and in greater amounts when infected with a virus; this "priming" increases the number of IFN-protected cells at the site of an invading virus.

Viruses differ greatly in sensitivity to the antiviral effects of IFN. Many viruses have evolved specific mechanisms for overcoming the effects of IFN [13], but nevertheless, the replication of almost all viruses is inhibited to at least some extent in IFN-treated cells.

IFN have a major role in the early defence of the body against an invading virus. Their effects come into play soon after infection, and well before specific immunological defence mechanisms develop in a non-immune host. Their importance has been shown by treating mice with neutralizing antibodies to IFN before infection with a challenge virus: the infection was rendered much more lethal than in control animals [14].

IFN proteins are very potent: the usual human adult doses of 1–10 mega units (Mu), given by intramuscular or subcutaneous injection, corresponds to only 0.01–0.1 mg of IFN protein, and a total of 3–5 mg is sufficient to treat a patient with hepatitis C three times a week for a year. To ensure that all the IFN protein in a preparation for clinical use is active, it is assayed in terms of its biological activity, and the results expressed in International Units (IU) [15].

Interferon preparations

The first identified member of the IFN family was "the interferon", discovered in 1957 because of its antiviral properties [16]. It was a protein made by chick cells exposed to a virus, and when other chick cells were incubated in its presence, they became resistant to infection with all viruses out of the wide range that was tested.

Attempts to exploit the discovery for medical purposes initially encountered many difficulties. It was found that the cells of other animals similarly formed IFN when exposed to viruses *in vitro* or in vivo, but each IFN was distinct, being most active on cells from the homologous species. It was realised that IFN for clinical use must be derived from human cells. In 1967, so-called leucocyte IFN from human white blood cells was produced [17]. About 1 Mu of antiviral activity was obtained from the white blood cells separated from a single 600 ml transfusion blood donation.

HuIFN-α for clinical use are now made on an industrial scale in two ways, from mass cultures of human cells, or from transfected bacterial cells expressing a human interferon gene. The former category includes preparations of leucocyte IFN (e.g. Alferon, Interferon Sciences; Finnferon, Finnish Red Cross) and Namalwa cell lymphoblastoid IFN (Wellferon, Wellcome). These products derived from human cells contain many individual IFN-α subtype proteins.

The three single subtype recombinant IFN-α available for clinical use, IFN-α2a (Roferon, Roche); IFN-α2b (Intron, Schering-Plough) and IFN-α2c (Berefor, Boehringer-Ingelheim) are versions of the same gene product, IFN-α2, each differing from the other two by a single amino acid in the peptide chain. The gene corresponding to IFN-α2b is the one most commonly found in human cell DNA [18, 19].

Preparations of HuIFN-β for clinical use include those made from cultured human fibroblasts (e.g. Frone A, Ares-Serono and Fiblaferon, Rentschler), and recombinant proteins, such as interferon β-serine$_{17}$ (recHuIFN-βser$_{17}$, Betaseron, Berlex), in which the native lysine at position 17 in the peptide chain has been replaced by serine.

Interferons used as antiviral agents

Data from animal studies

In the earliest animal studies, IFN were shown to give local protection to the skin or eye of rabbits or monkeys against later challenge at the same site with vaccinia virus or herpes simplex virus (reviewed [20]).

When more potent animal IFN preparations became available, these were soon shown to be able to protect against systemic virus infections [20–22]. Mice were injected intramuscularly with mouse interferon and challenged 18–24 h later with an arbovirus that killed all control animals after 4–5 days. Those given IFN lived longer, or survived the infection altogether [23].

These and similar studies soon showed points likely to be relevant to the use of IFN in patients. The extent of protection appeared to be roughly proportional to the logarithm of the amount of IFN used [23, 24]. Moreover, the protective effect of IFN was dependend on the amount of virus injected. More IFN was needed when given 18–24 hours after infection rather than before infection with the same inoculum; and 30 hours after infection, even a large amount of IFN was ineffective. Nevertheless, in some less rapidly progressing infections, IFN still gave protection even when treatment was started several days after the infection [20, 25].

In tissue culture experiments, the antiviral effects of an IFN reach their maximum after about 6 hours, and may then persist for several days. Similarly in animals, the effects of IFN reach a peak in the first 24 hours, and then slowly wane over a time that depends on the dose of IFN and the amount of challenge virus. For example, a large dose of IFN protected mice for only 2 days against infection with 200 LD50 of an arbovirus, but seven times less still gave protection after 4–5 days against 1 LD50 [20, 23]. In experimental herpes keratitis in rabbits, a single drop of IFN, given each day, was as effective as treatment with the same dose two or three times a day [24].

The toxicity of interferons

As IFN are naturally formed *in vivo*, it was initially thought that an injected IFN would neither have toxic effects nor be antigenic in the species of origin. Indeed, prolonged administration of mouse IFN did not seem to cause problems in mice [27]. The side-effects observed in early clinical studies with leucocyte IFN were at first attributed to protein contaminants. Later, injections of various very highly purified IFN-α preparations were found to be accompanied by the same side-effects [28].

IFN produce both acute and chronic toxic effects (Table 1). The acute side-effects are dose-related, and they usually diminish in intensity when treatment is continued. They closely resemble the symptoms of influenza, which indeed may reflect the considerable amounts of IFN then present in the blood.

After treatment for several weeks or months, patients may complain of increasing fatigue, anorexia and weight loss, and may suffer from changes in mood or depression. These central nervous system effects are most severe in the elderly. Electro-encephalograms show slowing of the α rhythm, and appearance of dif-

Table 1. Some of the side-effects that often accompany the use of alpha interferon preparations (3–10 Mu, given intramuscularly or subcutaneously)

Acute side effects
influenza-like:
fever
chills
headache
muscle pain
anorexia
nausea
bone-marrow depression:
leucopenia
thrombocytopenia
Chronic side-effects
central nervous system effects
fatigue
lethargy
anorexia
depression
electro-encephalographic changes
weight loss

fuse slow waves. These chronic effects may necessitate dose reduction or cessation of treatment.

There are many other side effects which occur less commonly [28], or affect particular patient populations. For example, in one study, three renal transplant patients given prophylactic treatment with 36 Mu of HuIFN-α2a three times a week developed a transient nephrotic syndrome [29], but it is not clear whether this reflected the particular IFN-α preparation or patients involved, or the large doses given.

In early animal studies, it seemed that IFN preparations were unable to provoke the formation of antibodies but this merely reflected the minute amounts of IFN protein in these early preparation. When more concentrated and pure IFN became available, it proved easy to prepare neutralising antisera. Patients frequently form antibodies that bind to the human IFN preparation used for their treatment and some may also form neutralising antibodies.

Efficacy studies in man

From the results of animal studies, some predictions about the likely utility of IFN in human virus infections could be made. First, IFN therapy was most likely to be of benefit when given prophylactically, or during the course of slowly progressing or chronic virus infections. Also, because the antiviral state persists for some time after a dose of IFN, treatment each day might not be necessary. On the other hand, IFN might well prove to have no value in acute virus infections, since the infection may already be widespread at the moment that treatment is begun. Furthermore, it is likely that IFN formed at the sites of virus replication will provide much greater local concentrations than can be produced by injecting IFN at a remote site [26].

Early studies showed that IFN could inhibit the growth of at least some animal tumour viruses in cell cultures and also in animals. It was found that IFN also inhibited the growth of many other tumours, including some very unlikely to be caused by a virus. These results suggested that IFN might have a role in cancer therapy, and consequently, most of the early clinical studies with leucocyte IFN in the 1970's involved patients with various tumours. A few patients with virus infections were also treated, and these early studies did identify certain chronic virus infections in which IFN therapy seemed to be beneficial.

Chronic virus infection of the liver

Hepatitis B virus (HBV)

Most of those who become infected with HBV after the neonatal period recover completely, but a small proportion of patients become chronic virus carriers, and some of these develop chronic active hepatitis (CAH-B) that may lead to progressive liver damage, liver cirrhosis or hepatocellular carcinoma. World-wide, an estimated 1.5 million chronic carriers of HBV die each year from these long term consequences, and in spite of current HBV vaccination programmes, CAH-B will remain a very important medical problem for many years.

In early uncontrolled studies, small numbers of patients with CAH-B – only four in the very first study [30] – were given short courses of treatment with leucocyte or fibroblast IFN. Overall in all these early studies, there was an antiviral effect in some 30% of the patients as shown by decreased serum levels of liver transaminases, and reduced serum levels of HBV DNA polymerase or HBV DNA. However, all the patients relapsed when the treatment stopped. Indeed, after further small trials with relatively low doses of leukocyte interferon, many investigators concluded that the benefits of the treatment were too short-lived to justify the problems and cost.

When it became possible to carry out larger controlled studies, it was found that a relatively high dose of an IFN-α preparation should be used and treatment continued for at least 3 months. A regimen of 5–10 Mu given daily for the first month and then on a three times a week schedule leads to a statistically significant increase of 25–40% in the proportion of patients who recover from infection compared with untreated control patients. In those who respond, an early antiviral effect is seen soon after treatment starts, in terms of a fall in the blood levels of virus DNA. After 4–10 weeks, there is a transient flare of hepatitis, and thereafter, virus DNA and e antigen disappear from blood. Such patients develop antibodies to the e antigen, and an occasional patient also loses circulating HBV surface antigen. Histological study of liver biopsy samples reveals reduced inflammation and signs of repair.

The predominant effect of IFN therapy in this disease is probably to increase expression of HLA markers on the surface of infected liver cells. This leads to their recognition and destruction by cytotoxic T cells so that virus replication is terminated. IFN treatment is most likely to be effective in patients who have moderately elevated levels of serum transaminases.

Similar results have been obtained with IFN-β preparations, but treatment with IFN-γ has proved ineffective [31].

Hepatitis C virus (HCV)

HCV infections are quite often inapparent, and very much more common than had previously been realised. Many of those infected become chronic carriers and progress to chronic active hepatitis, with the long term consequences of liver cirrhosis or carcinoma.

There have been many trials of IFN-α preparations in patients with chronic HCV with essentially similar results [32]. The usual regimen has been a dose of 3 Mu, given three times a week, and continued for 6 to 12 months. In about 50% of those treated, the serum levels of liver transaminases fell to base-line levels, and amounts of HCV in the blood decreased. However, residual HCV could be detected by PCR in most of those who responded. About half of these soon relapsed when treatment stopped. Overall, only some 25–30% of IFN-treated patients were long-term responders; the histology of serial liver biopsy samples from these patients confirmed the benefits of the treatment.

Several serotypes of HCV have now been recognised; one report suggests that patients are more likely to respond to IFN-α therapy if they are infected with some serotypes rather than others [33]. There are also hints that some IFN-α preparations may give better results than others, as in the only study so far in which two preparations were compared [34]. Also, when patients who had failed to respond to IFN-α2a were later given lymphoblastoid IFN, 50% then responded [35].

Chronic infections with human papillomaviruses (HPV)

These viruses cause chronic infections in the skin and other epithelia, leading to the formation of warts, and these have been targets for IFN therapy. There are many serotypes of HPV, and some are found much more frequently at particular anatomical sites. Since HPV cannot yet be readily grown *in vitro*, it is not clear whether IFN influence warts through antiviral mechanisms, immunological processes, or by slowing the growth of the infected cells, or by a combination of these effects.

Chronic respiratory papillomatosis

In this very uncommon disease, warts grow in the region of the larynx, and may interfere with speech or breathing. The disease can be very distressing in young children (juvenile laryngeal papillomatosis, JLP), who may require frequent surgery.

During the 1970's, small studies by Strander and colleagues strongly suggested that injections of leucocyte interferon benefited children with JLP. There have since been two larger controlled studies, but unfortunately the results are somewhat conflicting. In one study involving 123 children [36], leucocyte IFN significantly reduced the rate of growth of the laryngeal warts during the first 6 months of treatment, but the improvement was not sustained in the next 6 months. In the other, a cross-over study in 66 JLP patients [37], all the patients improved while receiving lymphoplastoid IFN. At the end of the study, many elected to continue treatment, and when 59 of the patients were studied 4 years later, it was found that 87% had had a complete or partial remission [38]. Whether the different outcome of these two studies reflects their design, the IFN preparation used, or some other factor, is not clear.

Condyloma acuminata

Sexually transmitted HPV lead to condyloma acuminata in the genital region, a problem now commoner than genital herpes. Patients with poor responses to local treatment such as freezing, surgery or podophyllin have participated in trials with IFN-α and IFN-β preparations, which were either injected directly into the warts, or at a remote site. In some, the treatment appeared to be beneficial [39, 40], but in others no apparent benefit was seen [41]. These conflicting results may well reflect the very many variables involved in such studies, for example the sites and age of the condylomas, the dose, method and duration of treatment, the type of patients selected for study, and perhaps also the particular IFN preparation used.

Common skin warts

IFN has been tried in patients where repeated conventional treatments have failed. Injection of IFN directly into the base of recalcitrant warts, a manoeuvre that is briefly intensely painful, has been followed by a considerable measure of success [42, 43].

Thus overall, the use of IFN in these various HPV diseases has given conflicting results, and there is at present no consensus whether IFN treatment should or should not be used. Nevertheless, the fact that positive results have been obtained in some studies indicates that further work is needed, and in particular to try to identify the sub-sets of patients who are most likely to respond well, and other variables that may affect the response.

IFN used in other virus infections

HIV infection

Although IFN markedly inhibit the growth of HIV in blood monocytes treated *in vitro*, attempts to treat patients with AIDS by administering various IFN preparations, even at doses up to 50 Mu a day, have been uniformly unsuccessful, perhaps because HIV-infected individuals at this stage in their disease have a severely compromised immune system, and many already have substantial amounts of endogenously-formed IFN in their blood.

In vitro, combinations of IFN and various nucleoside drugs, including zidovudine [44] and dideoxsyinosine have strikingly synergistic antiviral effects against HIV, but as yet, no such combination has proved useful, even in patients treated relatively early in their disease. Further studies with IFN and combinations of antiviral drugs are in progress.

Large and quite toxic doses of IFN-α (30 Mu daily or more) have had some success in patients with the AIDS- associated lesions of Kaposi's sarcoma [45].

Disseminated herpes zoster

Merigan and colleagues [46] gave relatively large amounts (15–20 Mu) of leucocyte IFN to immunosuppressed patients when they developed herpes zoster. Those who started treatment after a delay of more than 1 day from the time of appearance of vesicles had progressively more disseminated lesions and more post-herpetic pain than those who started IFN within 24 hours.

The common cold

In the very first studies in man with leucocyte IFN, volunteers started to use nose drops containing IFN before experimental challenge with a rhinovirus: there was no effect on the incidence of colds [47]. Later, nose drops containing more concentrated leucocyte IFN did indeed prevent symptoms of a cold and reduce rhinovirus growth in volunteers; there was less effect against experimental colds resulting from a coronavirus, or against influenza virus [48]. IFN nose drops had no effect if started after infection.

These studies suggested that IFN might provide long term prophylaxis, but unfortunately, after about three weeks, the nose drops cause unacceptable local toxicity [49]. Nevertheless, short term treatment with IFN nose-drops did significantly reduce the incidence of rhinovirus colds in trials involving families: as soon as a child developed a clinical cold, the other members of that family started to treat themselves [50].

Herpes keratitis

Studies in rabbits with acute herpes virus infections of the eye showed that daily administration of a single eye-drop containing IFN-α gave good results, and was as effective as more frequent treatment [24]. The same regimen was tried in patients with herpes keratitis and gave comparable results [51, 52]. When patients were treated with both acycloguanosine (acyclovir) and IFN-α in combination, local pain was lost sooner and corneal healing was quicker than after acycloguanosine used on its own [53], and some ophthalmologists regularly used this combined treatment.

Prevention of virus infection in transplant patients.

The immunosuppressive drugs given to these patients frequently lead to reactivation of latent viruses such as cytomegalovirus (CMV) and herpes simplex virus. In a study in renal transplant patients, prophylactic IFN reduced the incidence of CMV infections, but had no effect on Epstein-Barr or herpes viruses [54]. Nevertheless, IFN prophylaxis has not so far been adopted as a routine procedure in these patients.

In patients undergoing liver transplant for chronic viral hepatitis, reinfection with the virus concerned is common. Attempts to prevent this by giving IFN have not been successful.

Problems with the antiviral use of interferons

The results so far obtained with IFN in virus infections may seem disappointing, especially when related to the extravagant hopes of 35 years ago: toxicity has proved a considerable problem; only some of those treated have responded; and of those responding, many have soon relapsed after the course of treatment. In fact, it is in some ways remarkable that IFN therapy has been of great benefit to some patients, for there are reasons why it might have had little effect.

One problem is that of timing: IFN cannot be given soon enough to be of use in an acute virus infection. Even in a chronic infection,it may be started too late to be effective, for in addition to the increasing virus burden, if a virus replicates for a prolonged period, there is a greater chance of some mutation making it less sensitive to IFN.

In mice, very large doses of IFN can produce striking antiviral effects, but IFN toxicity is not an obvious problem in this species. In contrast, patients seldom accept a dose greater than 5–10 Mu for long, and even 3–5 Mu may cause distressing side-effects. If these could be overcome in some way so that larger IFN doses could be used, much greater antiviral effects would undoubtedly result.

Different viruses, virus serotypes [e.g. 33], and strains of virus vary greatly in their sensitivity to IFN. Thus apart from the problem of IFN-resistant mutants, the particular virus that infects an individual may greatly influence the response to IFN therapy.

In some patients, the formation of specific IFN-neutralising antibodies may prevent or reverse the benefits of treatment. Such antibodies are found more commonly in those treated for more than a few weeks and with relatively large amounts of IFN. There has been much dispute about their clinical significance, and about the relative antigenicity of the different IFN-α preparations. Some patients have low levels of neutralising antibodies in their blood with no apparent impact on the response to the treatment. However, antibody concentrations exceeding a critical value are likely to lead to loss of all the biological and clinical effects of the IFN preparation concerned [55–58]. Antibodies are more frequent after the use of a recombinant IFN-α2 preparation, and especially IFN-α2a, than with a human cell derived IFN-α preparation [59]. In patients who form high titre antibodies to a recombinant IFN-α2 preparation, change in treatment to a multi-subtype IFN-α derived from human cells may provide or restore a clinical response [56, 57].

Neutralising antibodies seem not to have been a major clinical problem in patients with chronic hepatitis B, though high titres were associated with a relatively low response rate in Chinese patients treated with recombinant IFN-α2a [60, 61). They are much more common in patients with chronic hepatitis C, and have been associated with a significant rate of failure to treatment [55].

It is nevertheless encouraging that in some virus infections, the proportion of patients responding to IFN therapy justifies the side effects, the need for frequent injections, and the not insignificant cost of treatment. An important objective must be to try to identify quickly those patients likely to respond, and equally importantly, those who are likely not to respond, so that their treatment can be stopped at an early stage. Some recent results suggest that this may indeed be possible [62].

Eventually, it may become possible to deliver large amounts of IFN selectively to the particular sites where they are actually needed, e.g. the dermis or liver, and thus provide much a greater antiviral effect without increased systemic toxicity. Meanwhile, one should not expect too much of IFN when used on their own; in the body they are a component, even if a key component, in a co-ordinated response to a virus infection which also involves cells, antibodies and other cytokines. To improve their therapeutic use, it may well prove best to use them in combination with antiviral drugs or with other cytokines.

Though not the universal remedy for virus infection once suggested, IFN can be of considerable value in some, particularly in certain chronic infections; they have also proved beneficial in some forms of cancer. So, despite thier side effects and other drawbacks, they will be used increasingly in the future in routine medical practice.

References

1. Finter N B, Chapman S, Dowd P, Johnston JM, Manna V, Sarantis N, Sheron N, Scott G, Phua S, Tatum PB. The use of Interferon-α in virus infections. Drugs 1991; 42: 749–765.
2. Trying SK. Introduction to the clinical uses of interferons. In: Baron S, Coppenhaver DH, Dianzani F, Fleischmann WR, Hughes TK, Klimpel GR, Niesel DW, Stanton GC, Tyring SK, eds. Interferon: principles and medical applications. Galveston, Tx: University of Texas Medical Branch 1992: 399–407.
3. Henco K, Brosius J, Fujisawa A, Fujisawa J-I, Haynes JR, Hochstadt J, Kovacic T, Pasek N, Schambock A, Schmid J, Todokoro K, Walchli M, Nagata S, Weissmann C. Structural relationship of human interferon alpha genes and pseudogenes. J Mol Biol 1985; 185: 227–260.
4. Diaz M, Allen G. Nomenclature of the human interferon genes. J interferon Res. 1993; 13: 61–62.
5. Weck P K, Apperson S, Hay L, Stebbing N. Comparison of the antiviral activities of various cloned human interferon-α subtypes in mammalian cell cultures. J Gen Virol 1981; 57: 233–237.
6. Zoon K, Zur Nedden DL, Enterline JC, Manischewitz JF, Dyer DR, Boykins RA, Bekisz J, Gerrard TL. Chemical and biological characterisation of natural human lymphoblastoid interferon alphas. In: Cantell K. Schellekens H, eds. The biology of the interferon system, 1986. Amsterdam: Martinus Nijhoff, 1987: 567–569.
7. Finter NB. Why are there so many subtypes of alpha-interferons? J Gen Virol 1991; 185–194.
8. Tanaka T, Taniguchi T. Cytokine gene regulation: regulatory cis-elements and DNA binding factors involved in the interferon system. Adv Immunol 1992; 52: 263–279.
9. Revel M, Chebath J. Interferon-activated genes. Trends in Biol Sci 1986; 11: 166–170.
10. Hovanessian AG. Interferon-induced and double stranded RNA-activated enzymes: a specific protein kinase and 2', 5' -Oligoadenylate synthetase. J Interferon Res 1991: 11: 199–205.
11. Pavlovic J, Staehli P. The antiviral potential of Mx proteins. J Interferon Res 1991; 11: 215–219.
12. Rhodes J. Ivanyi I, Cozens P. Antigen presentation by human monocytes: effects of modifying major histocompatability complex class II antigen expression and interleukin 1 production by using recombinant interferons and corticosteroids. Eur J Immunol 1986; 16: 370–375.
13. Gewert D, Finter NB. Antiviral effects of interferons: studies in animals and at the cellular level. In: Baron S, Coppenhaver DH, Dianzani F, Fleischmann WR, Hughes TK, Klimpel GR, Niesel DW, Stanton GC, Tyring SK, eds. Interferon: principles and medical applications. Galveston, Tx: University of Texas Medical Branch, 1992: 289–297.
14. Gresser I, Tovey MG, Bandu MT, Maury C, Brouty-Boye D. Role of interferon in the pathogenesis of virus disease as demonstrated by the use of anti-interferon serum. 1. Rapid evolution of encephalomyocarditis virus infection. J Exp Med 1976; 144: 1305–1315.
15. Standardization of interferons. Geneva: World Health Organisation Technical report series 1983: No. 687 Annex 1: 35–60. 1985: No. 725: 28–64. 1988: No. 771: 37–87.
16. Isaacs A, Lindenmann, J. Virus interference. I. The interferon. Proc Roy Soc ser B 1957; 147: 258–267.
17. Strander H, Cantell K. Production of interferon by human leukocytes in vitro. Ann Med Exp Biol Fenn 1966; 44: 265–273.
18. Hosai H, Miyake K, Yamanaka M. The interferon a2 gene in Japanese patients with chronic viral hepatitis who developed antibodies after recombinant a2A treatment. Abstr Sci Mtg Internatl. Assoc. for the study of the Liver, Brighton, 1992; June 3–6, 113.
19. Gewert D, Salom C, Barber K, Macbride S, Cooper H, Lewis A, Wood J, Crowe S. Analysis of interferon-$\alpha 2$ sequences in human genomic DNA. J Interferon Res 1993; 13: 27–231.
20. Finter N B. Interferons and inducers in vivo: I. antiviral effects in experimental animals. In: Finter NB, ed. Interferons and interferon inducers. Amsterdam: North-Holland, 1973: 295–362.
21. Gresser I, Bourali C, Thomas MT, Falcoff E. Effect of repeated inoculation of interferon preparations on infections of mice with encephalomyocarditis virus. Proc Soc Exp Biol Med 1968; 127: 491–496.
22. Hilfenhaus J, Polastri GD. Antiviral effects of interferons in animals. In: Finter NB and Oldham PK, eds. Interferon 4. Amsterdam: Elsevier, 1973: 3–21.
23. Finter NB. Interferon as an antiviral agent in vivo: quantitative and temporal aspects of the protection of mice against Semliki forest virus. Brit J Exp Pathol 1966; 47: 361–371.
24. McGill JI, Collins P, Cantell K, Jones BR, Finter NB. Optimal schedules for use of interferon in the corneas of rabbits with herpes simplex keratitis. J Infect Dis 1976; 133: A13–A19.
25. Gresser I, Tovey MG, Maury C. Efficacy of exogenous treatment with interferon after the onset of multiplication of vesicular stomatitis virus in the brains of mice. J Gen Virol 1975; 27: 395–403.
26. Heremans H, Billiau A, De Somer P. Interferon in experimental viral infections in mice: tissue interferon levels resulting from the virus infection and from exogenous interferon therapy. Infect Immun 1980; 30: 513–522.
27. Gresser I, Coppey J, Bourali C. Interferon and mouse leukemia. VI. The effect of interferon preparations on the lymphoid leukemia of AKR mice. J Nat Cancer Instit 1969; 43: 1083–1089.
28. Bottomley J M, Toy J L. Clinical side effects and toxicities of interferons. In: Finter NB and Oldham RK, eds. Interferon 4. Amsterdam: Elsevier, 1973: 155–180.
29. Kramer P, Ten Kate FWJ, Bijenen AB, Jeekel J, Weimar W. Recombinant leukocyte interferon A induces steroid-resistant acute vascular rejection episodes in renal transplant recipients. Lancet 1984; i: 989–990.
30. Greenberg HB, Pollard R, Lutwick L, Gregory P, Robinson W, Merigan TC. Effect of human leukocyte interferon on hepatitis B virus infection in patients with chronic active hepatitis. N Engl J Med 1976; 295: 517–522.
31. Di Bisceglie AM, Rustgi VK, Kassianides C, Lisker-Melman M, Park Y, Waggoner JG, Hoofnagle J. Therapy of chronic hep-

atitis B with recombinant alpha and gamma interferon. Hepatol 1990; 11: 266–270.
32. Hoofnagle JH. Interferon therapy of viral hepatitis. In: Baron S, Coppenhaver DH, Dianzani F, Fleischmann WR, Hughes TK, Klimpel GR, Niesel DW, Stanton GC, Tyring SK, eds. Interferon: principles and medical applications. Galveston, Tx: University of Texas Medical Branch 1992: 433–462.
33. Kanai K, Kako M, Okamoto H. HCV genotypes in chronic hepatitis C and response to interferon. Lancet 1992; 339: 1543.
34. Ideo, G., Bellati, G., Pedraglio, E., Leandro, G. One year of therapy of non A, non B/C chronic hepatitis with recombinant α-2a interferon (r-IFN) or lymphoblastoid α interferon (L-IFN). Abstr. 25th meeting Europ Assoc Study of Liver Dis. J Hepatol 1990; 14 suppl 2: S31.
35. Cimino L, Citarella C, Nardone G, Budillon G. Lymphoblastoid interferon in chronic hepatitis C patients, 'non-responders' to recombinant interferon-α (rIFN-α). Hepatol 1992; 14: 419–420.
36. Healy GB, Gelber RD, Trowbridge AL, Grundfast KM, Ruben RJ, Price KN. Treatment of recurrent respiratory papillomatosis with human leucocyte interferon. N Engl J Med 1988; 319: 401–407.
37. Kashima HK, Leventhal BG, Dedo H, Gardiner L, McCabe BF, Richardson M, Whisnant J, Clark K, Donovan D, Goepfert H, Mounts P, Singleton G, Wold D, Cohen F, Fearon B, Lusk R, Muntz H, Weck P, Yonkers A. Interferon-alfa N1 (Wellferon) in juvenile onset recurrent respiratory papillomatosis: results of a randomized study in twelve collaborative institutions. Laryngoscope 1988; 98: 334–340.
38. Leventhal BG, Kashima HK, Mounts P, Thurmond L, Chapman S, Buckley S, Wold D, and the Papilloma Study Group. Long-term response of recurrent respiratory papillomatosis to treatment with lymphoblastoid interferon Alfa-N1. N Engl J Med 1991; 325: 613–617.
39. Gall SA, Hughes RN, Mounts P, Segriti A, Weck PK, Whisnant JK. Efficacy of human lymphoblastoid interferon in the therapy of resistant condyloma acuminata. Obstet Gynecol 1986; 67: 643–651.
40. Friedman-Kien AE, Eron LJ, Conant M, Growdon W, Badiak H, Bradstreet PW, Fedorczyk MS, Trout JR, Plasse TF. Natural interferon alfa for treatment of condylomata acuminata. J Am Med Assoc 1988; 259: 533–538.
41. Condyloma international collaborative study group. Recurrent condyloma acuminata treated with recombinant interferon alfa-2a: a multicenter double-blind placebo controlled clinical trial. J Am Med Assoc 1991; 265: 2684–2687.
42. Gibson JR. The treatment of viral warts. J Antimicrob Chemother 1988; 21: 391–393.
43. Berman B, Davis-Reed L, Silverstein L. Treatment verruca vulgaris with an $\alpha 2$ interferon. J Infect Dis 1986; 154: 328–330.
44. Hartshorn, K L, Vogt MW, Chou TC, et al. Synergistic inhibition of human immune virus in vitro by azidothymidine (AZT) and recombinant alpha-A interferon. Antimicrob Agents Chemother 1987; 31: 168–172.
45. De Wit R. Kaposi's sarcoma and AIDS. In: Baron S, Coppenhaver DH, Dianzani F, Fleischmann WR, Hughes TK, Klimpel GR, Niesel DW, Stanton GC, Tyring SK, eds. Interferon: principles and medical applications. Galveston, Tx: University of Texas medical Branch 1992: 475–485.
46. Merigan TC, Gallagher JG, Pollard RB, Arvin AM. Short-course human leukocyte interferon in treatment of herpes zoster in patients with cancer. Antimicrob Agents Chemother 1981; 19: 193–195
47. Scientific Committee on Interferon. Experiments with interferon in man. Lancet 1965; i: 505–506.
48. Merigan TC, Reed SE, Tyrrell DAJ. Inhibition of respiratory virus infection by locally applied interferon. Lancet 1973; i: 563–567.
49. Hayden FG, Mills SE, Johns ME. Human tolerance and histopathologic effects of long term administration of intranasal interferon-alpha 2. J Infect Dis 1983; 148: 914–921.
50. Douglas RB, Moore BW, Miles HB. Prophylactic efficacy of intranasal alpha$_2$ interferon against rhinovirus infections in the family setting. N Engl J Med 1986; 314: 65–70.
51. Jones BR, Coster DJ, Falcon MG, Cantell K. Topical therapy of ulcerative herpetic keratitis with human interferon. Lancet 1976; ii: 128.
52. Sundmacher R, Neumann-Haefelin D, Cantell K. Interferon treatment of dendritic keratitis. Lancet 1976; i: 1406–1407.
53. De Koning EWJ, van Bijsterveld OP, Cantell K. Combination therapy for dendritic keratitis with acyclovir and α-interferon. Arch Ophthalm 1983; 101: 1866–1868.
54. Hirsch MS, Schooley RT, Cosimi AB, Russell PS, Delmonico FL, Tolkoff-Rubin NE, Herrin JT, Cantell K, Farrell M-L, Rota TR, Rubin RH. Effects of interferon-alpha on cytomegalovirus reactivation syndromes in renal-transplant recipients. N Engl J Med 1983; 308: 1489–1493.
55. Milella M, Antonelli A, Santantonio T, Currenti M, Monno L, Mariano N, Angarano G, Dianzani F, Pastore G. Neutralising antibodies to recombinant alpha-interferon and response to therapy in chronic hepatitis C virus infection. Liver 1993; 13: 146–150.
56. Von Wussow P, Jakschies D, Freund M, Hehlman R, Brockhaus F, Hochkeppel H. Treatment of anti-recombinant interferon-alpha 2 antibody positive CML patients with natural interferon-alpha. Br J Haematol 1991; 78: 210–216.
57. Von Wussow P, Pralle H, Hochkeppel H-K, Jakschies D, Sonnen S, Schmidt H, Muller-Rosenau D, Franke M, Haferlach T, Zwingers T, Rapp U, Deicher H. Effective natural interferon-α therapy in recombinant interferon-α-resistant patients with hairy cell leukaemia. Blood 1991; 78: 38–43.
58. McSweeney EN, Giles FJ, Worman CP, Jewel AP, Tsakona CP, Hoffbrand AV, Mehta AB, Newland AC, Cawley JC, Galvani D, Singer CDJ, Grant IR, Norfolk DR, Goldstone AH. Recombinant interferon alfa 2a in the treatment of patients with early stage B chronic lymphocytic leukaemia. Brit J Haematol 1993; 85: 77–83.
59. Antonelli G, Currenti M, Turriziani O, Dianzani F. Neutralising antibodies to interferon-α: relative frequency in patients treated with different interferon preparations J Infect Dis 1991; 163: 882–885.
60. Lok ASF, Lai C-L. Incidence, neutralising activity and clinical significance of interferon antibodies in chronic hepatitis B patients receiving recombinant a-interferons. In: Hollinger FB. Margolis HS, eds. Viral hepatitis and liver disease. Baltimore: Williams and Wilkins, 1991: 643–645.
61. Lok ASF, Lai C-L, Leung EK-Y. Interferon antibodies may negate the antiviral effects of recombinant α-interferon treatment in patients with chronic hepatitis B virus infection. Hepatol 1990; 12: 1266–1270.
62. Gianelli G, Antonelli G, Fera G, Dianzani F, Schiraldi 0. 2', 5'-Oligoadenylate synthetase activity as a responsive marker during interferon therapy for chronic hepatitis C. J Interferon Res 1993; 13: 57–60.

Biotherapy 7: 161–167, 1994.

Interleukin-1 and related pro-inflammatory cytokines in the treatment of bacterial infections in neutropenic and non-neutropenic animals

Jos W. M. van der Meer, Maria T.E. Vogels & Bart-Jan Kullberg
Department of Medicine, University Hospital Nijmegen, The Netherlands

Key words: Host defense, immunotherapy, bacterial infections, sepsis, granulocytopenia, interleukin, tumor necrosis factor, colony-stimulating factors

Abstract

Bacterial infections in the immunocompromized host cause considerable mortality, and even the recently developed antimicrobial strategies often fail to cure these infections, especially in granulocytopenic patients. Cytokines and hematopoietic growth factors have been shown to stimulate host defense mechanisms *in vitro* and *in vivo*. We discuss the possible role of the pro-inflammatory cytokines interleukin-1, tumor necrosis factor-α, interleukin-6 and interleukin-8 as modulators of host resistance to bacterial infections. Interleukin-1 has been shown effective in various animal models of potentially lethal bacterial infection, even during severe granulocytopenia. The protective mechanism of interleukin-1 may be mediated via downregulation of cytokine receptors and cytokine production, and via induction of acute phase proteins. Moreover, in subacute and chronic infections interleukin-1 interferes with microbial outgrowth, via mechanisms that have only been partially elucidated.

Abbreviations: G-CSF: granulocyte colony-stimulating factor; M-CSF: monocyte colony-stimulating factor; GM-CSF: granulocyte-monocyte colony-stimulating factor; IFN-γ: interferon-gamma; IL: interleukin; LAK: lymphokine-activated killer; LPS: lipopolysaccharide; TNF: tumor necrosis factor

Introduction

Despite the development of potent new antibacterial agents, bacterial infections still meet with considerable morbidity and mortality, especially in patients with impaired host defense. This is particularly true for the situation in which the number of polymorphonuclear granulocytes is low. Such a granulocytopenic state is usually due to bone-marrow insufficiency induced by intensive anticancer chemotherapy given for the treatment of hematological malignancy. Especially when the numbers of granulocytes fall below 100/μl the risk for life-threatening bacterial and fungal infections is greatly increased, and the outcome of treatment is strongly dependent on the recovery of the granulocytopoiesis [1].

The discovery of molecules capable of stimulating and regulating host defense systems creates new possibilities for treatment. Molecules such as the interleukins, interferons, hematopoietic growth factors are being produced by biotechnology industry and become available for clinical use in this particular area. Hematopoietic growth factors such as granulocyte colony stimulating factor (G-CSF), granulocyte-macrophage colony stimulating factor (GM-CSF) and macrophage colony stimulating factor (M-CSF) are already used extensively in clinical medicine to accelerate bone marrow recovery and to stimulate the function of granulocytes and mononuclear phagocytes [2]. The use of these hematopoietic growth factors is beyond the scope of this review; in this paper we will focus on the potential use of proinflammatory cytokines for treatment of infections in the neutropenic host.

Cytokines and host defense

The pro-inflammatory cytokines are polypeptides of 8–26 kilodaltons, which are primarily produceded during the infectious and non-infectious inflammatory response. The major proinflammatory cytokines are interleukin-1 alpha (IL-1α) and beta (IL-1β), tumor necrosis factor a (TNFa, cachectin), interleukin-6 (IL-6), and interleukin-8 (IL-8). Apart from their deleterious role in sepsis and organ failure, these cytokines also have beneficial effects in the responses of the host. Such beneficial effects, which seem to be aimed mainly at upregulation of humoral as well as cellular host defense, are more prominent when these molecules act locally in the inflammatory field, whereas the above-mentioned deleterious effects tend to occur with high circulating concentrations [3].

Interleukin-1

Interleukin-1 is the collective name for two 17 kD proteins, IL-1α and IL-1β, that are produced by a wide variety of cells, of which mononuclear phagocytes and possibly vascular endothelial cells are the most important. These molecules exert a wide array of inflammatory, metabolic, physiologic, hematopoietic, and immunologic activities [4–6]. Although IL-1α and IL-1β have little amino acid homology, they bind to the same cell surface receptors and their biologic activities are similar [7]. IL-1α remains mostly cell-associated and acts mainly via cell-cell contact, whereas IL-1β is released and acts more as a soluble mediator [8]. Injection of either IL-1α or IL-1β into animals or humans leads to fever, synthesis of a variety of hepatic acute-phase proteins, and an increase in the number of leukocytes [5, 6, 9]. These effects of IL-1 are considered essential to the host in the response to tissue damage or infection. It was a logical step to investigate whether the administration of recombinant IL-1 to experimental animals could influence the course of for instance a life-threatening bacterial infection. It turned out that low dosages of IL-1 were able to modify the course of lethal infections caused by a variety of pathogens in a beneficial sense (Table I); the beneficial effects were present in normal as well as in neutropenic animals. In addition, it was found that IL-1 protected against injection of a lethal amount of endotoxin [10, 11].

The mechanisms of the protective effect of IL-1 in neutropenic and in non-neutropenic animals have not been elucidated [12]. It has been demonstrated that IL-1 did not exert antimicrobial activity or enhanced the effect of antimicrobial drugs *in vitro* [13, 14]. In contrast, IL-1 can be utilized as a growth factor by pathogenic bacteria [15].

Table 1. Bacteria susceptible to IL-1-enhanced host resistance.

Type of infection	References
Pseudomonas aeruginosa	[13, 67–71]
Klebsiella pneumoniae	[10, 67–69, 71, 72]
Salmonella typhimurium	[68, 73, 74]
Escherichia coli	[75]
Staphylococcus aureus	[68, 72, 76]
Streptococcus pneumoniae	[68]
Listeria moncytogenes	[34, 69, 77–80]

Therefore, indirect mechanisms of protection against lethal pathogens are to be considered, and these are depicted in Table II. As mentioned above, phagocytic cells (granulocytes, monocytes, and macrophages) play a key role in the defense against bacterial and fungal pathogens, but it has been questioned whether the protective effect of IL-1 is due to increased production, recruitment or activation of these cells. Although IL-1 has an effect on the production and release of granulocytes [16, 17], the protective effect of IL-1 is also present in mice with severe granulocytopenia [13, 18], or complete agranulocytosis after total body irradiation [18]. In this respect, it is of importance that the treatment with IL-1 does not lead to increased numbers of phagocytic cells either in the peripheral blood or at the site of infection in these experimental models [19]. A major argument against a role of neutrophils in the IL-1-induced non-specific resistance is the observation that IL-8, a cytokine which is induced by IL-1 and is considered a major chemoattractant and activator of neutrophils, does not protect against infection, and may even be detrimental [20]. In addition, IL-1 does not directly activate granulocytes [21, 22], and it is not capable to activate macrophages to a measurable extent either [13, 23].

The beneficial effect of IL-1 in lethal infection does not seem to be mediated by lipid mediators like prostaglandins, leukotrienes and platelet activating factors, since inhibitors of these mediators do not influence the IL-1 effect [24].

Early administration of IL-1 could interfere with the action of cytokines (TNF-α, IL-1β, IL-6, IL-8,

Table 2. Possible mechanisms of IL-1-enhanced host resistance.

Possible mechanism	Experimental results	References
direct antimicrobial effect	not demonstrable	[13, 14]
changed distribution of organisms	not demonstrable	[18]
accelerated bone marrow recovery	contributes in some settings	[17]
increased neutrophil accumulation	not demonstrable	[18, 19]
neutrophil activation	not demonstrable	[21, 22]
macrophage activation	not demonstrable	[13, 23]
mediation by eicosanoids	not demonstrable	[13, 18, 24]
mediation by hypoferremia	not demonstrable	[75]
mediation by IL-6	minor effect	[59]
mediation by IL-8	not demonstrable	[20]
mediation by PAF	not demonstrable	[24]
mediation by TNF-α	minor effect	[24]
mediation by GM-CSF	not demonstrable	[24]
mediation by corticosteroids	not demonstrable	[81]
mediation by acute phase proteins	some effect	[35]
inhibition of cytokine production	present	[27, 28, and Vogels, submitted]
inhibition of cytokine receptor expression	present	[Vogels, submitted]

IFN-γ) that have been shown to contribute to death from severe infections [25, 26], a condition that we have named 'lethal cytokinemia' [10]. IL-1 could do so in a variety of ways. First, IL-1 may downregulate the production of the deleterious cytokines during the lethal phase of infection (Vogels and Van der Meer, manuscript in preparation), or induce the production of anti-inflammatory substances like the IL-1 receptor antagonist, a physiological inhibitor of IL-1. Secondly, IL-1 could induce a downregulation of the receptors for IL-1 and TNF-α, a phenomenon which was first observed *in vitro* [27, 28]. Recently, it has been confirmed that administration of IL-1 *in vivo* downregulates the expression of mRNA for the IL-1 receptor type I in the spleens of mice (Vogels and Van der Meer, submitted). Interference with the harmful effects of cytokines as a mechanism of IL-1 protection could also apply to other beneficial effects of exogenous IL-1, such as described in radiation protection [29], and protection against oxygen damage [30], against ischemia reperfusion damage [31], against IL-2 toxicity [32], and against alopecia induced by cancer chemotherapy [33]. Although interference with deleterious cytokine action might explain the IL-1-induced survival of mice with an acute potentially lethal infection, it does not explain the inhibitory effect of IL-1 on the outgrowth of microorganisms in the target organs during less acute infections like those caused by *Listeria monocytogenes* and *Candida albicans* [18, 34]. Other mechanisms probably play an additional role, and it has recently been shown that induction of synthesis of acute phase proteins by IL-1 contributes to survival of lethally infected mice [35]. Interestingly, synthesis of acute phase proteins by IL-6 did not lead to significant protection [35].

Tumor necrosis factor-α

TNF-α is a 17-kDa protein secreted predominantly by macrophages after a variety of stimuli [36]. It is a major pro-inflammatory and pyrogenic cytokine, and induces production of IL-1 [37]. Largely based on protection experiments with monoclonal antibodies against TNF-α, the deleterious role of TNF-α in sepsis has been established [25, 38–42]. In contrast to these potentially lethal effects of TNF-α circulating during sepsis, small amounts of TNF-α are essential for host resistance against infection. TNF-α causes recruitment and activation of neutrophils at the site of infection [43–45]. These effects are largely beneficial to the host because they enable the neutrophil to eliminate microorganisms. On the other hand, production of reactive molecules like chloramines by activated neutrophils may lead to damage at the tissue level [46]. Endogenously produced TNF-α plays an essential role as a mediator in host defense against infections caused by

Table 3. Bacteria susceptible to TNF-α-enhanced host resistance.

Type of infection	References
Chlamydia trachomatis	[82]
Escherichia coli	[83, 84]
Klebsiella pneumoniae	[83, 85]
Pseudomonas aeruginosa	[10]
Staphylococcus aureus	[86]
Listeria monocytogenes	[85, 87, 88]
Salmonella typhimurium	[89]
Legionella pneumophila	[52]
Mycobacterium spp.	[49, 90, 91]

facultative intracellular bacteria such as *Listeria monocytogenes* and *Mycobacterium spp.*, and administration of neutralizing antibody to TNF-α accelerates death in animals with such granulomatous infections, as well as in animals with peritoneal abscesses [47–50].

The protective effect of exogenous recombinant TNF-α has been demonstrated *in vitro* and *in vivo* in infections with a wide range of microorganisms (Table III). In our experiments in neutropenic mice with *Pseudomonas* infection and in normal mice with *Klebsiella* infection, recombinant human TNF-α is much less protective against lethality than IL-1 [10, 51]. To some extent, this is due to greater species specifity of TNF-α than of IL-1, since murine recombinant TNF-α is more protective than human TNF-α, albeit still not as protective as IL-1 [51]. The exact mechanism of this TNF-α-induced protection has not been clarified. Probably several cellular and non-cellular mechanisms are involved, some of which may be shared with the above-mentioned mechanisms of protection induced by IL-1. However, some mechanisms appear to differ from those of IL-1. For instance, TNF-α-enhanced killing of organisms by neutrophils has been found in a number of models, such as experimental legionellosis [52] and disseminated candidiasis [53, 54].

Similarly to IL-1, TNF-α is known to induce other cytokines like IL-1, IFN-γ, IL-6 and colony stimulating factors, which in turn could enhance aspecific protective mechanisms in the host [37]. TNF-α might induce reduced sensitivity of target cells to TNF-α in the phase of lethal cytokinemia by downregulation of TNF receptors [27], or protect cells by inducing shedding of TNF receptors, which then may act as TNF-antagonists [55].

Related cytokines

Production of the 26-kDa cytokine IL-6 is induced by IL-1, and IL-6 mediates a variety of the effects of IL-1, such as the synthesis of acute phase proteins [56]. Therefore, IL-6 could be responsible for the protective effect of IL-1 on the course of infections. The results of studies with administration of recombinant IL-6 in models of *Listeria monocytogenes* infection are contradictory [57, 58]. It has been demonstrated that IL-6 offers no protection against lethal *P. aeruginosa* infection in mice [35, 59]. Taken together, there is little evidence that IL-6, whether endogenous or administered, in itself has a beneficial effect on the course of infections.The 8 kDa polypeptide IL-8 was originally known as neutrophil-activating factor, and the effects of IL-8 on neutrophil granulocytes include chemotaxis as well as activation [60]. For example, IL-8-activated granulocytes are able to kill ingested *Candida albicans* and mycobacteria more efficiently [61, 62]. The production of IL-8 is induced by IL-1, TNF-α and LPS [63]. In a series of experiments, we investigated whether IL-8 could provide protection in lethal bacterial infection in neutropenic and normal animals. Some protection was found against *Klebsiella* infection in normal mice [20]. However, in infected neutropenic mice survival appeared to be diminished by IL-8 [20]. Histologically, endothelial damage was prominent in these animals, and such observations are in agreement with the finding that IL-8 contributes to endothelial damage, and with clinical observations that IL-8 concentrations in alveolar lavage fluid correlate with severity of adult respiratory distress syndrome [64, 65].

Concluding remarks

The experiments reviewed in this paper indicate beneficial effects of administration of interleukin-1 and related cytokines in bacterial infections. These experiments have increased our insight in the pathophysiology of lethal bacterial infection. Although the relative contribution of the various mechanisms to the beneficial effects is not entirely clear, the mechanisms can be divided into two categories: 1) interference with the inflammatory response, and 2) interference with microbial growth. The interference with the inflammatory reponse comprises modulation of cytokine responses (downregulation of cytokine production and receptor modulation) and production of acute phase proteins.

Interference with microbial growth seems to occur predominantly in subacute or chronic infections, by mechanisms not well understood as yet.

An important question is whether treatment with proinflammatory cytokines will have future clinical application in treatment of serious infection. So far, successful treatment in animals is rather prophylactic than therapeutic. Another limitation for therapeutic application are the potential side effects, although these can probably be largely prevented by pretreatment with cyclooxygenase inhibitors [10]. Trials with relatively low dosages of IL-1 to enhance platelet recovery after cancer chemotherapy in patients with neoplastic disease have met with acceptable side effects and therefore should encourage the design of studies in infection in humans [66].

References

1. Bodey GP, Buckley M, Sathe YS, Freireich EJ. Quantitative relationships between circulating leukocytes and infections in patients with leukemia. Ann Intern Med 1966; 64: 328–340.
2. Lieschke GJ, Burgess AW. Drug therapy: Granulocyte colony-stimulating factor and granulocyte-macrophage colony-stimulating factor (first of two parts). N Engl J Med 1992; 327: 28–35.
3. Dinarello CA. Role of interleukin-1 in infectious diseases. Immunol Rev 1992; 127: 119–146.
4. Oppenheim JJ, Kovacs EJ, Matsushima K, Durum SK. There is more than one interleukin-1. Immunol Today 1986; 7: 45–56.
5. Dinarello CA, Cannon JG, Wolff SM. New concepts on the pathogenesis of fever. Rev Infect Dis 1988; 10: 168–189.
6. Dinarello CA, Cannon JG, Mier JW, Bernheim HA, LoPreste G. Multiple biological activities of human recombinant interleukin-1. J Clin Invest 1986; 77: 1734–1739.
7. Dinarello CA. Interleukin-1. FASEB J 1988; 2: 108–115.
8. Dinarello CA. Interleukin-1 and interleukin-1 antagonism. Blood 1991; 77: 1627–1652.
9. Dinarello CA. Interleukin-1 and the pathogenesis of the acute-phase response. N Engl J Med 1984; 311: 1413–1419.
10. Van der Meer JWM. The effects of recombinant interleukin-1 and recombinant tumor necrosis factor on non-specific resistance to infection. Biotherapy 1988; 1: 19–25.
11. Alexander HR, Doherty GM, Fraker DL, Block MI, Swedenborg JE, Norton JA. Human recombinant interleukin-1α protection against the lethality of endotoxin and experimental sepsis in mice. J Surg Res 1991; 50: 421–424.
12. Vogels MTE, Van der Meer JWM. Use of immune modulators in nonspecific therapy of bacterial infections. Antimicrob Agents Chemother 1992; 36: 1–5.
13. Van der Meer JWM, Barza M, Wolff SM, Dinarello CA. A low dose of recombinant interleukin 1 protects granulocytopenic mice from lethal Gram-negative infection. Proc Natl Acad Sci USA 1988; 85: 1620–1623.
14. Van 't Wout JW, Van der Meer JWM, Barza M, Dinarello CA. Protection of neutropenic mice from lethal *Candida albicans* infection by recombinant interleukin 1. Eur J Immunol 1988; 18: 1143–1146.
15. Porat R, Clarck BD, Wolff SM, Dinarello CA. Intrleukin-1 enhances the growth of virulent strains of *Escherichia coli* via a specific receptor-like interaction. Science 1991; 254: 430–432.
16. Stork LC, Peterson VM, Rundus CH, Robinson WA. Interleukin-1 enhances murine granulopoiesis *in vivo*. Exp Hematol 1988; 16: 163–167.
17. Fibbe WE, Van der Meer JWM, Falkenburg JHF, Hamilton MS, Kluin PM, Dinarello CA. A single low dose of human recombinant interleukin 1 accelerates the recovery of neutrophils in mice with cyclophosphamide-induced neutropenia. Exp Hematol 1989; 17: 805–808.
18. Kullberg BJ, Van 't Wout JW, Van Furth R. Role of granulocytes in enhanced host resistance to *Candida albicans* induced by recombinant interleukin-1. Infect Immun 1990; 58: 3319–3324.
19. Kullberg BJ, Van 't Wout JW, Van Furth R. No effect of recombinant human interleukin-1 on the numbers of peripheral blood and peritoneal leukocytes during an acute inflammation. Inflammation 1991; 15: 457–470.
20. Vogels MTE, Lindley IJD, Curfs JAHJ, Eling WMC, Van der Meer JWM. Effects of interleukin-8 on non-specific resistance to infection in neutropenic and normal mice. Antimicrob Agents Chemother 1993; 37: 276–280.
21. Georgilis K, Schaeffer C, Dinarello CA, Klempner MS. Human recombinant interleukin-1β has no effect on intracellular calcium or on functional responses of human neutrophils. J Immunol 1987; 138: 3403–3407.
22. Yoshimura T, Matsushima K, Oppenheim JJ, Leonard EJ. Neutrophil chemotactic factor produced by lipopolysaccharide (LPS)-stimulated human blood mononuclear leukocytes: Partial characterization and separation from interleukin-1 (IL1). J Immunol 1987; 139: 788–793.
23. Langermans JAM, Van der Hulst MEB, Nibbering PH, Hiemstra PS, Fransen L, Van Furth R. IFN-γ-induced L-arginine-dependent toxoplasmastatic activity in murine peritoneal macrophages is mediated by endogenous tumor necrosis factor-α. J Immunol 1992; 148: 568–574.
24. Vogels MTE, Hermsen CC, Huys HLPG, Eling WMC, Van der Meer JWM. Roles of tumor necrosis factor alpha, granulocyte-macrophage colony-stimulating factor, platelet-activating factor, and arachidonic acid metabolites in interleukin-1-induced resistance to infection in neutropenic mice. Infect Immun 1944; 62: 2065–2070.
25. Cannon JG, Thompkins RG, Gelfand JA, *et al.* Circulating interleukin-1 and tumor necrosis factor in septic shock and experimental endotoxin fever. J Infect Dis 1990; 161: 79–84.
26. Waage A, Brandtzaeg P, Halstensen A, Kierulf P, Espevik T. The complex pattern of cytokines in serum from patients with meningococcal septic shock. Association between interleukin 6, interleukin 1, and fatal outcome. J Exp Med 1989; 169: 333–338.
27. Holtmann H, Wallach D. Down regulation of the receptors for tumor necrosis factor by interleukin-1 and 4β-phorbol-12-myristate-13-acetate. J Immunol 1987; 139: 1161–1167.
28. Ye K, Clark BD, Dinarello CA. Interleukin-1 downregulates gene and surface expression of interleukin-1 receptor type I by destabilizing its mRNA, whereas interleukin-2 increases its expression. Immunol 1992; 75: 427–434.
29. Neta R, Oppenheim JJ, Douches SD. Interdependence of the radioprotective effects of human recombinant interleukin-1α, tumor necrosis factor-α, granulocyte colony-stimulating factor, and murine recombinant granulocyte macrophage colony-stimulating factor. J Immunol 1988; 140: 108–114.

30. White CW, Ghezzi P. Protection against pulmonary oxygen toxicity by interleukin-1 and tumor necrosis factor. Role of antioxydant enzymes and effect of cyclooxygenase inhibitors. Biotherapy 1989; 1: 361–366.
31. Brown J, White CW, Terada LS, *et al.* Interleukin-1 pretreatment decreases ischaemia reperfusion injury. Proc Natl Acad Sci USA 1990; 87: 5026–5030.
32. Puri RK, Travis WD, Rosenberg SA. Decrease in interleukin 2-induced leakage in the lungs of mice by administration of recombinant interleukin-1α *in vivo*. Cancer Res 1989; 49: 969–976.
33. Jimenez JJ, Wong GHW, Yunis AA. Interleukin 1 protects from cytosine arabinoside-induced alopecia in the rat model. FASEB J 1991; 5: 2456–2458.
34. Czuprynski CJ, Brown JF, Young KM, Cooley AJ, Kurtz RS. Effects of murine recombinant interleukin 1 alpha on the host response to bacterial infection. J Immunol 1988; 140: 962–968.
35. Vogels MTE, Cantoni L, Carelli M, Sironi M, Ghezzi P, Van der Meer JWM. Role of acute phase proteins in interleukin-1-induced resistance to bacterial infection in mice. Antimicrob Agents Chemother 1993; 37: 2527–2533.
36. Beutler B, Cerami A. Cachectin/tumor necrosis factor: an endogenous mediator of shock and inflammation. Immunol Res 1986; 5: 281–293.
37. Dinarello CA, Cannon JG, Wolff SM. Tumor necrosis factor (cachectin) is an endogenous pyrogen and induces production of interleukin-1. J Exp Med 1986; 163: 1433–1450.
38. Beutler B, Milsark IW, Cerami AC. Passive immunization against cachexin/tumor necrosis factor protects mice from lethal effect of endotoxin. Science 1985; 229: 869–871.
39. Cerami A, Beutler B. The role of cachectin/TNF in endotoxic shock and cachexia. Immunol Today 1988; 9: 28–31.
40. Tracey KJ, Lowry SF, Fahey TJ, Albert JD, Fong Y, Hesse D. Cachectin/tumor necrosis factor induces lethal shock and stress hormone responses in the dog. Surg Gynecol Obstet 1987; 164: 415–422.
41. Tracey KJ, Beutler B, Lowry SF. Shock and tissue injury induced by recombinant human cachectin. Science 1986; 234: 470–474.
42. Opal SM, Cross AS, Kelly NM, *et al.* Efficacy of a monoclonal antibody directed against tumor necrosis factor in protecting neutropenic rats from lethal infection with *Pseudomonas aeruginosa*. J Infect Dis 1990; 161: 1148–1152.
43. Figari IS, Mori NA, Palladino MA Jr. Regulation of neutrophil migration and superoxide production by recombinant tumor necrosis factors-α and -β: comparison to recombinant interferon-γ and interleukin-1α. Blood 1987; 70: 979–984.
44. Ulich TR, del Castillo J, Guo K, Souza L. The hematologic effects of chronic administration of the monokines tumor necrosis factor, interleukin-1, and granulocyte-colony stimulating factor on bone marrow and circulation. Am J Pathol 1989; 134: 149–159.
45. Steinbeck MA, Roth JA. Neutrophil activation by recombinant cytokines. Rev Infect Dis 1989; 11: 549–568.
46. Weiss SJ. Tissue derstruction by neutrophils. N Engl J Med 1989; 320: 365–376.
47. Nacy CA, Meierovics AI, Belosevic M, Green SJ. Tumor necrosis factor-α: central regulatory cytokine in the induction of macrophage antimicrobial activities. Pathobiol 1991; 59: 182–184.
48. Nakane A, Minagawa T, Kato K. Endogenous tumor necrosis factor (cachectin) is essential to host resistance against *Listeria monocytogenes* infection. Infect Immun 1988; 56: 2563–2569.
49. Kindler V, Sappino AP, Grau GE, Piguet PF, Vassali P. The inducing role of tumor necrosis factor in the development of bactericidal granulomas during BCG infection. Cell 1989; 56: 731–740.
50. Echtenacher B, Falk W, Mannel DN, Krammer PH. Requirement of endogenous tumor necrosis factor/cachectin for recovery from experimental peritonitis. J Immunol 1990; 145: 3762–3766.
51. Vogels MTE, Van der Meer JWM. Comparison of the capacity of murine tumor necrosis factor and human interleukin-1 to prolong survival in lethal bacterial infection. Eur Cytokine Netw 1992; 2: 221.
52. Blanchard DK, Djeu JY, Klein TW, Friedman H, Stewart WE. Protective effect of tumor necrosis factor in experimental *Legionella pneumophila* infections of mice via activation of PMN function. J Leukocyte Biol 1988; 43: 429–435.
53. Djeu JY, Blanchard DK, Halkias D, Friedman H. Growth inhibition of *Candida albicans* by human polymorphonuclear neutrophils: activation by interferon-γ and tumor necrosis factor. J Immunol 1986; 137: 2980–2984.
54. Ferrante A. Tumor necrosis factor alpha potentiates neutrophil antimicrobial activity: Increased fungal activity against *Torulopsis glabrata* and *Candida albicans* and associated increases in oxygen radical production and lysosomal enzyme release. Infect Immun 1989; 57: 2115–2122.
55. Seckinger P, Isaaz S, Dayer JM. A human inhibitor of tumor necrosis factor α. J Exp Med 1988; 167: 1511 –1516.
56. Neta R, Vogel SN, Sipe JD, Wong GG, Nordan RP. Comparison of *in vivo* effects of human recombinant IL 1 and human recombinant IL 6 in mice. Lymphokine Res 1988; 7: 403–412.
57. Czuprynski CJ, Haak-Frendscho M, Maroushek N, Brown JF. Effects of recombinant human interleukin-6 alone and in combination with recombinant interleukin-1α and tumor necrosis factor-alpha on antibacterial resistance in mice. Antimicrob Agents Chemother 1992; 36: 68–70.
58. Liu Z, Simpson RJ, Cheers C. Recombinant interleukin-6 protects mice against experimental bacterial infection. Infect Immun 1992; 60: 4402–4406.
59. Van der Meer JWM, Helle M, Aarden L. Comparison of the effects of recombinant interleukin 6 and recombinant interleukin 1 in nonspecific resistance to infection. Eur J Immunol 1989; 19: 413–416.
60. Peveri P, Walz A, Dewald B, Baggiolini M. A novel neutrophil-activating factor produced by human mononuclear phagocytes. J Exp Med 1988; 167: 1547–1559.
61. Djeu JY, Matsushima K, Oppenheim JJ, Shiotsuki K, Blanchard DK. Functional activation of human neutrophils by recombinant monocyte-derived neutrophil chemotactic factor/IL-8. J Immunol 1990; 144: 2205–2210.
62. Nibbering PH, Pos O, Stevenhagen A, Van Furth R. Interleukin-8 enhances nonoxidative intracellular killing of *Mycobacterium fortuitum* by human granulocytes. Infect Immun 1993; 61: 3111–3116.
63. Lohmann-Matthes ML. Interaction of macrophages and cytokines. Curr Opinion Immunol 1989; 2: 33–38.
64. Chollet-Martin S, Montravers P, Gibert C, *et al.* High levels of interleukin-8 in the blood and alveolar spaces of patients with pneumonia and adult respiratory distress syndrome. Infect Immun 1993; 61: 4553–4559.
65. Donnelly SC, Strieter RM, Kunkel SL, *et al.* Interleukin-8 and development of adult respiratory distress syndrome in at-risk patient groups. Lancet 1993; 341: 643–647.

66. Smith JW, Longo DL, Alvord WG, *et al.* The effects of treatment with interleukin-1α on platelet recovery after high-dose carboplatin. N Engl J Med 1993; 328: 756–761.
67. Ozaki Y, Ohashi A, Minami A, Nakamura S. Enhanced resistance of mice to bacterial infection induced by recombinant human interleukin-1α. Infect Immun 1987; 55: 1436–1440.
68. Minami A, Fujimoto K, Ozaki Y, Nakamura S. Augmentation of host resistance to microbial infections by recombinant human interleukin-1α. Infect Immun 1988; 56: 3116–3120.
69. Morikage T, Mizushima Y, Sakamoto K, Yano. S. Prevention of fatal infections by recombinant human interleukin-1α in normal and anticancer drug-treated mice. Cancer Res 1990; 50: 2099–2104.
70. Campanile F, Binaglia L, Boraschi D, Tagliabue A, Fioretti MC, Puccetti P. Antibacterial resistance induced by recombinant interleukin-1 in myelosuppressed mice: effect of treatment schedule and correlation with colony-stimulating activity in the bloodstream. Cell Immunol 1990; 128: 250–260.
71. Nakamura S, Minami A, Fujimoto K, Kojima T. Combination effect of recombinant human interleukin-1α with antimicrobial agents. Antimicrob Agents Chemother 1989; 33: 1804–1810.
72. McIntyre KW, Unowsky J, DeLorenzo W, Benjamin W. Enhancement of antibacterial resistance of neutropenic bone marrow-suppressed mice by interleukin-1α. Infect Immun 1989; 57: 48–54.
73. Kampschmidt RF, Pulliam LA. Stimulation of antimicrobial activity in the rat with leukocyte endogenous mediator. J Reticuloendothel Soc 1975; 17: 162–169.
74. Morrissey PJ, Charrier K. Interleukin-1 administration to C3H/HeJ mice after but not prior to infection increases resistance to *Salmonella typhimurium*. Infect Immun 1991; 59: 4729–4731.
75. Pelkonen S, Pluschke G. Recombinant interleukin-1 stimulates clearance of *Escherichia coli* bacteremia. Microb Pathogen 1989; 6: 415–424.
76. Gladue R, Girard A, Newborg M. Enhanced antibacterial resistance in neutropenic mice treated with human recombinant interleukin-1 beta. Agents Actions 1988; 24: 130–136.
77. Czuprynski CJ, Brown JF. Purified human and recombinant murine interleukin-1 induced accumulation of inflammatory peritoneal neutrophils and mononuclear phagocytes: possible contributions to antibacterial resistance. Microb Pathogen 1987; 3: 377–386.
78. Czuprynski CJ, Brown JF. Recombinant murine interleukin-1α enhancement of nonspecific antibacterial resistance. Infect Immun 1987; 55: 2061–2065.
79. Kurtz RS, Young KM, Czuprynski CJ. Separate and combined effects of recombinant interleukin-1α and gamma interferon on antibacterial resistance. Infect Immun 1989; 57: 553–558.
80. Kurtz RS, Roll JT, Czuprynski CJ. Recombinant human interleukin 1 alpha enhances anti-*Listeria* resistance in both genetically resistant and susceptible strains of mice. Immunol Lett 1988; 18: 289–292.
81. Vogels MTE, Sweep CGJ, Hermus ARMM, Van der Meer JWM. Interleukin-1-induced nonspecific resistance to bacterial infection in mice is not mediated by glucocorticosteroids. Antimicrob Agents Chemother 1992; 36: 2785–2789.
82. Williams DM, Magee DM, Bonewald LF, *et al.* A role *in vivo* for tumor necrosis factor alpha in host defense against *Chlamydia trachomatis*. Infect Immun 1990; 58: 1572–1576.
83. Alexander HR, Sheppard BC, Jensen JC, *et al.* Treatment with recombinant human tumor necrosis factor-alpha protects rats against the lethality, hypotension, and hypothermia of Gram-negative sepsis. J Clin Invest 1991; 88: 34–39.
84. Cross AS, Sadoff JC, Kelly N, Bernton E, Gemski P. Pretreatment with recombinant murine tumor necrosis factor α/cachectin and murine recombinant interleukin-1α protects mice from lethal bacterial infection. J Exp Med 1989; 169: 2021–2027.
85. Parant F, Tavernier J, Fiers W, Parant M. Comparative activity of human and murine tumor necrosis factor in toxicity and anti-infectious assays in mice. Microb Pathogen 1990; 8: 143–149.
86. Vaudaux P, Grau GE, Huggler E, *et al.* Contribution of tumor necrosis factor to host defense against staphylococci in a guinea pig model of foreign body infections. J Infect Dis 1992; 166: 58–64.
87. Havell EA. Production of tumor necrosis factor during murine listeriosis. J Immunol 1987; 139: 4225–4231.
88. Desiderio JV, Kiener PA, Lin FP, Warr GA. Protection of mice against *Listeria monocytogenes* infection by recombinant human tumor necrosis factor. Infect Immun 1989; 57: 1615–1617.
89. Nauciel C, Espinasse-Maes F. Role of gamma-interferon and tumor necrosis factor alpha in resistance to *Salmonella typhimurium* infection. Infect Immun 1992; 60: 450–454.
90. Bermudez LEM, Young LS. Tumor necrosis factor, alone or in combination with IL-2, but not IFN-γ, is associated with macrophage killing of *Mycobacterium avium* complex. J Immunol 1988; 140: 3006–3013.
91. Bermudez LEM, Stevens P, Kolonoski P, Wu M, Young LS. Treatment of experimental disseminated *Mycobacterium avium* complex infection in mice with recombinant IL-2 and tumor necrosis factor. J Immunol 1989; 143: 2996–3000.

Address for correspondence: J.W.M. van der Meer, M.D., Ph.D., Division of General Internal Medicine, University Hospital Nijmegen, P.O. Box 9101, 6500 HB Nijmegen, The Netherlands

Biotherapy 7: 169–178, 1994.

Cytokines and the host defense against *Listeria monocytogenes* and *Salmonella typhimurium*

Jan A.M. Langermans & Ralph van Furth
Department of Infectious Diseases, University Hospital Leiden, the Netherlands

Key words: Cytokines, macrophages, intracellular pathogens, activation, deactivation, hepatocytes

Abstract

The host defense against intracellular pathogens depends largely on activation of phagocytes and is regulated by a complex network of cytokines. Modulation of this cytokine network might lead to new or additional therapies in the treatment of infections with intracellular pathogens. Therefore, insight in the role of various cytokines in the host defense against these pathogens is required. The present contribution summarizes the results of various studies on the role of different cytokines in the host defense against the intracellular bacteria *Listeria monocytogenes* and *Salmonella typhimurium.*

Abbreviations: ROI: reactive oxygen intermediates; IFNγ: interferon γ; TNF: tumor necrosis factors; IL: interleukin; CSF: colony-stimulating factor; CF: cerebrospinal fluid

Introduction

The host defense against intracellular pathogens, such as *Listeria monocytogenes* and *Salmonella typhimurium*, is mainly cell-mediated and requires the cooperation of various effector cells, such as T lymphocytes, granulocytes, and monocytes/macrophages. The functional activities of these cells are regulated by a complex network of cytokines [1].

During the first few days of an infection with intracellular bacteria, limitation of bacterial proliferation depends mainly on resident tissue macrophages and the influx of inflammatory phagocytes, i.e. granulocytes and exudate macrophages, that migrate rapidly to the site of infection [2, 3]. Intracellular bacteria have the capacity to survive and proliferate within nonactivated macrophages and other host cells like hepatocytes [4]. Microorganisms residing in host cells other than phagocytes are liberated by lysis of the cells by cytotoxic T lymphocytes, NK cells or granulocytes and are subsequently phagocytosed and killed by activated macrophages [5]. Eradication of intracellular bacteria is thought to depend mainly on the enhanced antimicrobial activity of activated macrophages. Our understanding of the involvement of resident, non-activated and activated macrophages in cell-mediated immunity originates from the studies of Mackaness and others [6–11], who demonstrated that mice injected with a sublethal number of *L. monocytogens* or *Mycobacterium tuberculosis* exhibit increased resistance to (re)infections with these pathogens; this increased resistance is accompanied by a decrease in the capacity of intracellular pathogens to survive in macrophages. The term activated macrophage is used to distinguish macrophages in which proliferation of intracellular pathogens is reduced from macrophages in which these pathogens can proliferate. In general, there are two phases in the host defense against intracellular pathogens: one is immunologically specific and involves T lymphocytes; the other, i.e. expression of macrophage activation is not specific.

In the sixties and seventies, several groups discovered that factors in the supernatant of stimulated T lymphocytes are able to activate macrophages [12, 13]. Independently of these findings, others demonstrated the presence of a protein with antiviral activity in the supernatant of stimulated T lymphocytes [14], which is now known to be interferon-γ (IFN-γ). It was not until the isolation and cloning of IFN-γ that the antiviral protein was found to be identical to the macrophage-activating factor in the lymphocyte supernatant [15, 16]. Originally, $CD4^+$ T lymphocytes were considered to be the major producers of IFN-γ. It is now clear that in addition to these cells, other cells of the immune system also produce substantial amounts of IFN-γ, e.g. $CD8^+$ T lymphocytes, NK cells and $\gamma\delta$ T lymphocytes [17–20]. Since the discovery of IFN-γ several other cytokines have been identified as being involved in the modulation of macrophage functions and host resistance against intracellular pathogens. In the present contribution, the role of various cytokines in the host defense against infections with *L. monocytogenes* and *S. typhimurium* will be reviewed.

Macrophages and host defense against *L. monocytogenes* and *S. typhimurium*

L. monocytogenes is a gram-positive bacterium which is abundantly present in nature; it is a facultative intracellular microbe and is often used as a model to study the host defense against intracellular bacteria. Infections of mice with *S. typhimurium*, a gram-negative bacterium, are often regarded as a disease analogous to human typhoid fever. The initial phase of host defense against *L. monocytogenes* is mediated by granulocytes and exudate macrophages whereas resident tissue macrophages control the initial proliferation of *S. typhimurium* [21, 22]. The initial phase of host defense against *L. monocytogenes* and *S. typhimurium* is followed by a phase in which activated macrophages are assumed to be the most important effector cells [23]. It has been demonstrated that macrophages become activated during an infection of mice with BCG or *L. monocytogenes*, as determined by various criteria, and that these activated macrophages kill *L. monocytogenes* faster than nonactivated macrophages [24]. These results indicate that activated macrophages are involved in the elimination of *L. monocytogenes in vivo*. In contrast, *S. typhimurium* is not killed more efficiently by macrophages that have become activated during a BCG or *L. monocytogenes* infection of mice [24]. Although macrophages become activated during an infection of mice with *S. typhimurium*, as judged by the inhibition of the intracellular proliferation of *Toxoplasma gondii*, the enhanced production of reactive oxygen intermediates (ROI) and the enhanced expression of Ia antigen on these cells, these activated macrophages do not kill *S. typhimurium* more efficiently than resident macrophages [25, 26]. During a secondary infection of mice with *S. typhimurium* , the bacteria do not proliferate in their liver. Together, these findings indicate that eradication of *S. typhimurium* from mice is not due to enhanced killing of these microorganisms by activated macrophages. Various functional and histological studies have demonstrated that *S. typhimurium* is readily killed by granulocytes, exudate macrophages and resident tissue macrophages [3, 27].

Role of IFN-γ

During an infection with *L. monocytogenes*, IFN-γ is produced in two phases; early in the infection this cytokine is produced by NK cells and in a later phase IFN-γ is produced by T lymphocytes [19]. In 1985, Buchmeier and Schreiber demonstrated that endogenous IFN-γ is essential in the limitation of the proliferation of *L. monocytogenes* in mice [28]. Convincing evidence on the protective role of IFN-γ against infections with *L. monocytogenes* has been provided in studies with mice that lack the receptors for IFN-γ [29]. In addition, various groups showed that treatment of mice with IFN-γ protected them against infections with *L. monocytogenes* [30, 31]. More recently, it has been shown that IFN-γ also mediates protection of mice against *S. typhimurium* [32] and is essential in the innate resistance against this bacterium [33]. One of the effects of IFN-γ is activation of macrophages, which results in a variety of biochemical and functional changes of these cells. However, different effects of IFN-γ on the antibacterial activity of macrophages against *L. monocytogenes* and *S. typhimurium* have been described. Various groups have reported that IFN-γ-activated macrophages kill *L. monocytogenes* and *S. typhimurium* more efficiently than non-activated macrophages [30, 34]. Others, however, failed to demonstrate an enhanced microbicidal activity against these bacteria upon activation of macrophages with IFN-γ [31, 35, 36]. Also *in vivo*, divergent results on the effect of IFN-γ on the course of an infection with *L. monocytogenes* and *S. typhimurium* have been reported [25, 30, 35, 37]. Recently, we found that the different effects of IFN-γ on the proliferation of *L. monocytogenes* could be attributed to variations in the number of injected bacteria [31]. I.v. injection of rIFN-γ resulted in inhibition of *L. monocytogenes* proliferation and marked decrease in tissue damage in the liver when the mice received an i.v. injection of less than 10 LD_{50} *L.*

monocytogenes, but not when 10 LD_{50} bacteria were injected [31, 38]. These results might explain the contradictory findings on the effect of rIFN-γ on the proliferation of *L. monocytogenes*. The rIFN-γ-induced inhibition of bacterial proliferation was not observed for the spleen [31]. IFN-γ-treatment of mice infected with various numbers of *S. typhimurium* did not result in a decreased proliferation of *S. typhimurium* in the liver and spleen [25].

These findings suggest that the inhibition of *L. monocytogenes* proliferation in the liver of rIFN-γ-treated mice is not directly due to an enhanced listericidal activity of rIFN-γ-activated macrophages. It has been demonstrated that *L. monocytogenes* escape from the phagolysosomes of naive macrophages but not from those of rIFN-γ-activated macrophages [39]; it is possible that a similar mechanism occurs *in vivo*. When *L. monocytogenes* are contained within the phagolysosomes of activated macrophages they remain exposed to the bactericidal activities of these cells; in this way cell-to-cell spreading within the liver is prevented. In naive mice, *L. monocytogenes* that have escaped from the phagolysosomes of macrophages penetrate hepatocytes and proliferate in these cells. It has been demonstrated recently that IFN-γ activates hepatocytes to limit the proliferation of *L. monocytogenes* in these cells [40]. The possible involvement of hepatocytes in the IFN-γ-induced protection against *L. monocytogenes* might explain the observed differences with respect to the effect of this cytokine on the bacterial proliferation in the liver and spleen [31]. It is not known whether similar mechanisms might be involved in the host defense against infections with *S. typhimurium*. Together, these results demonstrate that rIFN-γ by itself is not sufficient to stimulate enhanced bactericidal activity of macrophages against *L. monocytogenes* and *S. typhimurium*. The inhibition of *L. monocytogenes* proliferation by IFN-γ is most likely mediated by mechanisms other than enhancement of the antibacterial activity of macrophages.

Role of TNF

During the past few years it has become clear that besides IFN-γ, tumor necrosis factor-α (TNF) is an essential mediator in the immune response against a variety of microorganisms. One of the mechanisms by which TNF might benificially influence the host defense against infections with intracellular bacteria is by its involvement in the induction of IFN-γ. Bancroft *et al.* have demonstrated that in mice with severe combined immunodeficiency (SCID) TNF, which is produced by macrophages, is essential in the induction of IFN-γ production by NK cells during the early phase of an infection with *L. monocytogenes* [41, 42]. *In vitro*, TNF is also an essential mediator in the activation of macrophages against various intracellular pathogens, such as *Leishmania major* and *Toxoplasma gondii* [43, 44]. *In vivo*, TNF is involved in the innate resistance against infections with *L. monocytogenes* [45, 46] and *S. typhimurium* [34]. Treatment of mice with TNF protects them against infections with *L. monocytogenes* [44]; this effect is enhanced by interleukin-1 [48]. The importance of TNF in infections with *L. monocytogenes* is underscored by recent findings that mice that lack the 55 kD TNF receptor rapidly succumb to infections with these pathogens [49]. Treatment of mice with neutralizing antibodies against TNF makes them more susceptible to infections with *L. monocytogenes* and *S. typhimurium* [34, 45, 46]. Neutralization of endogenous TNF also abrogates the IFN-γ-induced inhibition of *L. monocytogenes* proliferation in the liver [50].

The mechanisms by which endogenous TNF mediates the resistance against infections with *L. monocytogenes* and *S. typhimurium* are not yet understood. In mice treated with anti-TNF and infected with *S. typhimurium* a decreased number of granulocytes was observed in the liver, indicating that during this infection endogenous TNF is involved in the recruitment of granulocytes to the site of infection [51]. TNF has also been reported to be involved in the recruitment of granulocytes and monocytes to inflammatory sites in infections with BCG [52] and *L. monocytogenes* [53]. Treatment of mice with anti-TNF antibodies inhibits the migration of granulocytes and monocytes from the bone marrow to the circulation and from the circulation to the peritoneal cavity during a sterile inflammatory reaction [53a].

It is also possible that TNF mediates activation of both macrophages and hepatocytes in the liver, and that these activated cells limit bacterial proliferation. Activated macrophages probably inhibit the escape of *L. monocytogenes* from the phagolysosomes, but the elimination of *S. typhimurium* is most likely mediated by other mechanisms [24, 25]. Induction of enhanced listericidal activity of macrophages obtained from *L. monocytogenes* infected mice requires TNF [46] and *in vitro* incubation of macrophages with this cytokine enhances their listericidal activity [54].

During an infection of mice with *S. typhimurium* or *L. monocytogenes* many bacteria can be found in the hepatocytes where they proliferate [3, 55] and these cells are activated by factors produced by macrophages, e.g. TNF [56]. Such activated hepatocytes have been shown to inhibit the intracellular proliferation of *Plasmodium berghei* [57]. *L. monocytogenes* are eliminated from hepatocytes of *L. monocytogenes*-immune mice faster than from the hepatocytes of nonimmune mice [58].

In sum, endogenous TNF is essential for the defense against infections with *L. monocytogenes* and *S. typhimurium* in mice; this cytokine is probably involved in the activation and/or recruitment of various types of cells.

Role of interleukins

Interleukin-1

Interleukin (IL)-1 is a collective name for two different proteins, IL-1α and IL-1β. Although these two proteins are structurally dissimilar, they bind to the same receptors and share many biological functions [59]. Administration of IL-1 has a beneficial influence on the host defense against a number of pathogens, such as various bacteria, the yeast *Candida albicans* and the parasite *Plasmodium berghei* [60–65]. Treatment of mice with IL-1α inhibits the proliferation of *S. typhimurium* and *L. monocytogenes* in their organs [66–68]. Evidence that IL-1 plays an essential role in the early resistance against *L. monocytogenes* was obtained by treatment of mice with antibodies that block the type I IL-1 receptor. By blocking the action of IL-1α and β this way, increased bacterial proliferation in these mice was seen [69]. Also SCID mice, in which NK cells play an essential role in the control of *L. monocytogenes* infections, become highly susceptible to infections with *L. monocytogenes* upon treatment with antibodies against the type I IL-1 receptor [70]. The mechanisms by which IL-1 exerts its protective functions against infections are not known. It has been reported that administration of neutralizing antibodies against IL-1α and IL-1β together with antibodies against the type I IL-1 receptor inhibits the elaboration of activated macrophages [70]. However, IL-1 is not directly involved in the induction of enhanced microbicidal activity of murine macrophage *in vitro* [44].

Interleukin-2

One of the functions of IL-1 is the activation of T lymphocytes, which then produce various cytokines including IL-2. IL-2 is directly involved in the activation of various functional activities of mononuclear phagocytes, e.g. enhancement of the cytotoxic activity of human monocytes [71]. In combination with IFN-γ, IL-2 enhances resistance to *Leishmania major* in murine macrophages *in vitro* [72]. Exogenously added IL-2 synergizes *in vitro* with IL-12 and TNF and with heat-killed *L. monocytogenes* in the induction of IFN-γ production by NK cells [73]. *In vivo*, IL-2 enhances the resistance of mice against *L. monocytogenes* [74]. However, during an infection of mice with *L. monocytogenes*, no increase in the amount of IL-2 mRNA in the liver is observed during the early phase of the infection, i.e. within the first 3 days of a primary infection [75], and enhanced IL-2 production by spleen cells is not observed until day 5 of a primary infection [76].

Interleukin-6

In mice infected with *L. monocytogenes*, high levels of IL-6 are detectable in the serum [77]. This IL-6 production is independent of TNF and IFN-γ [77, 78]. *In vitro*, IL-6 enhances the listericidal activity of infected murine bone marrow derived macrophages [54]. Whether IL-6 can induce protection against infections with *L. monocytogenes* is not clear. Liu *et al.* have reported that administration of IL-6 can protect mice against infections with *L. monocytogenes* [79]. However, others reported that IL-6 by itself or in combination with suboptimal concentrations of TNF or IL-1 has no effect on an infection of mice with *L. monocytogenes* [80].

Interleukin-12

IL-12 is a cytokine that has been cloned recently. It is produced by macrophages and is a potent inducer of IFN-γ production by NK cells and various T lymphocytes [74, 81]. Since it has been described that NK cells play an essential role in the host defense against *L. monocytogenes* by producing IFN-γ very early in the infection [19, 82], IL-12 may have an important role in here. Heat-killed *L. monocytogenes* induces the production of IL-12 by splenocytes and peritoneal macrophages [74, 83] and IL-12 has been demonstrated to be involved in the induction of IFN-γ by splenocytes from SCID mice [74]. Together, these data provide convincing evidence that IL-12 has an important role in the early phase of the host defense against infections with *L. monocytogenes*. Since NK cells also have been indicated to play an important role in the host defense against *S. typhimurium* [84], IL-12 might be involved in the host defense against these bacteria.

Role of hematopoietic growth factors

Hematopoietic growth factors, also called colony-stimulating factors (CSF), are glycoproteins that stimulate clonal growth of hematopoietic progenitor cells and *in vivo* increase the number of bone marrow-derived cells. Interestingly, several of these factors also affect various functional activities of mature macrophages and of granulocytes.

In vitro, granulocyte-macrophage CSF (GM-CSF) activates macrophages to inhibit the intracellular proliferation of *Leishmania donovani*, *Leishmania tropica* and *Trypanosoma cruzi* [85–87], induces an enhanced respiratory burst [87] and stimulates the release of IL-1 and TNF by human mononuclear cells [88]. Treatment of mice with GM-CSF protects them against lethal infections with *S. typhimurium* [89]. It is possible that the GM-CSF-induced resistance is mediated by an increased production of mononuclear phagocytes by the bone marrow [90].

Macrophage-CSF (M-CSF) enhances antibody-dependent cell-mediated cytotoxicity [91]; this mechanism might play a role in the lysis of cells infected with intracellular bacteria. Early during an infection of mice with *L. monocytogenes*, elevated levels of M-CSF are detected in the serum and liver tissue [92]. Neutralization of endogenous M-CSF results in a large increase in the number of *L. monocytogenes* in the liver of mice [93] and administration of M-CSF inhibits the proliferation of *L. monocytogenes* in mice [94]. Granulocyte-CSF (G-CSF) influences various functions of granulocytes [95] but does not have any effect of macrophages. Granulocytes play an essential role in the initial defense against infections with *L. monocytogenes* and *S. typhimurium*, probably by their capacity to lyse hepatocytes in which these pathogens reside [96, 97]. Enhanced concentrations of G-CSF are observed in mice during the onset of an infection with *L. monocytogenes* [98] and treatment of mice with G-CSF enhances their resistance against infections with *L. monocytogenes* [99, 100]. The effects of G-CSF on infections with intracellular bacteria are probably due to enhanced recruitment of granulocytes and by augmentation of their functional activities, e.g. the oxidative burst, phagocytosis and bactericidal activity [101].

Role of deactivating cytokines

Host defense against intracellular pathogens, such as *L. monocytogenes* and *S. typhimurium*, is a controlled process. To limit detrimental effects on the host by mediators that are released by enhanced production of cytokines, e.g. TNF and IFN-γ, a number of anti-inflammatory cytokines are produced. Cytokines that have been demonstrated to downregulate the host defense against *L. monocytogenes* and *S. typhimurium* include interleukin-4 and interleukin-10.

Interleukin-4

Although IL-4 has been reported to activate macrophages [102, 103], suppression of various functional activities of macrophages by this cytokine has also been reported [104–107]. IL-4 inhibits the production of several macrophage-derived cytokines, such as IL-1 and TNF, that are involved in the host defense against *L. monocytogenes* and *S. typhimurium* [105, 106]. Moreover, it has been demonstrated recently that IL-4 also induces the production of the IL-1 receptor antagonist, the natural inhibitor of IL-1 [107]. Although different findings on the induction of IL-4 mRNA in the spleen of *L. monocytogenes*-infected mice have been published [75, 92], it has been demonstrated that neutralization of endogenous IL-4 by monoclonal antibodies enhances the resistance of mice against infections with *L. monocytogenes* [108]. In the host defense against *S. typhimurium*, IL-4 probably inhibits the activation of macrophages; the immunosuppression that is normally observed in *S. typhimurium*-infected mice is reversed by IL-4 [109].

Interleukin-10

IL-10 is a potent inhibitor of various macrophage functions [110–115]. IL-10 was originally defined as a product of T_H2 lymphocytes but it is now clear that mononuclear phagocytes are major producers of this cytokine [110]. IL-10 inhibits the production of IFN-γ by NK cells from SCID mice stimulated with heat-killed *L. monocytogenes*, either by inhibiting the ability of NK cells to respond to TNF and IL-12 [74] or by inhibiting the synthesis of these two cytokines by *L. monocytogenes*-stimulated macrophages [74, 83]. Whether IL-10 inhibits the elimination of intracellular bacteria *in vivo* is not known. Mice suffering from meningitis with *L. monocytogenes* contain high levels of IL-10 in the cerebrospinal fluid (CF) and the CF from these mice inhibits the listericidal activity of macrophages *in vitro* [113]. It is postulated that the unrestricted bacterial growth in the CF despite the presence of large numbers of leukocytes is due to the presence of high amounts of IL-10. The relevance of this finding is illustrated by the observation that the CF of children suffering from bacterial meningitis contain high levels of IL-10 [113].

Conclusion

With respect to the involvement of cytokines in the host defense against *L. monocytogenes* and *S. typhimurium*, the following model is proposed (Figure 1). In infections with *L. monocytogenes*, the first step of activation is the induction of IL-12 and TNF by infected macrophages [74, 83]. These two cytokines induce the production of IFN-γ by NK cells, already early during the infection [41, 42, 74]. Next, IFN-γ activates macrophages and this results in the prevention of the escape of *L. monocytogenes* from the phagolysosomes of these cells, thus limiting the cell-to-cell spread of these bacteria [39, 116]. However, some *L. monocytogenes* are able to invade hepatocytes where they proliferate. This proliferation is limited by granulocytes that invade the liver and lyse infected hepatocytes [96, 97]. In a later phase of the infection, activated T lymphocytes also produce large amounts of IFN-γ. Probably the most important mechanism to limit the proliferation of *L. monocytogenes* in the hepatocytes is the activation of these cells by IFN-γ and by various factors that are released by activated macrophages, such as TNF. IFN-γ also activates hepatocytes to limit proliferation of *L. monocytogenes* in these cells [40].

In the host defense against *S. typhimurium* the situation is somewhat different: these bacteria are easily killed by naive macrophages and activation of macrophages does not seem to be essential for their elimination [3, 25]. However, some of the bacteria enter hepatocytes before they are ingested by macrophages and proliferate in these cells [3]. Large numbers of granulocytes are present in the livers of *S. typhimurium*-infected mice and are probably involved in the lysis of infected hepatocytes [97]. Other cells

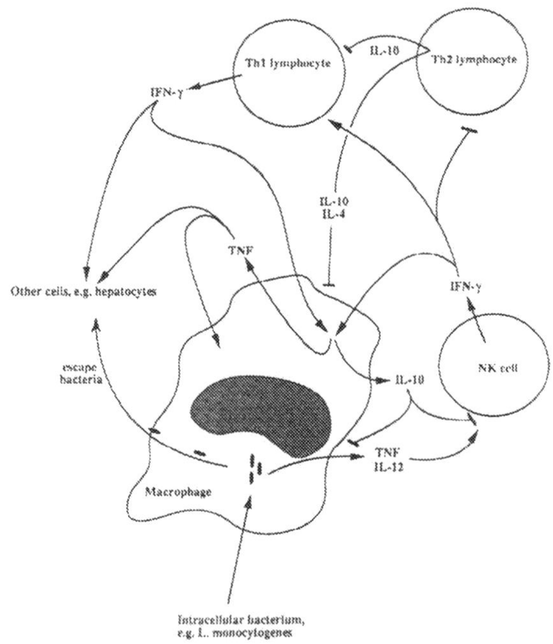

Fig. 1. Hypothetical model on the interactions between various cytokines and cells in the host defense against *L. monocytogenes*. Details on the involvement of the various cytokines in the regulation of the host defense are mentioned in the text. →: activating pathways; <⊣>: inhibiting pathways.

involved in the resistance against *S. typhimurium* include natural killer cells [84] that may also lyse infected hepatocytes. It is possible that activation of hepatocytes by macrophage-derived factors, such as TNF, plays an essential role in the limitation of the proliferation of *S. typhimurium* in the liver, as has been suggested for *L. monocytogenes* (see above).

Together, these findings suggest that in the host defense against infections with *L. monocytogenes* and *S. typhimurium* a complex network of cytokines is involved and that the main function of activated macrophages, which are suggested to be the major cells involved in this defense, is the release of a variety of factors that stimulate other cells, e.g. hepatocytes, which results in the inhibition of bacterial proliferation.

Acknowledgements

The authors thank Drs. J.N. Samsom and A.M. Buisman for critical reading of the manuscript and for helpful discussions.

References

1. Langermans JAM, Nibbering PH, van der Hulst MEB, van Furth R. Macrophage activation by recombinant cytokines. In: van Furth R, ed. Mononuclear phagocytes. Biology of monocytes and macrophages. Dordrecht, Boston, London: Kluwer Academic Publishers, 1992: 602–617.
2. Mitsuyama M, Takeya K, Nomoto K, Shimotori S. Three phases of phagocyte contribution to resistance against Listeria monocytogenes. J Gen Microbiol 1978; 106: 165–171.
3. Hsu H. Pathogenesis and immunity in murine salmonellosis. Microbiol Rev 1989; 53: 390–409.
4. Wood S, Maroushek N, Czuprynski CJ. Multiplication of Listeria monocytogenes in a murine hepatocyte cell line. Infect Immun 1993; 61: 3068–3072.
5. Mielke ME, Hahn H. T-cell-phagocyte interactions induced by Listeria monocytogenes In: Van Furth R, ed. Mononuclear phagocytes. Biology of monocytes and macrophages. Dordrecht, Boston, London, Kluwer Academic Publishers, 1992: 577–584.
6. Mackaness GB. Resistance to intracellular infection. J Infect Dis 1971; 123: 439–445.
7. Mackaness GB. Cellular resistance to infection. J Exp Med 1962; 116: 381–417.
8. Mackaness GB. The immunological basis of acquired resistance. J Exp Med 1964; 120: 105–120.
9. Collins FM. Vaccines and cell-mediated immunity. Bact Rev 1975; 38: 371–402.
10. Blanden RV, Mackaness GB, Collins FM. Mechanisms of aquired resistance in mouse typhoid. J Exp Med 1966; 124: 585–600.
11. North RJ. Introduction to macrophage activation. Lymphokines 1981; 3: 1–10.
12. Simon HB, Sheagren JN. Enhancement of macrophage bactericidal activity by antigenically stimulated lymphocytes. Cell Immunol 4: 163–174.
13. Fowles RE, Fajardo IM, Leibowitch JL, David JR. The enhancement of macrophage bacteriostasis by products of activated lymphocytes. J Exp Med 1973; 138: 952–964.
14. Wheelock EF. Interferon-like virus-inhibitor induced in human leukocytes by phytohemagglutinin. Science 1965; 149: 310–311.
15. Gray PW, Goeddel DV. Structure of the human immune interferon gene. Nature 1982; 298: 859–863.
16. Gray PW, Goeddel DW. Cloning and expression of murine interferon cDNA. Proc Natl Acad Sci USA 1983; 80: 5842–5846.
17. Hiromatsu K, Yoshikai Y, Matsuzaki G, Ohga S, Muramori K, Matsumoto K, Bluestone JA, Nomoto K. A protective role of γ/δ T cells in primary infection with Listeria monocytogenes in mice. J Exp Med 1992; 175: 49–56.
18. Garcia-Penarrubia P, Koster FT, Kelley RO, McDowell TD, Bankhurst AD. Antibacterial activity of natural killer cells. J Exp Med 1989; 169: 99–113.
19. Dunn PL, North RJ. Early gamma interferon production by natural killer cells is important in defense against murine listeriosis. Infect Immun 1991; 59: 2892–2900.
20. Follows GA, Munk ME, Gatrill AJ, Conradt P, Kaufmann SHE. Gamma interferon and interleukin 2, but not interleukin 4, are detectable in γ/δ T-cell cultures after activation with bacteria. Infect Immun 1992; 60: 1229–1231.
21. Skamene E. Genetic regulation of host resistance to bacterial infection. Rev Infect Dis 1983; 5: S823–S832.
22. Sluiter W, Elzenga-Claasen I, van der Voort van der Kley-van Andel A, van Furth R. Differences in the response of inbred mouse strains to the factor increasing monocytopoiesis. J Exp Med 1984; 159: 524–536.
23. Hahn H, Kaufmann SHE. The role of cell-mediated immunity in bacterial infections. Rev Infect Dis 1981; 3: 1221–1250.
24. Van Dissel JT, Stikkelbroeck JJM, van den Barselaar MTh, Sluiter W, Leijh PCJ, van Furth R. Divergent antimicrobial activity after immunologic activation of mouse peritoneal macrophages. J Immunol 1987; 139: 1665–1672.
25. Langermans JAM, Nibbering PH, van der Hulst MEB, van Furth R. Microbicidal activities of Salmonella typhimurium- and interferon-gamma-activated mouse peritoneal macrophages. Pathobiol 1991; 59: 189–193.
26. Langermans JAM, van der Hulst MEB, Nibbering PH, van Furth R. Activation of mouse peritoneal macrophages during infection with Salmonella typhimurium does not result in enhanced intracellular killing. J Immunol 1990; 144: 4340–4346.
27. Lin FR, Hsu HS, Mumaw VR, Moncure CW. Confirmation of destruction of salmonellae within murine peritoneal exudate cells by immunocytochemical technique. Immunology 1989; 67: 394–400.
28. Buchmeier NA, Schreiber RD. Requirement of endogenous interferon-gamma production for resolution of Listeria monocytogenes infection. Proc Natl Acad Sci USA 1985; 82: 7404–7408.
29. Huang S, Hendriks W, Althage A, Hemm S, Bluethmannn H, Kamijo R, Vilcek J, Zinkernagell RM, Aguet M. Immune response in mice that lack the interferon-γ recepor. Science 1993; 259: 1742–1745.
30. Kiderlen AF, Kaufmann SHE, Lohmann-Matthes ML. Protection of mice against the intracellular bacterium L. monocytogenes by recombinant immune interferon. Eur J Immunol 1984; 14: 964–967.
31. Langermans JAM, van der Hulst MEB, Nibbering PH, van der Meide PH, van Furth R. Intravenous injection of interferon-γ inhibits the proliferation of Listeria monocytogenes in the liver but not in the spleen and peritoneal cavity. Immunology 1992; 77: 354–361.
32. Matsumura H, Onozuka K, Terada Y, Nakano Y, Nakano M. Effect of murine recombinant interferon-γ in the protection of mice against Salmonella. Int J Immunopharmacol 1990; 12: 49–56.
33. Nauciel C, Espinasse-Maes F. Role of gamma interferon and tumor necrosis factor alpha in resistance to Salmonella typhimurium. Infect Immun 1992; 60: 450–454.
34. Kagaya K, Watanabe K, Fukazawa Y. Capacity of recombinant gammma interferon to activate macrophages for Salmonella-killing activity. Infect Immun 1989; 57: 609–615.
35. Van Dissel JT, Stikkelbroeck JJM, Michel BC, van den Barselaar MTh, Leijh PCJ, van Furth R. Inability of recombinant interferon-γ to activate the antibacterial activity of mouse peritoneal macrophages against Listeria monocytogenes and Salmonella typhimurium. J Immunol 1987; 139: 1673–1678.
36. Campbell PA, Canono BP, Cook JL. Mouse macrophages stimulated by recombinant gamma interferon to kill tumor cells are not bactericidal for the facultative intracellular bacterium Listeria monocytogenes. Infect Immun 1988; 56: 1371–1375.
37. Edwards III CK, Ghiasuddin SM, Yunger LM, Lorence RM, Arkins S, Dantzer R, Kelley KW. *In vivo* administration of recombinant growth hormone or gamma interferon activates macrophages: enhanced resistance to experimental Salmonel-

la typhimurium infection is correlated with generation of reactive oxygen intermediates. Infect Immun 1992; 60: 2514–2521.
38. Langermans JAM, Mayanski DM, Nibbering PH, van der Hulst MEB, van de Gevel JS, van Furth R. Effect of IFN-γ and endogenous TNF-α on the histopathological changes in the liver of L. monocytogenes-infected mice. Immunology, 1994; 81: 192–197.
39. Portnoy DA, Schreiber RD, Connelly P, Tilney LG. γ Interferon limits access of Listeria monocytogenes to the macrophage cytoplasm. J Exp Med 1989; 170: 2141–2146.
40. Gregory SH, Wing EJ. IFN-γ inhibits the replication of Listeria monocytogenes in hepatocytes. J Immunol 1993; 151: 1401–1409.
41. Bancroft GJ, Sheehan KCF, Schreiber RD, Unanue ER. Tumor necrosis faactor is involved in the T cell-independent pathway of macrophage activation in SCID mice. J Immunol 1989; 143: 127–130.
42. Wherry JC, Schreiber RD, Unanue ER. Regulation of gamma interferon production by natural killer cells in scid mice. Roles of tumor necrosis factor and bacterial stimuli. Infect Immun 1991; 59: 1709–1715.
43. Green SJ, Crawford RM, Hockmeyer JT, Meltzer MS, Nacy CA. Leishmania major amastigotes initiate the L-arginine-dependent killing mechanism in IFN-γ-stimulated macrophages by induction of tumor necrosis factor α. J Immunol 1990; 145: 4290–4297.
44. Langermans JAM, van der Hulst MEB, Nibbering PH, Hiemstra PS, Fransen L, van Furth R. IFN-γ-induced L-arginine-dependent toxoplasmastatic activity in murine peritoneal macrophages is mediated by endogenous tumor necrosis factor α. J Immunol 1992; 148: 568–574.
45. Havell EA. Evidence that tumor necrosis factor has an important role in antibacterial resistance. J Immunol 1989; 143: 2894–2899.
46. Nakane A, Minagawa T, Kato K. Endogenous tumor necrosis factor (cachectin) is essential to host resistance against Listeria monocytogenes infection. Infect Immun 1988; 56: 2563–2569.
47. Desiderio JV, Kiener PA, Lin PF, Warr GA. Protection of mice against Listeria monocytogenes infection by recombinant tumor necrosis factor alpha. Infect Immun 1989; 57: 1615–1617.
48. Roll JT, Young KM, Durtz RS, Czuprynski CJ. Human rTNF-α augments anti-bacterial resistance in mice; potentiation of its effects by recombinant human rIL-α. Immunology 1990; 69: 316–322.
49. Pfeffer K, Matsuyama T, Kündig TM, Wakeham A, Kishihara K, Shahinian A, Wiegmann K, Ohashi PS, Krönke M, Mak TW. Mice deficient for the 55 kd tumor necrosis factor receptor are resistant to endotoxic shock, yet succum to L. monocytogenes infection. Cell 1993; 73: 457–467.
50. Langermans JAM, van der Hulst MEB, Nibbering PH, van Furth R. Endogenous tumor necrosis factor alpha is required for enhanced antimicrobial activity against Toxoplasma gondii and Listeria monocytogenes in gamma-interferon-treated mice. Infect Immun 1992; 60: 5107–5112.
51. Langermans JAM. The cytokine network, macrophage activation, and enhanced antimicrobial activity. A central role for TNF-α. Thesis Rijksuniversity Leiden, The Netherlands. 1992; 95–101.
52. Kindler V, Sappino AP, Grau GE, Piguet PF, Vassali P. The inducing role of tumor necrosis factor in the development of bactericidal granulomas during BCG infection. Cell 1989; 56: 731–740.
53. Mielke MEA, Rosen H, Brocke S, Peters C, Hahn H. Protective immunity and granuloma formation are mediated by two distinct but TNF-α and IFN-γ-dependent T cell-phagocyte interactions in murine listeriosis. Dissociation on the basis of phagocyte adhesion mechanisms. Infect Immun 1992; 60: 1875–1882.
53a. Van Furth R, Van Zwet Th. L., Buisman AM, Van Dissel JT. Anti-tumor necrosis factor antibodies inhibit the influx of granulocytes and monocytes into an inflammatory exudate and enhance the growth of Listeria monocytogenes in various organs. J. Infect. Dis. 1994; 170: 234–237.
54. Denis M. Growth of listeria monocytogenes in murine macrophages and its modulation by cytokines; activation of bactericidal activity by interleukin-4 and interleukin-6. Can J Microbiol 1991; 37: 253–257.
55. Rosen H, Gordon S, North RJ. Exacerbation of murine listeriosis by a monoclonal antibody specific for the type 3 complement receptor of myelomonocytic cells. J Exp Med 1989; 170: 27–37.
56. Curran RD, Billiar TR, Stuehr DJ, Hofmann K, Simmons RL. Hepatocytes produce nitrogen oxides from L-arginine in response to inflammatory products from Kupffer cells. J Exp Med 1989; 170: 1769–1774.
57. Mellouk S, Green SJ, Nacy CA, Hoffman SL. IFN-γ inhibits development of Plasmodium berghei exoerythrocytic stages in hepatocytes by an L-arginine-dependent effector mechanism. J Immunol 1991; 146: 3971–3976.
58. Gregory SH, Barczynski LK, Wing EJ. Effector function of hepatocytes and Kupffer cells in the resolution of systemic bacterial infections. J Leuk Biol 1992; 51: 421–424.
59. Dinarello CA. Interleukin-1 and interleukin-1 antagonism. Blood 1991; 77: 1627–1652.
60. Ozaki SJ, Ohashi T, Minami A, Nakamura S-I. Enhanced resistance of mice to bacterial infection induced by recombinant interleukin-1α. Infect Immun 1987; 55: 1436–1440.
61. Van der Meer JWM, Barza M, Wolff SM, Dinarello CA. A low dose of recombinant interleukin 1 protects granulocytopenic mice from lethal gram-negative infection. Proc Natl Acad Sci USA 1988; 85: 1620–1623.
62. Minami A. Fujimoto K, Ozaki Y, Nakamura S. Augmentation of host resistance to microbial infections by recombinant interleukin-1α. Infect Immun 1988; 56: 3116–3120.
63. Van 't Wout JW, van der Meer JWM, Barza M, Dinarello CA. Protection of neutropenic mice from lethal Candida albicans infections by recombinant interleukin 1. Eur J Immunol 1988; 18: 1143–1146.
64. Curfs JHA, van der Meer JWM, Sauerwein RW, Eling WMC. Low dosages of interleukin 1 protect mice against lethal cerebral malaria. J Exp Med 1990; 172: 1287–1291.
65. Kullberg BJ, van 't Wout JW, van Furth R. Role of granulocytes in increased host resistance to Candida albicans induced by recombinant interleukin-1. Infect Immun 1990; 58: 3319–3324.
66. Morrissey PJ, Charrier K. Interleukin-1 administration to C3H/HeJ mice after but not prior to infection increases resistance to Salmonella typhimurium. Infect Immun 1991; 59: 4729–4731.
67. Czuprinsky CJ, Brown JF, Young KM, Cooley AJ, Kurtz RS. Effects of murine recombinant interleukin 1α on the host response to bacterial infection. J Immunol 1988; 140: 962–968.

68. Czuprynski CJ, Brown JF. Recombinant murine interleukin-1α enhancement of nonspecific antibacterial resistance. Infect Immun 1987; 55: 2061–2065.
69. Havell EA, Moldawer LL, Helfgott D, Kilian P, Sehgal PB. Type I IL-1 receptorblockade exacerbates murine listeriosis. J Immunol 1992; 148: 1486–1492.
70. Rogers HW, Sheehan KCF, Brunt LM, Dower SK, Unanue ER, Schreiber RD. Interleukin-1 participates in the development of anti-Listeria responses in normal and SCID mice. Proc Natl Acad Sci USA 1992; 89: 1011–1015.
71. Malkovský M, Loveland B, North M, Asherson GL, Gao L, Ward P, Fiers W. Recombinant interleukin-2 directly augments the cytotoxicity of human monocytes. Nature 1987; 325: 262–265.
72. Belosovic M, Finbloom DS, Meltzer MS, Nacy CA. IL-2, a cofactor for induction of activated macrophage resistance to infection. J Immunol 1990; 145: 831–839.
73. Haak-Frendscho M, Young KM, Czuprinsky CJ. Treatment of mice with human recombinant interleukin-2 augments resistance to the facultative intracellular pathogen Listeria monocytogenes. Infect Immun 1989; 57: 3014–3021.
74. Tripp CS, Wolf SF, Unanue ER. Interleukin-12 and tumor necrosis factor α are costimulators of interferon γ production by natural killer cells in severe combined immunodeficiency mice with listeriosis, and interleukin 10 is a physiological antagonist. Proc Natl Acad Sci USA 1993; 90: 3725–3729.
75. Iizawa Y, Brown JF, Czuprynski CJ. Early expression of cytokine mRNA in mice infected with Listeria monocytogenes. J Immunol 1992; 60: 4068–4073.
76. Kratz SS, Kurlander R. Characterization of the pattern of inflammatory cell influx and cytkoine production during the murine host response to Listeria monocytogenes. J Immunol 1988; 141: 598–606.
77. Havell EA, Sehgal PB. Tumor necrosis factor-independent IL-6 production during murine listeriosis. J Immunol 1991; 146: 756–761.
78. Nakane A, Numatta A, Minagawa T. The role of TNFin listeriosis. In: van Furth R, ed. Mononuclear phagocytes. Biology of monocytes and macrophages. Dordrecht, Boston, London: Kluwer Academic Publishers, 1992: 626–630.
79. Liu Z, Simpson RJ, Cheers C. Recombinant interleukin-6 protects mice against experimental bacterial infection. Infect Immun 1992; 60: 4402–4406.
80. Czuprynski CJ, Haak-Frendscho M, Maroushek N, Brown JF. Effects of recombinant human interleukin-6 alone and in combination with recombinant interleukin-1α and tumor necrosis factor alpha on antibacterial resistance in mice. Antimicrobial Agents Chemother 1992; 36: 68–70.
81. Manetti R, Parronchi P, Giudizi MG, Piccini MP, Maggi E, Trinchieri G, Romagnani. Natural killer cell stimulatory factor (Interleukin-12 [IL-12]) induces T helper type 1 (Th1)-specific immune responses and inhibits the development of IL-4 producing Th cells. J Exp Med 1993; 177: 1199–1204.
82. Nakane A, Numata A, Asano M, Konahawa M, Chen Y, Minagawa T. Evidence that endogenous gamma interferon is produced early in Listeria monocytogenes infection. 1990; 58: 2386–2388.
83. Hsieh CS, Macatonia SE, Tripp CS, Wolf SF, O'Garra A, Murphy KM. Development of T_H1 $CD4^+$ T cells through IL-12 produced by Listeria-induced macrophages. Science 1993; 260: 547–549.
84. Schafer R, Eisenstein TK. Natural killer cells mediate protection induced by a Salmonella aroA mutant. Infect Immun 1992; 60: 791–797.
85. Weiser WY, van Niel A, Clark SC, David JR, Remold HG. Recombinant human granulocyte/macrophage colony-stimulating factor activates intracellular killing of Leishmania donovani by human monocyte-derived macrophages. J Exp Med 1987; 166: 1436–1446.
86. Handman E, Burgess AW. Stimulation by granulocyte-macrophage colony stimulating factor of Leishmania tropica killing by macrophages. J Immunol 1979; 122: 1134–1137.
87. Reed SG, Nathan CF, Pihl DL, Rodricks P, Shanebeck K, Conlon PJ, Grabstein KH. Recombinant granulocyte/macrophage colony-stimulating factor activates macrophages to inhibit Trypanosoma cruzi and release hydrogen peroxide. J Exp Med 1987; 166: 1734–1746.
88. Sisson SD, Dinarello CA. Production of interleukin-1α, interleukin 1β and tumor necrosis factor by human mononuclear cells stimulated with granulocyte-macrophage colony-stimulating factor. Blood 1988; 72: 1368–1374.
89. Morrisey PJ, Charrier K. GM-CSF administration augments the survival of ITY-resistant A/J mice, but not ITY-susceptible C57Bl/6 mice, to a lethal challenge with Salmonella typhimurium. J Immunol 1990; 144: 557–561.
90. Metcalf D. The granulocyte-macrophage colony-stimulating factors. Science 1985; 229: 16–22.
91. Mufson RA, Aghajanian J, Wong G, Woodhouse C, Morgan AC. Macrophage colony-stimulating factor enhances monocyte and macrophage antibody-dependent cell-mediated cytotoxicity. Cell Immunol 1989; 119: 182–192.
92. Ehlers S, Mielke MEA, Blankenstein T, Hahn H. Kinetic analysis of cytokine gene expression in the livers of naive and immune mice infected with Listeria monocytogenes. The immediate early phase in innate resistance and acquired immunity. J Immunol 1992; 149: 3016–3022.
93. Gregory SH, Wing EJ, Tweardy DJ, Shadduck RK, Lin HS. Primary listerial infections are exacerbated in mice administered neutralizing antibody to macrophage colony-stimulating factor. J Immunol 1992; 149: 188–193.
94. Kayashima S, Tsuru S, Shinomiya N, Katsura Y, Motoyoshi K, Rokutanda M, Nagata N. Effects of macrophage colony-stimulating factor on reduction of viable bacteria and survival of mice during Listeria monocytogenes infection: characteristics of monocyte subpopulations. Infect Immun 1991; 59: 4677–4680.
95. Cohen AM, Hines DK, Korach ES, Ratzkin BJ. *In vivo* activation of neutrophil function in hamsters by recombinant human granulocyte colony-stimulating factor. Infect Immun 1988; 56: 2861–2865.
96. Conlan JW, North RJ. Neutrophil-mediated dissolution of infected host cells as a defense strategy against a facultative intracellular pathogen. J Exp Med 1991; 174: 741–744.
97. Conlan JW, North RJ. Early pathogenesis of infection in the liver with the facultative intracellular bacteria Listeria monocytogenes, Francisella tularensis, and Salmonella typhimurium involves lysis of infected hepatocytes by leukocytes. Infect Immun 1992; 60: 5164–5171.
98. Cheers C, Haigh AM, Kelso A, Metcalf D, Stanley ER, Young AM. Production of colony-stimulating factors (CSFs)during infection. Separate determinations of macrophage-, granulocyte-, granulocyte-macrophage-, and multi-CSFs. Infect Immun 1988; 56: 247–251.
99. Shinomiya N, Tsuru S, Katsura Y, Kayashima S, Nomoto K. Enhanced resistance against Listeria monocytogenes achieved by pretreatment with granulocyte colony-stimulating factor. Infect Immun 1991; 59: 4740–4743.

100. Serushago A, Yoshikai Y, Handa T, Mitsuyama M, Muramori K, Nomoto K. Effect of recombinnant human granulocyte colony-stimulating factor (rhG-CSF) on murine resistance against Listeria monocytogenes. Immunology 1992; 75: 475–480.
101. Dale DC. Granulocyte colony-stimulating factor in infectious diseases. Current Opinion in Infectious Diseases 1993; 6: 369–373.
102. Wirth JJ, Kierzenbaum F, Zlotnick A. Effects of IL-4 on macrophage functions: increased uptake and killing of a protozoan parasite (Trypanosoma cruzi). Immunol 1989; 66: 296–302.
103. Stenger S, Solbach W, Röllinghoff M, Bogdan C. Cytokine interaction in experimental cutaneous leishmaniasis II. endogenous tumor necrosis factor-α production by macrophages is induced by the synergistic action of interferon-(IFN)-γ and interleukin (IL) 4 and accounts for the antiparasitic effect mediated by IFN-γ and IL-4. Eur J Immunol 1991; 21: 1669–1675.
104. Abramson SL, Gallin JI. IL-4 inhibits superoxide production by human mononuclear phagocytes. J Immunol 1990; 144: 625–630.
105. Te Velde AA, Huijbens RJF, Heije K, de Vries JE, Figdor CG. Interleukin 4 (IL-4) inhibits secretion of IL-1β, tumor necrosis factor α and IL-6 by human monocytes. Blood 1990; 76: 1392–1397.
106. McBride WH, Economou JS, Nayersina R, Comora S, Essner R. Influence of interleukin 2 and 4 on tumor necrosis factor production by murine mononuclear phagocytes. Cancer Res 1990; 50: 2949–2952.
107. Vannier E, Miller LC, Dinarello CA. Coordinated antiinflammatory effects of interleukin 4: Interleukin 4 suppresses interleukin 1 production but up-regulates gene expression and synthesis of interleukin 1 receptor antagonist. Proc Natl Acad Sci USA 1992; 89: 4076–4080.
108. Haak-Frendscho M, Brown JF, Iizawa Y, Wagner RD, Czuprynski CJ. Administration of anti-IL-4 monoclonal antibody 11B11 increases the resistance of mice to Listeria monocytogenes infection. J Immunol 1992; 148: 3978–3985.
109. Al-Ramadi BK, Chen YW, Meissler JJ Jr, Eisenstein TK. Immmunosuppression induced by attenuated Salmonella. Reversal by IL-4. J Immunol 1991; 147: 1954–1961.
110. De Waal-Malefyt R, Abrams J, Bennett B, Figdor C, de Vries JE. IL-10 inhibits cytokine synthesis by human monocytes: an autoregulatory function of IL-10 produced by monocytes. J Exp Med 1991; 174: 1209–1220.
111. Fiorentino DF, Zlotnik A, Mosmann TR, Howard M, O'Garra A. IL-10 inhibits cytokine production by activated macrophages. J Immunol 1991; 147: 3815–3822.
112. Bogdan C, Vodovotz Y, Nathan C. Macrophage deactivation by interleukin 10. J Exp Med 1991; 174: 1549–1555.
113. Frei K, Nadal D, Pfister HW, Fontana A. Listeria meningitis: identification of a cerebrospinal fluid inhibitor of macrophage listericidal function as interleukin-10. J Exp Med 1993; 178: 1255–1261.
114. Silva JS, Morrisey PJ, Grabstein KH, Mohler KM, Anderson D, Reed S. Interleukin 10 and interferon γ regulation of experimental Trypanosoma cruzi infection. J Exp Med 1992; 175: 169–174.
115. Gazzinelli RT, Oswald IP, James SL, Sher A. IL-10 inhibits parasite killing and nitrogen oxide production by IFN-γ-activated macrophages. J Immunol 1992; 148: 1792–1796.
116. Tilney LG, Portnoy DA. Actin filaments and the growth, movement and spread of the intracellular bacterial parasite, Listeria monocytogenes. J Cell Biol 1989; 109: 1597–1608

Address for correspondence: J.A.M. Langermans, Department of Infectious Diseases, Building 1, C5P, University Hospital, P.O. Box 9600, 2300 RC Leiden, The Netherlands

Biotherapy 7: 179–186, 1994.

Cytokines and legionellosis

Thomas F. Byrd
West Los Angeles Veterans Affairs Medical Center, Wilshire and Sawtelle, Building 500, Room 4469, W111F, Los Angeles, California 90073, U.S.A.

Key words: ferritin, interferon gamma, iron, lactoferrin, monocyte, transferrin

Abstract

Recent studies have led to an enhanced understanding of the role of cell-mediated immunity and cytokines in Legionnaires' disease. In particular, the effect of interferon gamma on human mononuclear phagocyte iron metabolism and the role of iron availability in *Legionella pneumophila* intracellular multiplication in human monocytes has been elucidated. With this knowledge it is now possible to develop treatment strategies for Legionnaires' disease using interferon gamma and/or agents affecting human mononuclear phagocyte iron metabolism.

Abbreviations: M-CSF: Macrophage colony stimulating factor

Introduction

Legionnaires' disease occurs worldwide in epidemic and endemic forms. It is a leading cause of pneumonia, causing an estimated 100,000 cases annually in the U.S., and it affects all age groups. It causes a substantial proportion of deaths from hospital-acquired pneumonia. It is important cause of pneumonia in immunosuppressed patients occurring most often in patients receiving corticosteroids, patients with neoplasms and patients who have had renal transplants [1].

Although adequate antibiotic therapy exists for Legionnaires' disease, case-fatality ratios up to 25% have been reported in immunosuppressed patients in spite of receiving appropriate antibiotics [1]. This highlights the recognized importance of the cell-mediated immune response to this disease. The major mediators of the cell-mediated immune response are cytokines. Recent studies have advanced our understanding of important cytokines in host defense against *Legionella pneumophila*, as well as the mechanisms wherebey these cytokines activate effector cells against this pathogen.

Cell-mediated immunity

There is substantial evidence indicating a central role for the cell-mediated immune response in *L. pneumophila* infection.

Pathologic findings show that mononuclear phagocytes and polymorphonuclear leukocytes both respond to *L. pneumophila* infection in the lung. The role of polymorphonuclear leukocytes in host defense against *L. pneumophila* is unclear, although there is some evidence that polymorphonuclear leukocyte effector functions against *L. pneumophila* may be augmented by cytokines. *L. pneumophila* has been found to be resistant to killing by polymorphonuclear leukocytes, even in the presence of specific antibody [2]. However, it has been shown that polymorphonuclear leukocytes activated with interferon gamma and tumor necrosis factor alpha have enhanced bactericidal activity against *L. pneumophila*, suggesting that under certain conditions, polymorphonuclear leukocytes may play a role in the elimination of *L. pneumophila* during the course of infection [3].

Animal models of infection support the important role of the cell-mediated immune response to *L. pneumophila*. Guinea pigs exposed to various *L. pneumophila* antigens develop strong cell-mediated immune responses that are manifested by cutaneous delayed-type hypersensitivity and *in vitro* lymphocyte proliferation in response to these antigens. These guinea pigs are protected from lethal *L. pneumophila* aerosol challenge. In addition, lymphocytes from patients who have recovered from Legionnaires's disease respond to *L. pneumophila* antigens with proliferation and the production of cytokines capable of activating human monocytes [4].

In vitro studies indicate that the major contribution of cell-mediated immunity to host defense against *L. pneumophila* is to inhibit bacterial multiplication rather than to kill the pathogen [5].

Activating cytokines in *L. pneumophila* infection

Cytokines reported to activate mononuclear phagocyte antimicrobial mechanisms against *L. pneumophila* include macrophage colony stimulating factor (M-CSF) and interferon gamma.

Granulocyte-macrophage colony stimulating factor has been reported to have no activating effect on human alveolar macrophages or peripheral blood monocytes against *L. pneumophila* [6]. In another study a modest activating effect of human M-CSF on guinea pig alveolar macrophages was noted against *L. pneumophila* [7]. However, more important than direct mononuclear phagocyte activating effects against *L. pneumophila*, colony stimulating factors may increase the number of polymorphonuclear leukocytes and monocytes at sites of *L. pneumophila* infection where these cells can be activated by interferon gamma and tumor necrosis factor. In a recent case report, a neutropenic patient with Legionnaires' disease who failed to clear his pneumonia with appropriate antibiotics, responded to granulocyte-macrophage colony stimulating factor with increased neutrophils and resolution of pneumonia [8].

Interferon gamma activation and *L. pneumophila* infection

The most extensively studied cytokine with activity against *L. pneumophila* is interferon gamma. It is induced *in vitro* and *in vivo* by *L. pneumophila*. Interferon gamma activates human mononuclear phagocytes to inhibit the intracellular multiplication of, but not kill *L. pneumophila* [9]. This suggests that the major contribution of cell-mediated immunity to host defense against *L. pneumophila* in humans may be to limit bacterial multiplication rather than to kill the pathogen.

Interferon gamma and mononuclear phagocyte iron metabolism

Recently a new hypothesis has been proposed for a mechanism by which interferon gamma-activated human monocytes inhibit the intracellular multiplication of *L. pneumophila*. This hypothesis centers around the availability of iron for *L. pneumophila* intracellular growth.

L. pneumophila has a definite metabolic requirement for iron, reflected by an inability to grow on agar medium in the absence of iron supplementation or in broth medium to which iron chelators, including apotransferrin, enterochelin, or deferoxamine have been added [10]. Unlike most gram-negative bacteria, *L. pneumophila* does not produce siderophores, soluble iron-chelating compounds that would allow it to remove iron *in vivo* from high affinity iron-binding compounds such as transferrin [11]. *L. pneumophila* multiplication is thus restricted to environments in which iron is readily available and not bound to high affinity iron-binding compounds. The distinctive ribosome-lined phagosome in which *L. pneumophila* multiplies intracellularly is presumably one such environment in mononuclear phagocytes.

Mononuclear phagocytes play a central role in iron processing in the human body. These cells acquire iron via transferrin receptors on their surface. The transferrin receptor is thought to be comprised of two identical polypeptide chains each capable of binding a diferric transferrin molecule at neutral pH. The transferrin receptor- transferrin complex is endocytized, after which the endocytic vesicle is acidified. As the pH decreases, ferric ions dissociate from transferrin and are distributed intracellularly. The apotransferrin remains bound to the transferrin receptor until the receptor recycles back to the cell surface, whereupon apotransferrin dissociates from the receptor [12]. The internalized iron enters the so-called labile iron pool of the cell [13]. In addition to transferrin, mononuclear phagocytes internalize the iron binding protein lactoferrin released by polymorphonuclear leukocytes at sites of inflammation. In contrast to transferrin, lactoferrin is felt to donate its iron to the cell by a different mechanism. Lactoferrin receptors are located on the surface of the cell. In contrast to transferrin receptors, lactoferrin receptors have similar affinity for iron saturated and unsaturated lactoferrin. In addition, one molecule of lactoferrin is felt to bind to one lactoferrin receptor. The lactoferrin-lactoferrin receptor complex is endocytized into an acidic endocytic vesicle. In contrast to transferrin, iron remains tightly bound to lactoferrin even under the acidic conditions of the endocytic vesicle and iron is not released. In the case of lactoferrin, a significant proportion of the molecules are recycled back to the cell membrane [14]. However, a certain proportion of lactoferrin molecules enter the lysosomal compartment where the lactoferrin/lactoferrin receptor complex is degraded and the iron is released to the intermediate iron pool. The iron in the intermediate iron pool is used for metabolic processes or is bound to the iron storage protein ferritin. Some studies have provided evidence that the size of the intermediate iron pool is influenced by the quantity and type of ferritin found within the cell.

In view of the above considerations, it was hypothesized that *L. pneumophila* requires intracellular iron to multiply in human mononuclear phagocytes, and that it obtains intracellular iron from an intermediate labile iron pool. Consistent with this hypothesis, deferoxamine, an iron chelator that chelates intracellular iron in what has been characterized as the labile iron pool, completely inhibits the intracellular multiplication of *L. pneumophila*. Moreover, the effect of deferoxamine is completely reversed by the addition of iron-saturated transferrin but not by apotransferrin [15]. In addition, chloroquine, a lysosomotropic weak base which raises the intravesicular pH in eucaryotic cells and interferes with the unloading of iron from transferrin, lactoferrin and ferritin, inhibits *L. pneumophila* multiplication by an iron-dependent mechanism [16].

It was then hypothesized that iron may play an important role in monocyte activation against *L. pneumophila*. To explore this, the influence of iron transferrin on *L. pneumophila* multiplication in interferon gamma-activated monocytes was studied. Iron transferrin neutralized the effect of interferon gamma-activation against *L. pneumophila* in a dose-dependent fashion (Figure 1). In addition, apotransferrin at the highest concentration of iron-saturated transferrin studied, had only a minimal effect on *L. pneumophila* multiplication in activated monocytes. One way that activated monocytes might limit the availability of intracellular iron is by downregulating transferrin receptors on their surface. To examine this possibility, transferrin receptor expression on activated and non-activated monocytes cultured *in vitro* for 5 days was

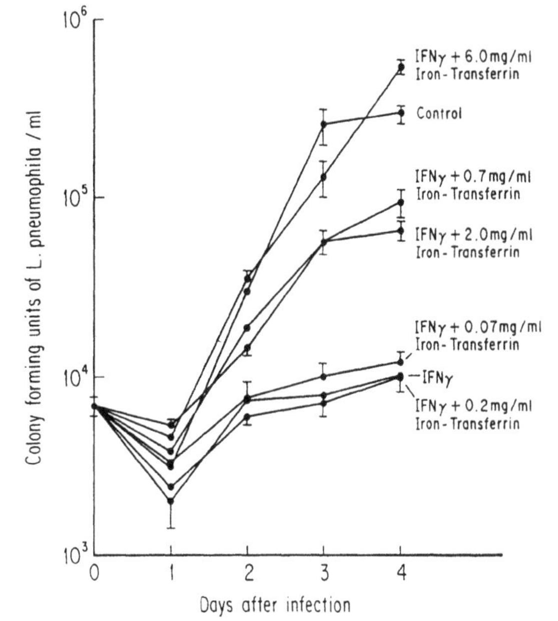

Fig. 1. Dose dependent reversal of interferon gamma-mediated inhibition of *L. pneumophila* multiplication in human monocytes by iron-saturated transferrin. Monocytes were incubated in medium alone (control) or activated by incubation with interferon gamma. At the same time, the interferon gamma-treated monocytes were incubated with various concentrations of iron-saturated transferrin ranging from 0.07 to 6.0 mg/ml. After 24 h, all cultures were infected with *L. pneumophila*. Colony forming units (CFU) of *L. pneumophila* was determined daily. Data are mean ± SEM for triplicate cultures.

investigated. By fluorescence-activated flow cytometry, activated monocytes exhibited markedly fewer transferrin receptors than nonactivated monocytes. By Scatchard analysis of 125I-transferrin binding to monocytes, nonactivated monocytes had 38,300 ± 12,700 (mean ± SEM) transferrin binding sites, whereas activated monocytes had 10,300+1,600, a reduction of 73% (Table 1). These results suggested an important role for the transferrin/transferrin receptor pathway as a mediator of the interferon gamma effect of iron limitation against *L. pneumophila* [15].

Next, the role of lactoferrin in *L. pneumophila*-monocyte interaction in both nonactivated and interferon gamma-activated monocytes was explored. Lactoferrin is an iron-binding protein with a high degree of homology to transferrin. It is found in the specific granules of neutrophils and in mucosal secretions including bronchial secretions. In its unsaturated form, it has been found to have either a bacteriostatic or a bactericidal effect against a variety of extracellular bacteria *in vitro*. At sites of inflammation, such as occurs at infect-

Table 1. Transferrin Receptor Number is Decreased on IFN γ-Activated Monocytes

Subject	Status of Monocytes	Number of Transferrin Binding Sites Per Monocytes (Mean±SD)	Kd (nM) (Mean±SD)	% Decrease in Transferrin Binding Sites Per Monocyte with Activation
1	Nonactivated	69,000± 4,800	1.92±1.03	82%
	Activated	12,300± 100	2.16±0.97	
2	Nonactivated	48,500± 9,600	2.39±0.73	75%
	Activated	11,900± 600	2.28±0.08	
3	Nonactivated	22,600± 800	1.81±0.35	49%
	Activated	11,600± 800	1.54±0.10	
4	Nonactivated	13,100± 3,600	1.23±0.67	57%
	Activated	5,600± 4,200	1.38±1.32	
		Mean±SEM	Mean±SEM	
Total	Nonactivated	38,300±12,700	1.84±0.24	73%
	Activated	10,300± 1,600	1.84±0.22	

Transferrin binding sites on nonactivated and IFNγ-activated monocytes were measured twice on each of 4 subjects in 8 independent experiments by Scatchard analysis of ^{125}I - transferrin equilibrium binding. Data are the mean and SD of the two measurements of transferrin binding sites and Kd (dissociation constant) for each subject, and the mean and SEM of transferrin binding sites and Kd for all 4 subjects.

ed sites in the body, unsaturated lactoferrin is released by the specific granules of neutrophils into the extracellular environment where is able to bind free iron. It is subsequently taken up by mononuclear phagocytes via receptors with specificity for lactoferrin. To determine the effect of apolactoferrin on *L. pneumophila* intracellular multiplication, monocytes were infected in the presence or absence of this molecule. At a concentration of 2.0 mg/ml, apolactoferrin markedly inhibited *L. pneumophila* intracellular multiplication. The inhibitory effect was not due to a toxic effect of apolactoferrin on monocytes because apolactoferrin-treated monocyte monolayers were intact after 4 days of culture and the monocytes were viable by trypan blue exclusion [17].

The inhibitory effect of apolactoferrin was dependent upon its iron-unsaturated state. In contrast to apolactoferrin, iron-saturated lactoferrin at a concentration of 6 mg/ml had no effect on *L. pneumophila* multiplication [17].

Since interferon gamma-activated monocytes inhibit *L. pneumophila* multiplication by limiting the availability of iron to the bacterium, it was determined whether iron lactoferrin could supply iron to *L. pneumophila* and reverse the inhibitory effect of activation. Similar to iron transferrin, iron lactoferrin reversed interferon gamma-activation against *L. pneumophila* in dose-dependent fashion. Whereas iron lactoferrin reversed the inhibitory effect of activation, apolactoferrin had no such effect and in fact enhanced the inhibitory effect of interferon gamma (Figure 2). In these experiments, the apolactoferrin-treated monolayers remained intact throughout the course of infection, and the monolayers were viable at 4 days by trypan blue exclusion [17]. This enhancement of the inhibitory effect of interferon gamma-activation against *L. pneumophila* is not seen when apotransferrin is added to activated monocytes. This may reflect more efficient endocytosis of lactoferrin because the affinity of the lactoferrin receptor for apolactoferrin is much greater than the affinity of the transferrin receptor for apotransferrin. In addition, whereas interferon gamma activation downregulates the expression of monocyte transferrin receptors, recent data suggest that interferon gamma has no effect on lactoferrin receptor expression [18]. These results show that apolactoferrin inhibits the intracellular multiplication of *L. pneumophila* in nonactivated monocytes and enhances the inhibitory effect of activation on *L. pneumophila* intracellular multiplication.

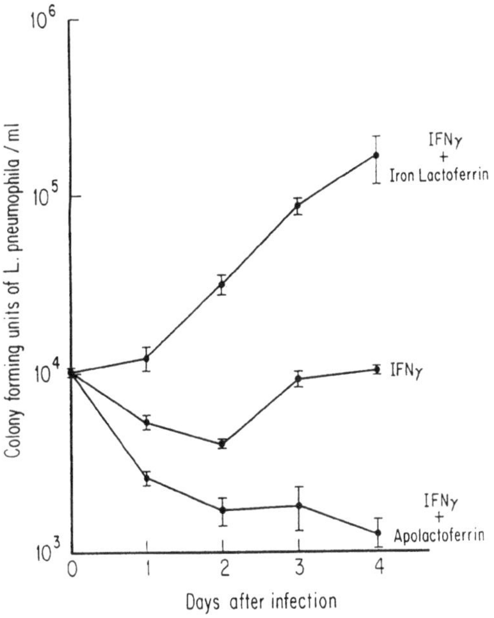

Fig. 2. Iron-saturated lactoferrin reverses and apolactoferrin enhances the capacity of interferon gamma-activated monocytes to inhibit *L. pneumophila* intracellular multiplication. Monocytes were activated with interferon gamma and, at the same time, they were incubated with control medium (RPMI containing 20% NHS), iron-saturated lactoferrin (2 mg/ml), or apolactoferrin (2 mg/ml). After 24 h, all cultures were infected with *L. pneumophila*, and CFU were determined daily. Data are mean ± SEM for triplicate cultures.

Since tumor necrosis factor alpha has been shown to be induced in mononuclear phagocytes by *L. pneumophila* our results suggest a possible role for tumor necrosis factor alpha and apolactoferrin in polymorphonuclear phagocyte – mononuclear phagocyte cooperation against *L. pneumophila* infection: a)release of tumor necrosis factor alpha by *L. pneumophila*-infected monocytes, b)Tumor necrosis factor alpha acting on polymorphonuclear leukocytes in the immediate vicinity resulting in degranulation of specific neutrophil granules with release of apolactoferrin, c)uptake of apolactoferrin by *L. pneumophila*-infected mononuclear phagocytes and d)binding of labile intracellular iron in the infected mononuclear phagocyte with subsequent inhibition of *L. pneumophila* multiplcation.

In addition to transferrin and lactoferrin, the other major iron-binding protein felt to play an important role in intracellular iron homeostasis is ferritin. Ferritin is the major iron storage protein in the human body and represents a form of iron that can be mobilized within cells. Human monocytes synthesize ferritin, and it is also found in human alveolar macrophages, with the alveolar macrophages of cigarette smokers who have increased susceptibility to Legionnaires' disease, having significantly more ferritin than the alveolar macrophages of nonsmokers. Iron bound to ferritin is felt to be in equilibrium with iron in the intermediate labile iron pool. Thus, the concentration of intracellular ferritin may influence the size of the intermediate labile iron pool and consequently iron availability to *L. pneumophila*. To determine whether interferon gamma affects monocyte ferritin content, the ferritin content of 5 day nonactivated and interferon gamma-activated monocytes was measured twice in each of four subjects in eight independent experiments. By radioimmunoassay, the mean ferritin content of nonactivated monocytes was 361 ± 107 fg/monocyte (mean ± SEM) whereas the mean content of interferon gamma-activated monocytes was 64 ± 13 fg/monocyte, an 82% reduction with activation [19](Table 2). Consistent with its downregulating effect on these iron proteins, interferon gamma treatment also resulted in decreased iron incorporation. Interferon gamma-activated monocytes incorporated 33% less iron from 59 Fe-transferrin than nonactivated monocytes ($p<0.05$)[19]. Gel filtration chromatography revealed that incorporated iron is located primarily in ferritin in both nonactivated and interferon gamma-activated monocytes [19](Figure 3). Ferritin in interferon gamma-activated monocytes is saturated with approximately three times as much ^{59}Fe as ferritin in nonactivated monocytes [19]. In a previous study, it was found that iron-saturated transferrin reverses the inhibitory effect of interferon gamma activation on *L. pneumophila* intracellular multiplication. Therefore the effect of iron-transferrin on transferrin receptor expression and intracellular ferritin content was explored. We found that iron transferrin markedly upregulates both transferrin receptor expression and intracellular ferritin content in both nonactivated (2.3 and 1.3 fold, respectively) and interferon gamma (3.4 and 2.9 fold, respectively) monocytes [19]. These studies demonstrate that transferrin receptor expression and intracellular ferritin content of human monocytes is coordinately downregulated by interferon gamma. The upregulation of transferrin receptors and intracellular ferritin by iron transferrin may partly explain the mechanism whereby this molecule reverses the inhibitory effect of interferon gamma against *L. pneumophila*. Iron transferrin appears to influence its own uptake via a positive feedback mechanism, i.e., by increasing transferrin receptor expression [19].

Table 2. Ferritin Levels are Decreased in IFNγ-Activated Human Monocytes

Subject	Intracellular Ferritin fg/Monocyte (mean± SD) Nonactivated	Activated	% Reduction with Activation
1	178± 3	38±16	79
2	421±13	84± 1	80
3	206±10	43± 4	79
4	638±37	89±25	86
Mean±SEM	361±107	64±13	82

Intracellular ferritin content of nonactivated and IFNγ-activated monocytes was measured by radioimmunoassay twice on each of four subjects in eight independent experiments. Data are the mean±SD of the two measurements of intracellular ferritin content for each subject, and the mean±SEM of ferritin content of all subjects. $p \leq 0.01$ by paired, two-tailed t test.

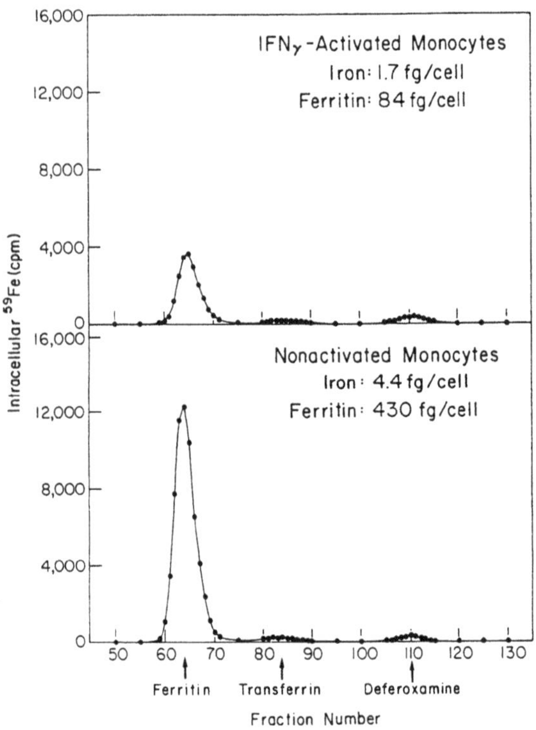

Fig. 3. Iron from iron transferrin is incorporated primarily into intracellular ferritin in both nonactivated and interferon gamma-activated monocytes. Nonactivated and interferon gamma-activated monocytes were incubated with Fe^{59} transferrin. After 5 d, the monocytes were lysed in the presence of deferoxamine, and the lysates run on a precalibrated ACA-34 gel filtration column. Radioactivity of each of the fractions was measured using a gamma counter. The locations where ferritin, transferrin, and deferoxamine come off the column are indicated.

Cytokine therapy of *L. pneumophila* infection

With knowledge of the important activating cytokines in *L. pneumophila* infection, it is possible to develop treatment strategies using these cytokines. Cytokine therapy of *L. pneumophila* infection may have its greatest utility in treating infection in the immunosuppressed host where it is likely that there are specific defects in the cell-mediated immune response which may be overcome by administration of cytokines. Aerosolized interferon gamma acting on alveolar macrophages and polymorphonuclear leukocytes might prove to be an effective cytokine therapy. Combination therapy may abe even more effective. The findings presented in this review suggest that agents such as deferoxamine, chloroquine, and apolactoferrin which decrease mononuclear phagocyte intracellular iron availability may be a useful adjunct to interferon gamma therapy against *L. pneumophila* infection. Aerosolized interferon gamma and tumor necrosis factor acting alveolar macrophages and polymorphonuclear leukocytes respectively might be another useful combination. In the monocytopenic/granulocytopenic patient, a combination of aerosolized interferon gamma, and aerosolized tumor necrosis factor with intravenous colony stimulating factors might serve to get effector cells to the lung and activate them when they arrive.

Delivery of cytokines to sites of infection

Systemic interferon gamma therapy has been used in humans to treat leprosy. In addition, in animal models, it has been administered intravenously or via aerosol into the lung to study its ability to enhance mononuclear phagocyte function. Murine recombinant interferon gamma given intraperitoneally or intravenously to mice has been found to activate alveolar and peritoneal macrophages to inhibit the intracellular multiplication of Toxoplasma gondii [20]. This activity lasted for up to 3 days following a single intravenous injection. Another study found that aerosolized murine recombinant interferon gamma or recombinant human tumor necrosis factor alpha given to rats increased interleukin 1 production by both alveolar macrophages and blood monocytes for at least 5 days after administration. Murine recombinant interferon gamma also increased Ia expression on alveolar macrophages and human recombinant tumor necrosis factor alpha increased alveolar macrophage and blood monocyte-mediated tumor lysis. When given sequentially, these cytokines increased Ia expression on alveolar macrophages and monocytes over that seen with either cytokine alone. In addition, aerosolized tumor necrosis factor alpha produced high cytokine levels in the lung, but very low uptake into the circulation [21]. These studies form a rational basis for the delivery of cytokines to the *L. pneumophila*-infected host.

In conclusion, recent findings have elucidated the potential role of cytokines, particularly interferon gamma, in host defense against *L. pneumophila*. Evidence suggests that cytokine treatment of *L. pneumophila* infection may have beneficial effects on the outcome of infection. Further work with animal models followed by clinical trials in immunosuppressed patients needs to be done.

References

1. Meyer RD, Finegold SM. Legionnaires' Disease. Ann Rev Med 1980; 31: 219–232.
2. Horwitz, MA, Silverstein SC. Interaction of the Legionnaires' disease bacterium (*Legionella pneumophila*) with human phagocytes. I. *L. pneumophila* resists killing by polymorphonuclear leukocytes, antibody, and complement. J Exp Med 1981; 153: 386–397.
3. Blanchard DK, Friedman H, Klein TW, Djeu JY. Induction of interferon-gamma and tumor necrosis factor by *Legionella pneumophila*: Augmentation of human neutrophil bactericidal activity. Journal of Leukocyte Biology 1989; 45: 538–545.
4. Horwitz MA. Cell-mediated immunity in Legionnaires' disease. J Clin Invest 1983; 71: 1686–1697.
5. Horwitz MA, and SC Silverstein. Activated human monocytes inhibit the intracellular multiplication of Legionnaires' disease bacterium. J Exp Med 1981; 154: 1618–1635.
6. Jensen WA, Rose RM, Burke RH, Anton K, Remold HG. Cytokine activation of antibacterial activity in human pulmonary macrophages: Comparison of recombinant interferon gamma and granulocyte-macrophage colony-stimulating factor. Cellular Immunology 1988; 117: 369–377.
7. Owan I, Saito A. Effect of human urinary colony-stimulating factor on experimental *Legionella pneumophila* infection in guinea pigs. Journal of Antimicrobial Chemotherapy 1990; 26: 831–840.
8. Hollander A, Kluin-Nelemans HC, Haak HR, Stern AC, Willemze R, Fibbe WE. Correction of neutropenia associated with chronic lymphocytic leukaemia following treatment with granulocyte-macrophage colony-stimulating factor. Hematology 1991; 62: 32–34.
9. Bhardwaj N, Nash TW, Horwitz MA. Interferon-gamma-activated human monocytes inhibit the intracellular multiplication of *Legionella pneumophila*. J Immunol 1986; 137: 2662–2669.
10. Quinn FD, Weinberg ED. Killing of *Legionella pneumophila* by human serum and iron binding agents. Curr Microbiol 1988; 17: 111–116.
11. Reeves MW, Pine LP, Neilands JB, Balows A. Absence of siderophore activity in Legionella species grown in iron deficient media. J Bacteriol 1983; 154: 324–329.
12. Dautry-Varsat A, Ciechanover A, Lodish HF. pH and recycling of transferrin during receptor mediated endocytosis. Proc. Natl Acad Sci USA 1983; 80: 2258–2262.
13. Jacobs A. Ferritin: An interim review. Curr Topics Hematol 1985; 5: 25–62.
14. Moguilevsky N, Masson PL, Courtoy PJ. Lactoferrin uptake and iron processing into macrophages: a study in familial haemochromatosis. Br J Haematol 1987; 66: 129–136.
15. Byrd TF, Horwitz MA. Interferon gamma-activated human monocytes downregulate transferrin receptors and inhibit the intracellular multiplication of *Legionella pneumophila* by limiting the availability of iron. J Clin Invest 1989; 83: 1457–1465.
16. Byrd TF, Horwitz MA. Chloroquine inhibits the intracellular multiplication of *Legionella pneumophila* by limiting the availability of iron. A potential new mechanism for the therapeutic effect of chloroquine against intracellular pathogens. J Clin Invest 1991; 88: 351–357.
17. Byrd TF, Horwitz MA. Lactoferrin inhibits or promotes *Legionella pneumophila* intracellular multiplication in non-activated and interferon gamma-activated human monocytes depending upon its degree of iron saturation. Iron lactoferrin and nonphysiologic iron chelates reverse monocyte activation against *Legionella pneumophila*. J Clin Invest 1991; 88: 1103–1112.
18. Britigan BE, Serody JS, Hayek MB, Charniga GM, Cohen MS. Lactoferrin uptake by mononuclear phagocytes. J Immunol 1991; 147: 4271–4279.
19. Byrd TF, Horwitz MA. Regulation of transferrin receptor expression and ferritin content in human mononuclear phagocytes: Coordinate upregulation by iron-transferrin and downregulation by interferon gamma. J Clin Invest 1993; 91: 969–976.
20. Black CM, Catterall JR, Remington JS. *In vivo* and *in vitro* activation of alveolar macrophages by recombinant interferon gamma. J Immunol 1987; 138: 491–495.

21. Debs RJ, Fuchs HJ, Philip R, Montgomery AB, Brunette EN, Liggit D, Patton JS, Shellito JE. Lung-specific delivery of cytokines induces sustained pulmonary and systemic immunomodulation in rats. J Immunol 1988; 140: 3482–3488.

Biotherapy 7: 187–193, 1994.

The role of cytokines in mycobacterial infection

J.H. Champsi[1,2], L.E. Bermudez[1] & L.S. Young[1]
[1]*Kuzell Institute for Arthritis and Infectious Diseases, California Pacific Medical Center Research Institute, San Francisco, CA 94115;* [2]*Stanford University, Department of Infectious Diseases and Geographical Medicine, 300 Pasteur Drive, Stanford, CA 94305, USA.*

Key words: mycobacteria, cytokines, tuberculosis, leprosy, *Mycobacterium avium* complex

Abstract

Mycobacterial infections are a major cause of morbidity and mortality worldwide. The pathogenesis of infection and the mechanisms for the development of protective immunity are poorly known, but cytokines appear to play an important role in the modulation of the immune response. Evidence exists for the role of tumor necrosis factor (TNF-α), granulocyte macrophage colony stimulating factor (GM-CSF) and interferon-gamma (IFN-γ) in the host defense against mycobacteria. In this article we discuss recent findings about the role of cytokines in leprosy, tuberculosis and *Mycobacterium avium* infection, using *in vitro* and *in vivo* human and murine data.

Abbreviations: M.TB: *Mycobacterium tuberculois*; IFN-γ: interferon gamma; TNF-α: tumor necrosis factor-alpha; LAM: Lipoarabinomannam; IL-8: Interleukin-8; IL-6: Interleukin-6; IL-2: Interleukin-2; CMI: cell-mediated immunity; PPD: purified protein derivative of tuberculin; MAC: *Mycobacterium avium* complex; AIDS: Acquired Immunodeficiency Syndrome; GM-CSF: granulocyte macrophage colony stimulating factor; IL-10: Interleukin-10; TGFβ: transforming growth factor β_1

Introduction

Mycobacterial infections are a major cause of morbidity and mortality worldwide. Leprosy and tuberculosis are still widely prevelant infections in the Third World. Due to the AIDS pandemic, there has been an increased incidence of tuberculosis and disseminated infection caused by organisms of the *Mycobacterium avium-Mycobacterium intracellulare* complex. In the human host, mycobacteria are facultative intracellular pathogens which survive and multiply mainly within the macrophages. Cellular immunity plays a key role in protective immunity to mycobacterial infection, as evidenced by the increased incidence of disease observed in AIDS patients. The pathogenesis of infection and the mechanisms for the development of protective immunity are unclear, but cytokines appear to play an important role in the modulation of the immune response.

Cytokines are molecules which are involved in the recruitment of cells, communication among cells and activation of the immune response. Elucidation of the role that cytokines play in protective immunity to mycobacterial infection would contribute towards a better understanding of the pathogenesis of infection.

Tuberculosis

Current information about the pattern of cytokine synthesis in the course of tuberculosis and the role of cytokines in the host defense against *M. tuberculosis (M. TB)* is not well defined due to conflicting data obtained from patients, and studies in experimental animals and *in vitro* models.

Interferon gamma (IFNγ) is an important immunoregulatory cytokine which has been shown to enhance killing of several intracellular pathogens such as *Legionella* sp [1] *Leishmania* sp [2], and *Chlamydia* sp [3]; however, its ability to stimulate anti-tuberculosis activity in human and murine macrophages is still unproven. Douvas and colleagues described enhanced mycobacterial replication in human macrophages pretreated with IFNγ, when compared with untreated macrophages [4]. This finding was supported by Rook and colleagues, who found IFNγ treated human macrophages were permissive of mycobacterial growth [5]. In contrast, murine bone marrow macrophages when stimulated with recombinant IFNγ markedly reduced the growth of *M. TB* [6]. Rook and colleagues described similar antimycobacterial activity in murine peritoneal macrophages pretreated with IFNγ [5].

Denis reported that infusion of recombinant IFNγ led to improved survival and decreased viable bacterial organ counts in Balb/c mice infected with *M. TB* [7]. Furthermore, treatment of infected mice with anti-IFNγ antibody was associated with significant decreased in survival. In addition, anti IFNγ antibody prevented the development of protective immunity in previously treated infected mice [7].

The mechanism responsible for the inhibition of growth of *M. TB* within macrophages is believed to be partially dependent on the production of nitric oxide or another inorganic nitrogen oxide effector molecule. Chan and colleagues showed that murine macrophages activated with IFNγ and Tumor Necrosis Factor-alpha (TNFα) had anti-*M. tuberculosis* activity that was correlated with induction of L-arginine dependent generation of reactive nitrogen intermediates [8]. This finding was supported by Denis using murine peritoneal macrophages [9]. Unfortunately, there is no good evidence that human macrophages are able to produce reactive nitrogen intermediates. Hence, the differences observed when comparing studies carried out with mice macrophages and human macrophages could be related to the inability of human macrophages to produce nitric oxide when stimulated by IFNγ or TNFα.

TNFα is a pro-inflammatory, endogenous pyrogen that plays a role in the immune response to a wide range of infectious pathogens and in the actual manifestations of disease caused by these organisms. Valone and colleagues [10] have recently demonstrated that BCG and mycobacterial products are capable of directly stimulating monocytes and alveolar macrophages to produce TNFα *in vitro*. Infection of mice by BCG leads to granuloma formation which occurs coincidentally with an increase in local TNFα mRNA production. Infusion of anti-TNFα antibody leads to abrogation of granuloma formation and increased bacterial counts [11]. Studies in humans have shown that patients with tuberculosis pleuritis, usually a self-limited disease, have high levels of TNFα in the pleural fluid, and pleural monocytes of infected patients have been shown to secrete high levels of TNFα when compared to peripheral monocytes [12]. In contrast, monocytes obtained from patients with refractory chronic tuberculosis have depressed TNFα production when compared to monocytes from patients with recently diagnosed tuberculosis, suggesting that the bacteria possibly interferes with the signal transduction within macrophages [13].

In a recent report, Denis treated *M. TB* infected Balb/c mice with exogenous TNFα and observed an increased survival when compared to untreated infected controls [7]. Infusion of anti-TNFα antibody led to decreased survival suggesting that TNFα is involved in promoting host resistance to *M. TB*.

Lipoarabinomannam (LAM) is a major component of the mycobacterial cell wall. LAM which has been purified from the virulent Erdman strain of *M. TB* is different structurally when compared to LAM purified from an attenuated strain of *M. TB*, H37Ra. In a recent study by Chatterjee and colleagues, it was shown that LAM from the virulent strain did not stimulate murine macrophages to produce high levels of TNFα unlike the LAM from the attenuated strain which was a potent trigger for TNFα release [14]. This observation suggests that TNFα may have a beneficial effect in the host defense against *M. TB*, and that virulent strains can inhibit the release of TNFα by macrophages.

Interleukin–8 (IL–8) is a potent neutrophil and T cell chemotatic factor *in vitro*. IL–8 is believed to be important in granuloma formation. Friedland and colleagues reported that human monocytic cell lines (THP–1 and MonoMac 6) produced high levels of IL–8 after phagocytosis of *M. TB* [5]. Although, IL–8 secretion appeared to be independent of strain virulence [15], the elevated levels of IL–8 could be responsible for early granuloma formation seen in *M. TB* infection.

Interleukin–6 (IL–6), which is a B cell stimulatory factor has been shown to cause marked tuberculostatic activity when added to murine macrophages infected with *M. bovis*. In contrast, preincubation of murine and human macrophages with IL–6 prior to infection had no effect on the intracellular growth of *M. tuberculosis* [16]. IL–6 may provide a T-cell-independent mode of mycobacterial activity by macrophage activation.

Interleukin–2 (IL–2) is a T lymphocyte growth factor which is involved in T cell and monocyte activation [17]. Cells which interact with IL–2 require the presence of an IL–2 receptor on their surface. The IL–2 receptor is a heterodimer molecule. The 75 kDa β

chain of the IL–2 receptor, also known as TAC protein, is released in soluble form in several disease processes [18, 19]. Elevated soluble IL–2 receptor levels have been described in tuberculosis pleural effusions [20] and in the sera of patients with active pulmonary tuberculosis [21]. Elevated IL–2 soluble receptor levels probably represent T cell activation and on-going immune response. Peripheral monocytes isolated from patients with active pulmonary tuberculosis expressed IL–2 receptor on their surface and released soluble IL–2 receptor constitutively into the culture supernant [22]. It has been proposed that soluble IL–2 receptor may have a role in pathogenesis of disease by binding IL–2 in the sera and preventing it from interacting with cellular targets, thereby causing depressed cellular immunity leading to mycobacterial disease. However, the meaning of high levels of IL–2 receptor in tuberculosis is currently unknown.

Leprosy

Mycobacterium leprae is an intracellular organism preferentially infecting dermal macrophages and Schwann neural cells. Clinical presentation of leprosy is dependent on the host's immune response to infection. In tuberculoid leprosy, there is strong cell-mediated immunity (CMI) and low bacterial counts. In contrast, in lepromatous leprosy, a form of the disease which is characterized by large bacterial counts in the lesions, peripheral monocytes have no discernible underlying defect and have normal oxidative response after activation with recombinant IFNγ [23]. Lymphocytes from infected patients do not release IFNγ when exposed to *M. leprae* antigens *in vitro*. The same lymphocytes, however, proliferate in the presence of other antigens. This suggests that there is selective anergy to *M. leprae* antigen that leads to a lack of CMI and wide spread disease [24, 25].

Patients with lepromatous leprosy will react to purified protein derivative of tuberculin (PPD) in previously PPD positive hosts [26]. During the immune response to PPD antigen, local IFNγ production and clearance of *M. leprae* was noted [26]. Clinical trials in humans demonstrated that injection of recombinant IFNγ into the site of infection was associated with decrease in local bacterial burden. Furthermore, monocytes from IFNγ treated patients, when challenged with *M. leprae* antigen, showed improved H_2O_2 production compared to subnormal pretreatment levels of H_2O_2 [27]. These studies demonstrated a decrease in the number of bacilli in the lesion, but they failed to show if IFNγ-activated macrophages were ingesting and killing the bacteria. It is possible that activated peripheral monocytes increased the clearance of dead bacteria within the lesion. In more recent studies, administration of recombinant IFN-γ in sites distant from the lepromatous lesion appear to confirm the beneficial effect of the cytokine [28]. Marked intralesional accumulation of $CD3^+$, $CD4^+$, $CD8^+$ and CDa^+ T cells was observed with a dose of 10 to 30μg of recombinant IFNγ/m^2 [28], converting the lepromatous lesion into a tuberculoid lesion.

Work by Kaplan and colleagues showed that intradermal injections of IL–2 in patients with lepromatous leprosy caused recruitment of T cells into the site of injection and a decrease in bacillary load [29]. Peripheral blood monocytes from patients with lepromatous leprosy, normally unresponsive to *M. leprae* antigen were shown to be stimulated to proliferate *in vitro* by exogenous IL–2 [30].

In studies comparing cytokine profiles from draining lymph nodes from susceptible infected (CBA, Balb/C) mice and from resistant (C57BL/6) infected mice, resistant mice were found to have high levels of IL–2, IL–6 and IFN-γ. In contrast, susceptible mice did not produce IFNγ or IL–6 in response to *M. leprae* antigen [31], therefore suggesting IL–2, IL–6 and IFNγ have a role in protective immunity to *M. leprae*. The role of IL–2 and TNF in protective immunity is supported by an *in vivo* study where exogenous intraperitoneal infusion of IL–2, and TNF into infected susceptible Balb/c mice and resistant A/J mice lead to improved overall survival for both strains when compared to untreated controls. IFN-γ given intravenously did not have any effect on survival [32].

Yamamura examined cytokine expression in lepromatous skin biopsy specimens using polymerase chain reaction. There was elevated IL–2 and IFNγ in the tuberculoid leprosy skin biopsy specimens when compared to lepromatous leprosy [33]. This finding supports the protective role of IFNγ and IL–2 against *M. leprae* and is consistent with the good clinical prognosis seen in the tuberculoid form of the disease.

Mycobacterium avium complex (MAC)

MAC is a common pathogen of immunocompromised and Acquired Immunodeficiency Syndrome (AIDS) patients. In this population of individuals, MAC is associated with bacteremia and disseminated disease

Table 1. Activity *in vitro* against Mycobacteria

	Stimulates mycobacteriostatic activity			
Infection	yes	no effect	hinder	effector cell*
M. tuberculosis	IFNγ		IFNγ	
	GM-CSF			h Mo
	TNF		IL–1, IL–3	h Mono
	IFNγ			m Mo
		IFNγ		h Alv Mo
		IFNγ		m BM Mo
M. avium	TNF	IFNγ	IL–3	
	IFNγ		IL–1	
	GM-CSF		IL–6	h Mono
	TNF	IFNγ	M-CSF	
	GM-CSF		TGFβ	h Mono
	IFNγ			h Alv Mo
	IFnγ		IL–3	
	IL–4		IL–10	m Mo

* Mo = macrophage; Mono = monocytes; Alv Mo = alveolar macrophages; BM = bone marrow; m = murine; h = human

[34]. MAC is an intracellular pathogen found within the host's macrophages. The role of HIV–1 infection on the susceptibility of macrophages to MAC infection is presently unknown. A recent report by Johnson and colleagues showed preservation of monocyte effector function against *M. avium* when comparing monocytes from AIDS patients and normal volunteers [35]. Meyland and colleagues reported similar results using health donor macrophages which were infected *in vitro* with HIV–1 [36]. In contrast, Kallenius and colleagues reported that infection of macrophages by HIV–1 lead to increased *M. avium* growth *in vitro* [37].

A number of laboratories, including our own, have shown that stimulation of infected murine or human macrophages with recombinant granulocyte macrophage colony stimulating factor (GM-CSF) or TNF induces mycobacteriostatic/mycobactericidal activity [38–40]. This observation is supported by work carried out *in vivo* in which the administration of exogenous TNFα or GM-CSF to MAC infected beige mice lead to increased mycobactericidal activity [41]. IFNγ is a classic macrophage activator. In the case of MAC, the IFNγ mediated activation of macrophages to inhibit the growth or killing of intracellular bacteria appears to be strain and morphotype dependent. Colonial morphology of MAC is an important determinant of intracellular growth and drug susceptibility [42, 43]. Fresh isolates of MAC from AIDS patients are predominantly of flat and transparent colony morphotype and fully pathogenic in mice [44]. During successive passage *in vitro*, a transition to domed and opque colonies occurs and is associated with loss of virulence [45]. In fact, colony morphology of MAC seems to affect response of infected macrophage to cytokines and profiles of cytokine synthesis by macrophages exposed to MAC. The virulent smooth transparent morphotype appears to depress IL–1 and TNFα expression when compared to the less virulent smooth domed isogenic colonies of MAC [46]. We have observed that macrophages infected with smooth transparent morphotype for periods longer than 2 days are unable to produce TNF-α when properly stimulated [47]. Recently, we have observed that the IFN-γ mediated stimulation of mycobacteriostatic activity of macrophages against MAC appears to be dependent on the macrophage population. While INF-γ stimulated human monocyte-derived macrophages and murine peritoneal macrophages cannot inhibit the intracellular growth of MAC 101, stimulation of intestinal macrophages with INF-γ resulted in inhibition of intracellular growth of MAC [48].

The inability of infected macrophages to clear MAC infection could be related to the generation of "immunosupressive" cytokines. Transform-

Table 2. In vivo effect of cytokines in Mycobacterial infections

Infection	Activity yes	no effect	host
M. tuberculosis		IFNγ	human
	IFNγ		mouse
	TNF		mouse
M. leprae	IFNγ		human
	IL–6		human
	TNF		mouse
M. avium	GM-CSF		mouse
	TNF		mouse
	IL–2		mouse

ing growth factor-β 1 (TGFβ_1), interleukin–10 (IL–10) and interleukin–6 (IL–6) are immunosuppressive cytokines that have been shown to counteract the stimulatory effects of immunoactivating cytokines resulting in immunosuppresion and intracellular survival of the pathogenic organism. Barral-Netto and colleagues reported that murine peritoneal macrophages infected with *Leishmania amazonensis* increased TGFβ_1 production *in vitro*. [49]. Exogenous TGFβ_1 led to leishmania infection in genetically resistant mice and anti-TGFβ_1 arrested leishmania infection in susceptible mice [49]. Bermudez and colleagues found infection of macrophages with *Toxoplasma gondii* induced production and release of TGFβ_1 with down regulation of macrophage TNF receptors; this effect was partially reversed by anti-TGFβ_1 [50]. Similarly in MAC infection, human monocyte-derived macrophages secrete high levels of a potent suppressor of TNF production and macrophage activation [51]. Secretion of TGFβ_1 occurs early in the infection and appears to be dependent on the strain of MAC. TGFβ_1 impairs the macrophage response to stimulation with TNFα and use of anti-TGFβ_1 antibody is associated with improved response to TNFα and IFNγ. Therefore, these results indicate that unresponsiveness of MAC-infected macrophages to IFNγ is due to the induction of TGFβ_1 by some MAC strains. MAC infection also stimulates IL–6 release and down regulation of TNF receptors [52, 53]. IL–10 was initially described as cytokine synthesis inhibitory factor known to suppress many macrophage functions and to suppress cytokine production. Recently, our laboratory reported high levels of IL–10 in spleen cells isolated from MAC infected mice [54]. Administration of IL–10 antibody to infected mice lead to lower bacterial counts when compared to untreated controls. The presence of inhibitory cytokines like IL–6, IL–10, and TGFβ_1 may be responsible for MAC survival within the macrophage.

Cytokine interactions with various co-factors and drugs could enhance therapy of mycobacterial infection. For example, treatment of infected macrophage monolayers with Azithromycin and exogenous TNFα, IFNγ leads to increased drug uptake by the infected cells [55]. Treatment of MAC infection, in patients with AIDS, with Azithromycin and GM-CSF are presently in clinical trials. Other factors which may inhibit macrophage activation include ethanol which has been shown to impair macrophage activation by TNF and GM-CSF *in vitro* [56]. Administration of ethanol to mice infected with MAC was associated with a higher bacterial organ count when compared to infected untreated mice. Recent experiments in our laboratory have shown that exposure to ethanol induces a stress-like response in MAC with consequent upregulation of the synthesis of a number of bacterial proteins, which have been associated with the pathogenesis of infection.

Cytokine networks play an important role in the immune response to mycobacterial infection. The cytokine cascade initiated by infection is modulated by numerous factors including the colony morphology, strain of mycobacteria, host resistance and the presence or absence of other modifying cytokines and co-factors. In the studies discussed in this paper, there is quite diverse information utilizing various experimental conditions. Interpretation of the data available can be difficult because of conflicting results, depending on the experimental model used. *In vitro* data, as in the case of IFNγ and MAC, does not always reflect *in vivo* and patient data. In addition, we have to be aware that the concentration of cytokine production for optimal effect has not been determined; therefore the experimental data may not reflect physiological effects of the cytokine. Due to the complexity of cytokine interactions, the autocrine effects versus the paracrine effects of cytokines, application of cytokine therapy to patient population is challenging and fraught with difficulties. Elucidation and better understanding of the complex interactions involved in protective immunity will enable us to understand mycobacterial pathogenesis. Finally, recombinant cytokine therapy could be utilized clinically to modify the disease course in recalcitrant disease.

Acknowledgements

Dr. Champsi is supported by training grant AI–07089, from the National Institutes of Health and by the California Universitywide AIDS Research Program through the California Collaborative Treatment Group (CC93-SD-132).

References

1. Bhardwaj N, Nash T, Horwitz M. Interferon γ activated human monocytes inhibit the intracellular multiplication of *Legionella pneumophila*. J Immunol 1986 137: 2662–2669.
2. Murray H, Rubin B, Rothermel C. Killing of intracellular *Leishmania donovani* by lymphokine-stimulated human mononuclear phagocytes: Evidence that interferon γ is the activating lymphokine. J Clin Invest 1983 72: 1506–1510.
3. Rothermel C, Rubin B, Murray H. Interferon γ is the factor in lymphokines that activates human macrophages to inhibit intracellular *Chlamydia psittaci* replication. J Immunol 1983 131: 2542–2544.
4. Douvas GS, Looker DL, Vatter AE, Crowle AJ. Interferon-γ activates human macrophages to become tumoricidal and leishmanicidal but enhances duplication of macrophage-associated mycobacteria. Infect Immun 1985 50: 1–8.
5. Rook GAW, Steele J, Ainsworth M, Champion BR. Activation of macrophages to inhibit proliferation of *Mycobacterium tuberculosis*: comparison of the effects of recombinant gamma-interferon on human monocytes and murine peritoneal macrophage. Immunology 1986 59: 333–338.
6. Flesch I, Kaufmann SHE. Mycobacterial growth inhibition by interferon γ activated bone marrow macrophages and differential susceptibility among strains of *Mycobacterium tuberculosis*. J Immunol 1987 138: 4408–4413.
7. Denis M. Involvement of cytokines in determining resistance and acquired immunity in murine tuberculosis. J Leukocyte Biol 1991 50: 495–501.
8. Chan J, Xing, Magliozzo R, Bloom B. Killing of virulent *Mycobacterium tuberculosis* by reactive nitrogen intermediates produced by activated murine macrophages. J Exp Med 1992 175: 1111–1122.
9. Denis M. Interferon γ-treated murine macrophages inhibit growth of tubercle bacilli via the generation of reactive nitrogen intermediates. Cell Immunol 1991 132: 150–157.
10. Valone SE, Rich EA, Wallis RS, Ellner JJ. Expression of TNF *in vitro* by human mononuclear phagocytes stimulated with whole *M. bovis* BCG and mycobacterial antigens. Infect Immun 1988 56: 3313–3315.
11. Kindler V, Sappino A, Grau G, Piguet P, Vassalli P. The inducing role of tumor necrosis factor in the development of bactericidal granulomas during BCG infection. Cell 1989 56: 731–740.
12. Barnes PF, Fong SJ, Brennan PJ, et al. Local production of tumor necrosis factor and IFN-gamma in tuberculosis pleuritis. J Immunol 1990 145: 149–154.
13. Takashima T, Ueta C, Tsuyuguchi I, Kishimoto S. Production of tumor necrosis factor α by monocytes from patients with pulmonary tuberculosis. Infect Imm 1990 58: 3286–3292.
14. Roach T, Barton G, Chatterjee D, Blackwell J. Macrophage activation: Lipoarabinomannan from avirulent and virulent strains of *Mycobacterium tuberculosis* differentially induce the early genes c-fos, KC, JE and tumor necrosis factor-α. J Immunol 1993 150: 1886–1896.
15. Friedland J, Remick D, Shattock R, Griffin G. Secretion of interleukin–8 following phagocytosis of *Mycobacterium tuberculosis* by human monocyte cell lines. Eur J Immunol 1992 22: 1575–1578.
16. Flesch IEA, Kaufman SHE. Stimulation of antibacterial macrophage activities by β-cell stimulatory factor 2 (interleukin–6). Infect Immun 1990 58: 269–271.
17. Cantrell D, Smith K. Interleukin–2 T cell system: a new cell growth model. Science 1984 224: 1312–1316.
18. Hancock W, Muller W, Cotren R. Interleukin–2 receptors are expressed by alveolar macrophages during pulmonary sarcoidosis and are inducible by lymphokine treatment of normal human lung macrophages, blood monocytes and monocyte cell lines. J Immunol 1987 138: 185–191.
19. Reddy M, Grieco M. Elevated soluble interleukin–2 receptor levels in serum of human immunodeficiency virus-infected population. AIDS Res Hum Retrovir 1988 4: 115–120.
20. Ito M, Kojimo N, Shirasaka T, Moriwaki Y, Tachibana I, Kokubu T. Elevated levels of soluble Interleukin–2 receptors in tuberculous pleural effusions. Chest 1988 97: 1141–1143.
21. Brown A, Rieder K, Webster H. Prolonged elevations of soluble interleukin–2 in tuberculosis. Am Rev Resp Dis 1989 139: 1031–1038.
22. Tossi Z, Sedor JR, Lapurga JP, Ondash RJ, Ellner JJ. Expression of functional interleukin–2 receptors by peripheral blood monocytes from patients with active pulmonary tuberculosis. J Clin Invest 1990 85: 1777–1784.
23. Kaplan G, Nathan CF, Horwitz M, et al. Effect of recombinant gamma interferon on hydrogen peroxide-releasing capaciity of monocyte-derived macrophages from patients with lepromatous leprosy. J Immunol 1986 137: 983–987.
24. Nogueira N, Kaplan G, Levy E, et al. Defective interferon-γ production in leprosy: reversal with antigen and interleukin–2. J Exp Med 1983 158: 2165–2170.
25. Kaplan G, Weinstein D, Steinman RM, et al. An analysis of *in vitro* T cell responsiveness in lepromatous leprosy. J Exp Med 1985 162: 917–929.
26. Kaplan G, Laal S, Sheftel G, et al. The nature and kinetics of a delayed immune response to purified protein derivative of tuberculin in the skin of lepromatous leprosy patients. J Exp Med 1988 168: 1811–1824.
27. Nathan CF, Kaplan G, Levis WR, Nusrat A, et al. Local and systemic effects of intradermal recombinant interferon-γ in patients with lepromatous leprosy. N Engl J Med 1986 315 : 6–15.
28. Nathan CF, Squires K, Griffow W, Levis W, Varghese M, et al. Widespread intradermal accumulation of mononuclear leukocytes in lepromatous leprosy patients treated systemically with recombinant interferon γ. J Exp Med 1990 172: 1509–1512.
29. Nathan G, Briton WJ, Hancock GE, et al. Systemic influence of recombinant interleukin–2 on the manifestations of lepromatous leprosy. J Exp Med 1991 173: 993–1006.
30. Ottenhett T, Wondimu A, Reddy N. A comparative study on the effect of rIL–4, rIL–2, rINFγ, and TNFa or specific T cell non-responsiveness to mycobacterial antigens in lepromatous leprosy patients *in vitro*. Scand J Immunol 1990 31: 553–565.
31. Roch F, Bach M. Strain differences in mouse cellular responses to *Mycobacterium lepraemurium* and BCG subcutaneous infections. Clin Immunol Immunopath 1991 60: 443–454.
32. Denis M. Cytokine modulation of *Mycobacterium lepraemurium* infection in mice, important involvement of tumor necrosis

factor, interluekin–2, and dissociation from macrophage activation. J Immunopharmac 1991 13: 889–895.
33. Yamamura M, Uyemura K, Deans RJ, Weinberg K, et al. Defining protective responses to pathogens: cytokine profiles in leprosy lesions. Science 1991 256: 277–279.
34. Hawkins CC, Gold JW, Whimbey E, Kiehn TE, Brannon P, Cammarata R. *Mycobacterium avium* complex infections in patients with the acquired immunodeficiency syndrome. Ann Intern Med 1986 2: 184–188.
35. Johnson JL, Shiratsuchi H, Toba H, Ellner JJ. Preservation of monocyte effector functions against *Mycobacterium avium-Mycobacterium intracellulare* in patients with AIDS. Infect 1991 59: 3639–3645.
36. Meyland PRA, Munis JR, Richman DD, Kornbluth RS. Concurrent human immunodeficiency virus and mycobacterial infection of macrophages *in vitro* does not reveal any reciprocal effect. J Infect Dis 1992 165: 80–86.
37. Kallenius G, Koivula T, Rydgard KJ, Hoffner SE, et al. Human immunodeficiency virus type I enhances intracellular growth of *Mycobacterium avium* in human macrophages. Infect Immun 1992 60: 2453–2458.
38. Bermudez LE, Young LS. Recombinant granulocyte-macrophage colony stimulating factor (GM-CSF) activates human macrophages to inhibit growth or kill *Mycobacterium avium* complex. J Leukocyte Biol 1990
39. Bermudez LE, Young LS. Tumor necrosis factor, alone or in combination with IL–2 but not IFN-gamma, is associated with macrophage killing of *Mycobacterium avium* complex. J Immunol 1988 9: 3006–3013.
40. Denis M, Gregg E. Recombinant tumor necrosis factor-alpha decreases whereas recombinant interleukin–6 increases growth of a virulent strain of *Mycobacterium avium* in human macrophages. Immunol 1990 71: 139–141.
41. Bermudez LE, Stevens P, Kolonoski P, Wu M, Young LS. Treatment of disseminated *Mycobacterium avium* complex infection in mice with recombinant interleukin–2 and tumor necrosis factor. J Immunol 1989 143: 2996–3002.
42. Shiratuchi H, Johnson JL, Toba H, Ellner JJ. Strain and donor-related differences in the interaction of *Mycobacterium avium* with human monocytes and its modulation by interferon γ. J. Infect Dis 162: 932–936.
43. Saito H, Tomioka H. Susceptibilities of transparent, opaque and rough colonial variants of *Mycobacterium avium* to various fatty acids. Antimicrob Agents Chemother 32: 400–402.
44. Dunbar FP, Pejovich R, Cacciatore L, Peric-Golio L, Runyan EH. *Mycobacterium intracellulare* maintenance of pathogenicity in relationship to hypophilization and colony formation. Scand J Resp Dis 1968 49: 153–162.
45. Schaefer WB, Davis CL, Cohn ML. Pathogenicity of transparent, opaque and rough variants of *Mycobacterium avium* in chickens and mice. Am Rev Respir Dis 1970 102: 499–506.
46. Shiratsuchi H, Toosi Z, Mettler MA, Ellner JJ. Colonial morphotype as a determinant of cytokine expression by human monocytes with *Mycobacterium avium*. J Immunol 1993 150: 2945–2954.
47. Bermudez LE, Young LS. Killing of *Mycobacterium avium*: Insights provided by the use of recombinant cytokines. Research in Microbiol 1990 141: 241–245.
48. Hsu N, Young L, Bermudez L. Intestinal macrophages can be activated to kill *M. avium* complex but have variable ability to produce cytokines. In: Program and abstracts of the ASM General Meeting 1993 Atlanta, GA. Abstract U69.
49. Barral-Neto M, Barral A, Brownell CE, Skeiky YAW, Ellingsworth LR, Twardzik DR. Transforming growth factor-β in leishmanial infection: A parasite escape mechanism. Science 1992 257: 545–548.
50. Bermudez LE, Covaro G, Remington J. Infection of murine macrophages with *Toxoplasma gondii* is associated with release of TGFβ and downregulation of the expression of TNF receptors. Infect Immun 1993 61: 4126–4130.
51. Bermudez LE. Production of Transforming Growth Factor β by *Mycobacterium avium* infected macrophages is associated with unresponsiveness to Interferon-gamma. J Immunol 1993 150: 1838.
52. Bermudez LE, Wu M, Petrofsky M, Young LS. Interleukin–6 antagonizes tumor necrosis factor-mediated mycobacteriostatic and mycobactericidal activities in macrophages. Infect Immun 1992 60: 4245–4252.
53. Blanchard DK, Michelini-Norris MB, Pearson CA, Freitag CS, Djeu JY. *Mycobacterium avium-intracellulare* induces interleukin–6 from human monocytes and large granular lymphocytes. Blood 1991 77: 2218–2224.
54. Bermudez LE, Champsi J. Infection with *Mycobacterium avium* induces production of IL–10 and administration of anti–IL–10 antibody is associated with enhanced resistance to infection in mice. Infect Immun 1993 61: 3093–3096
55. Bermudez LE, Inderlied C, Young LS. Stimulation with cytokines enhances penetration of Azithromycin into human macrophages. Antimicrob Agents Chemother 1991 12: 2625–2629.
56. Bermudez LE, Young LS. Ethanol augments intracellular survival of *Mycobacterium avium* complex and impairs macrophage responses to cytokines. J Infect Dis 1991 63: 1286–1292.

Address for correspondence: Dr. Luiz E. Bermundez, Kuzell Institute, 2200 Webster St., Room 305, San Francisco, CA 94115

Biotherapy 7: 195–210, 1994.

Cytokines in the treatment of fungal infections

Bart-Jan Kullberg & Jan W. van 't Wout
Department of Medicine, University Hospital Nijmegen, The Netherlands, and Department of Infectious Diseases, University Hospital Leiden, The Netherlands

Key words: Invasive mycoses, *Candida, Aspergillus*, host defense, immunotherapy, interferon, interleukin, tumor necrosis factor, colony-stimulating factors

Abstract

The incidence of invasive fungal infections in the immunocompromized host has increased during the past decade. Even the recently developed antifungal drugs are unable to cure these infections in patients with severely impaired host defense mechanisms. Cytokines have great potential to augment host resistance and as adjunctive therapy of invasive mycoses. We discuss the mechanisms of host defense against invasive candidiasis, aspergillosis, and cryptococcosis, and review the use of cytokines and growth factors in this setting. Interleukin-1 has been shown effective in an animal model of disseminated candidiasis, even during severe granulocytopenia. Interferon-γ has been very effective as a modulator of resistance against a variety of fungal infections *in vitro*. The effect of interferon-γ against disseminated candidiasis has been demonstrated in a mouse model. Activation of neutrophils is the main mechanism by which interferon-γ enhances the elimination of *Candida*, and consequently the agent is not effective in severly granulocytopenic animals. Data on the role of colony-stimulating factors against fungal pathogens are accumulating, and trials with these agents for hematologic patients with invasive fungal infections are now being performed.

Abbreviations: CGD: chronic granulomatous disease; G-CSF: granulocyte colony-stimulating factor; M-CSF: monocyte colony-stimulating factor; GM-CSF: granulocyte-monocyte colony-stimulating factor; IFN-γ: interferon-gamma; IL: interleukin; LAK: lymphokine-activated killer; LPS: lipopolysaccharide; MDP: muramyl dipeptide; NK: natural killer; PMN: polymorphonuclear leukocytes; rh: recombinant human; ROI: reactive oxygen intermediates; TNF: tumor necrosis factor

Introduction

During the past decade, progress has been made in the treatment of patients with acute leukemia, and the proportion of patients achieving complete remission and longer survival has increased. A significant number of patients still fail to achieve long term survival, the most frequent cause of treatment failure being infection. Fungi, particularly *Candida* and *Aspergillus* species, are responsible for a majority of the fatal infections [1, 2]. Autopsy studies have revealed that 40 percent of the deceased cancer patients at the U. S. National Cancer Institute had a fungal infection [1, 3]. Among patients with hematologic malignancies the incidence of fungal infections is even substantially higher than among patients with solid tumors [1, 4, 5]. The incidence of nosocomial fungemia has increased five-fold in the United States between 1980 and 1990 [6], and *Candida* species now are the fourth most common isolates recovered from blood [7, 8]. In Europe and Japan the incidence of fungal infections may be lower than in the United States: a recent multinational autopsy survey revealed fungal infections in 25% of patients with leukemia or malignant lymphoma and 5% of patients with solid tumors in these countries [5]. Whereas patients with hematologic malignancies receiving anticancer chemotherapy are the main group at risk for disseminated candidiasis, the disease is also seen in other patient groups, such as organ transplant recipients [9] and intravenous drugs users. For invasive aspergillosis, profound and persistent granulocytopenia or functional defects of granulocytes, such as in patients with chronic granulomatous disease, constitute the major risk factors [10, 11]. Moreover, an increased susceptibility to *Aspergillus* infections has been described in patients treated with glucocorticosteroids and in those with AIDS [10, 12]. Infections with *Cryptococcus neoformans* are found predominantly in patients with impaired T-cell-mediated cellular immunity, and the AIDS epidemic has lead to a substantial rise of the incidence of cryptococcosis [13]. Moreover, cryptococcal infections are difficult to cure in these patients and residual infection often necessitates life-long antifungal treatment, underscoring the importance of intact host defense mechanisms against cryptococcosis.

For the divergent manifestations of *Candida* infection, various pathways of host resistance are involved, and therefore specific patient groups appear to be at risk for different types of candidiasis. Patients with markedly reduced numbers of circulating polymorphonuclear leukocytes (PMN), i. e.$< 0.5 \times 10^9$/l, are at high risk for acute and chronic disseminated candidiasis, indicating that PMN play an important role in host defense against invasive, deep-seated *Candida* infections. In contrast, disseminated candidiasis is highly unusual in patients with impaired T-cell-mediated cellular immunity, such as those with AIDS or chronic mucocutaneous candidiasis. These patients develop severe candidiasis of the skin, oropharynx, and esophagus. For *Candida*, impaired phagocytosis and killing by PMN and monocytes have been described in parenteral drug users with AIDS but not in other AIDS patients [14–17], indicating that phagocytic cells from patients with AIDS are functionally intact in respect to the phagocytosis and killing of *C. albicans*. These observations indicate that T-cell-mediated immunity is not of great importance in the host defense against disseminated candidiasis. Although PMN form the main defense against invasive candidiasis, their role is less important in superficial infections, in which T-cell-mediated immunity is the main mechanism for clearance of the *Candida*.

Effector cells in host defense to fungal infections

C. albicans

The concept that the phagocytosis and killing of *Candida* species by PMN and monocytes or macrophages play the most important role in the host defense against disseminated candidiasis is supported by abundant data from *in vitro* and *in vivo* experiments [18, 19]. Animals pretreated with agents that reduce the numbers of PMN are more susceptible to a systemic challenge with *C. albicans* [20–22]. In contrast, the results of *in vitro* studies on the killing of *C. albicans* by murine macrophages are divergent. Various investigators have reported that murine resident peritoneal and alveolar macrophages are unable to kill ingested *C. albicans in vitro* [23–27], although others have found opposite results [28, 29].

The mechanism by which phagocytic cells kill ingested *C. albicans* has only been partly elucidated. Activation of PMN and mononuclear phagocytes leads to the generation of reactive oxygen intermediates, which have long been considered crucial for the host defense against *C. albicans* [25, 30]. Oxidative intracellular killing is not the only mechanism by which phagocytic cells are able to kill *Candida*. Recently, it has been shown that defensins, isolated from azurophil granules in human PMN, are able to kill *C. albicans in vitro* [31, 32]. Moreover, both monocytes and PMN are able to kill *C. albicans* extracellularly by attachment to hyphae and degranulation of their fungicidal content into the immediate microenvironment without phagocytosis [32, 33]. Still another mechanism of extracellular killing of *C. albicans* has been described recently [34, 35]. Human PMN contain a cytoplasmic 30 kDa protein that is released only after death of the PMN [34]. Lysed neutrophils or the purified protein almost completely inhibit the growth of *C. albicans* [35]. It may be speculated that death and disintegration of large numbers of PMN on the battlefield of infection and release of this fungostatic substance thus serve as a second mechanism of defense when the classic system of oxidative and non-oxidative killing has failed.

Aspergillus species

Invasive aspergillosis in immunocompromized hosts develops after inhalation of *Aspergillus* conidia into the lungs. Pulmonary alveolar macrophages constitute the first line of defense against these conidia, as has been demonstrated by various studies *in vitro* and *in vivo* [36]. When the infection progresses, the *Aspergillus* conidia in the alveolar space germinate into hyphal forms. A rapid influx of PMN is seen at the site of infection, and opsonized *A. fumigatus* hyphae attach to PMN and stimulate their oxidative burst [37]. Thus, PMN form the second line of defense to invasive aspergillosis, being fungicidal for the mycelium of Aspergillus by secretion of oxidative and nonoxidative metabolites [36, 38]. These data from *in vitro* experiments have been supported by *in vivo* models, showing that the sensitivity to invasive aspergillosis is increased in neutropenic mice [39].

Cryptococcus neoformans

It is generally accepted that T-cell mediated immunity is the most important host defense mechanism against the encapsulated fungus *Cryptococcus neoformans* [40]. Cryptococcosis is strongly associated with disorders of lymphocyte function, such as AIDS and lymphoma, but it is unclear which lymphocyte populations and which effector mechanisms are essential for host defense to *C. neoformans*. In animal models, both $CD4^+$ and $CD8^+$ T-cells are required for the host resistance to cryptococcosis [41]. Depletion of NK-cells did not affect the course of experimental cryptococcosis [42] and the load of *C. neoformans* in the organs except for the lungs [43], indicating that NK cells play a limited and early role in the host defense to *C. neoformans* in the lung. In the early phase of infection, before activation of specific cell-mediated immunity, macrophages and PMN also play a role in host defense to *C. neoformans*. Following inhalation of the organism, pulmonary alveolar macrophages provide the first line of defense, rapidly followed by recruitment of PMN, which clear the organism from the inflammatory infiltrate [44].

Biological response modifiers

Many investigators have attempted to enhance the nonspecific resistance to infection by injection of microorganisms such as *Mycobacterium bovis* BCG [27, 45, 46], *Listeria monocytogenes* [47], *Salmonella typhimurium* [48], or *Candida albicans* [49–51]. A similar immunomodulatory effect is obtained by administration of a number of agents derived from microorganisms, such as bacterial endotoxin (lipopolysaccharide, LPS) [52] or muramyl dipeptides [53–55].

The mechanisms whereby these agents accomplish their protective effect vary. Injection of BCG, *L. monocytogenes*, or *S. typhimurium* into mice leads to activation of macrophages, which then become able to inhibit the proliferation of various intracellular microorganisms [47, 48, 56]. It has been demonstrated that *Listeria*-activated peritoneal macrophages are able to kill *C. albicans*, whereas resident macrophages do not kill *Candida* [57]. Moreover, these activated macrophages were able to inhibit the outgrowth of extracellular *C. albicans* hyphae almost completely via an oxygen-independent mechanism [57, 58]. Although not all investigators have found an effect of BCG on disseminated candidiasis [59], it has been reported that pretreatment of mice with BCG led to an increased survival after a lethal *C. albicans* challenge in granulocytopenic mice [46]. Moreover, BCG pretreatment reduces the outgrowth of *C. albicans* in the kidney, spleen and liver of *Candida*-infected mice [27, 60]. Macrophages of BCG-treated mice were better able to kill *C. albicans in vivo*, and inhibited the intracellular formation of germ tubes [27]. Whether or not activated macrophages are totally responsible for the beneficial effects observed *in vivo* is not clear, and it cannot be excluded that the *in vivo* effect of BCG on disseminated candidiasis is partly mediated by PMN or by still other mechanisms.

For a number of other agents that have been shown to enhance host resistance *in vivo*, such as LPS or muramyl dipeptide, the mechanism of action is even less well known. Several microorganisms and microbial products known to enhance host defense mechanisms, such as bacterial endotoxin, BCG, and muramyl peptides, stimulate the synthesis of interleukin-1 (IL-1), tumor necrosis factor-α (TNF-α), and interleukin-6 (IL-6) [55]. The immunomodulatory effects of such agents are at least partly mediated by the induction of these cytokines [61–63]. One of the biological response modifiers studied extensively is muramyl dipeptide (MDP).

Muramyl dipeptides

Synthetic MDP was originally identified as the minimal functional component of Freund's adjuvant [64]. In view of the effects on host defense of *Mycobacterium bovis* BCG, the main constituent of complete Freund's adjuvant, MDP and its structural variants have aroused interest as potential immunomodulatory agents [53, 65]. Several authors have shown that pretreatment with MDP enhances survival of mice with a lethal *C. albicans* infection [66, 67]. It has been suggested that the effect of MDP on host defense is mediated via activation of oxidative killing mechanisms of macrophages [66–68]. It has been shown that MDP induces production of IL-1 [69], IL-6 [70], TNF-α, M-CSF and GM-CSF [71]. Endotoxin, another bacterial cell wall product shown to enhance host defense against infections in several models [52, 72], is also a potent inducer of cytokines such as IL-1 [73], suggesting that the beneficial effect of MDP or endotoxin on the course of infections is due to induction of IL-1 and other cytokines.

Interleukin-1

The two proteins IL-1α and IL-1β possess a wide spectrum of inflammatory, metabolic, physiologic, hematopoietic, and immunomodulatory properties [63, 74, 75]. IL-1 was originally described in the 1940's as an endogenous pyrogen, a protein that produced fever in rabbits [76–78]. IL-1 is produced by blood monocytes, macrophages, granulocytes, vascular endothelial cells, and a variety of other cells [79, 80]. With the exception of skin keratinocytes and some epithelial cells, there is no evidence of mRNA coding for IL-1 in healthy subjects [73]. In contrast, there is a dramatic increase in IL-1 production in response to infection, microbial toxins, inflammatory agents, complement, and clotting factors.

Administration of IL-1 has been shown to influence beneficially the course of infection due to a large number of bacterial pathogens [81]. Pretreatment of mice with a single low dose of recombinant IL-1α or β induces protection against a lethal acute disseminated candidiasis [82]. Subsequent studies have demonstrated that treatment with IL-1α significantly decreases the number of *C. albicans* in the kidneys and spleens during disseminated candidiasis [22, 83]. This effect of IL-1 on disseminated candidiasis was not only present in normal mice, but also in mice under various forms of immunosuppression, such as treatment with cyclophosphamide, hydrocortisone acetate, or total body irradiation [22].

The mechanism responsible for the beneficial effect of IL-1 on disseminated candidiasis in these animals is not known. It has been suggested that IL-1 augments host defense through enhancement of the production of granulocytes, their release from the bone marrow, and subsequently their migration to the site of infection [84–86]. Indeed, neutrophilia is a prominent feature of IL-1 administration, both through direct effects and via induction of colony-stimulating factors [87–89]. In cyclophosphamide-treated mice, IL-1 accelerates recovery of the bone marrow [90]. However, in neutropenic infection models the protective effect of IL-1 was evident before neutrophil recovery [22, 82], and even during complete agranulocytosis after total body irradiation the outgrowth of *C. albicans* was reduced by IL-1. Histologic examination of the organs of mice infected with *C. albicans* did not show any differences in the numbers of granulocytes at the foci of infection between IL-1 treated mice and controls [22]. Moreover, IL-1 did not increase the number of granulocytes in the peripheral blood or at the site of infection in mice with a *C. albicans* peritonitis [91]. Taken together, these studies led to the conclusion that the favorable effect of IL-1 on the course of a systemic *C. albicans* infection is not mediated via PMN.

Although it has been suggested that IL-1 is able to activate macrophages *in vitro* for killing of *C. albicans* [92, 93], we have not been able to demonstrate an effect of IL-1 on the production of O_2^- [94], H_2O_2, NO_2^- [95] or on the toxoplasmastatic activity of peritoneal macrophages [95]. Furthermore, we have been unable to show enhanced intracellular killing of *C. albicans* by peritoneal macrophages of mice treated with IL-1 *in vivo* or by macrophages incubated with IL-1 *in vitro* (unpublished data). Another possibility is that IL-1 exerts its beneficial effect through downregulation of the receptors for IL-1 and TNF-α [96] or induction of IL-1 receptor antagonist, a physiological inhibitor of IL-1. Thus, pretreatment with IL-1 would prevent the subsequent lethal cascade of cytokines such as TNF-α, IL-1β, IL-6 in the circulation [97]. Indeed, it has been confirmed that administration of IL-1 downregulates the expression of mRNA for the IL-1 receptor type I in mice (MTE Vogels *et al.*, submitted). Although this mechanism might explain the IL-1-induced prolongation of survival of mice with lethal acute disseminated candidiasis, it is not clear how this hypothesis would explain the effect of IL-1 on the outgrowth of *C. albicans* in the target organs.

One of the phenomena that deserve further investigation is the effect of IL-1 on other cell types, such as endothelial cells. IL-1 has been shown to stimulate expression of adherence molecules on endothelial cells [98] and the permeability of endothelium [99]. In this way, IL-1 may indirectly activate PMN to exhibit enhanced antifungal activity by yet unspecified interactions between endothelial cells and PMN, as has recently been demonstrated for killing of *C. neoformans* [100]. Another possibility is that the effect of IL-1 on endothelial cells promotes the migration of humoral factors that contribute to the host resistance to the focus of infection. This hypothesis could explain why the effect of IL-1 on the numbers of *C. albicans* is already seen on the first day of infection, whereas the growth rate of the *Candida* does not differ much in IL-1-treated and control animals in later stages of the infection [22].

Tumor necrosis factor-α

The activity of a tumor necrosis factor in patients with a concurrent infection has already been described in 1890 [101] and has subsequently been demonstrated in mice challenged with endotoxin or the combination of BCG and endotoxin (reviewed in [102]). Two TNF's have now been described: TNF-α, a soluble 17-kDa protein secreted predominantly by macrophages upon stimulation with endotoxin, BCG, or IL-2, and TNF-β, also called lymphotoxin, a 25-kDa product of activated T-cells [102]. TNF-α is an important proinflammatory cytokine, acts as endogenous pyrogen, and induces production of IL-1 [103]. The massive production of TNF-α and release into the circulation during severe sepsis are responsible for shock, acidosis, neutrophil accumulation in the lungs, and death [104–107]. In contrast, small amounts of TNF-α appear to be essential for host resistance against infections. TNF-α causes neutrophilia [89], and increases neutrophil migration [108], adherence [109], degranulation, and respiratory burst [108, 110]. Activation of murine macrophages with IFN-γ leads to production of TNF-α [95, 111], which then serves as an intermediate for the intracellular killing of intracellular parasites [95, 112, 113]. Pretreatment with a low dose of recombinant TNF-α protects animals from lethal endotoxinemia or sepsis [114–116].

Until now, data on the role of TNF-α in experimental fungal infections have been scarce. Treatment of mice with monoclonal antibodies against TNF-α enhances the mortality to experimental systemic cryptococcosis and leads to increased numbers of yeasts in the brain and meninges as compared to control mice [117]. TNF-α has been demonstrated to enhance the complement-dependent phagocytosis of *C. neoformans* by murine macrophages *in vitro* [117], and neutralization of TNF-α *in vivo* may also impair other host defense mechanisms to cryptococcosis, such as the formation of reactive nitrogen intermediates [118, 119].

Injection of monoclonal antibodies against TNF-α also leads to an increased outgrowth of *C. albicans* during disseminated candidiasis in normal mice but not granulocytopenic mice [120]. These findings are in line with our own observation that an i.v. injection of a single dose of polyclonal rabbit anti-mouse-TNF-α simultaneously with the i.v. injection of 1×10^5 CFU *C. albicans* led to a significantly increased outgrowth of *C. albicans* in the kidneys and spleens of mice at day 1 and day 3 infection (unpublished data). Pretreatment of mice with pentoxifylline, an inhibitor of TNF-α production, led to lower levels of circulating TNF-α in neutropenic mice with disseminated candidiasis but did not influence survival of these mice [121]. The numbers of *C. albicans* in the organs of pentoxifylline-treated mice tended to be higher in this model, although the differences were not significant. Since TNF-α production was only partially suppressed in these experiments, these observations cannot be considered conclusive.

In vitro, incubation of human peripheral blood monocytes with TNF-α inhibits the intracellular outgrowth of *Coccidioides immitis* [122]. Incubation of human PMN with recombinant TNF-α increased the intracellular killing of *C. albicans* [28, 123] and *C. glabrata* [123]. TNF-α caused an increased release of both O_2^- and lysosomal enzymes from PMN [123]. These data, as well as our observation that recombinant TNF-α did not affect the capacity of murine peritoneal macrophages to kill intracellular *C. albicans in vitro* (unpublished data), suggest that the role of TNF-α in the host defense against candidiasis is mediated by granulocytes. This is in line with the observation that blocking TNF-α *in vivo* deteriorates disseminated candidiasis in normal mice but not in granulocytopenic mice [120].

In contrast, Diamond *et al.* have found that incubation of human PMN with TNF-α markedly impaired the capacity of PMN to kill *C. albicans* hyphae extracellularly, whereas rIFN-γ caused increased fungicidal activity [124]. In view of the still limited data and the different methods used *in vitro* by the various investigators [28, 123, 124], it is too early to speculate on a correlation of these divergent findings *in vitro* with *C. albicans* infections *in vivo*, e. g. to question whether the presence of blastospores versus hyphae or the timing and concentration of TNF-α determine the beneficial or detrimental effects of TNF-α *in vivo*. Nevertheless, the administration of monoclonal antibodies to TNF-α, as has recently been reported in patients with sepsis syndrome [125], should not be applied to patients with proven or suspected disseminated candidiasis.

Interferon-γ

IFN-γ is a product of activated T-lymphocytes and natural killer (NK) cells that exhibits pleiotropic biological activities, and there is abundant evidence that IFN-γ is the main lymphokine involved in macrophage activation [126, 127]. On granulocytes, a wide variety of effects of IFN-γ has been demonstrated, including migration and adherence [128], phagocytosis [129], and oxidative killing [124, 130]. Although most of the effects of IFN-γ on the inflammatory response are beneficial for the host, disparate effects have also been described. For instance, IFN-γ appears to be the pivotal mediator of the LPS-induced Schwartzman reaction and lethality [131, 132].

Administration to mice of antibodies to IFN-γ caused an inhibition of clearance of *L. monocytogenes* and a higher mortality rate [127]. Likewise, administration of recombinant IFN-γ beneficially influences the course of an experimental infection with a wide variety of intracellular pathogens [133–136]. The mechanism by which IFN-γ increases host resistance in these models has not been completely elucidated, and its mode of action may not be the same in all infections studied. In a number of models, activation of macrophages by IFN-γ has been shown to be responsible for the observed effects [137]. For other microorganisms such as *Mycobacterium fortuitum*, activation of PMN is the pathway through which IFN-γ augments host resistance [138].

IFN-γ is now widely used for patients with chronic granulomatous disease (CGD), an uncommon hereditary disorder characterized by the inability of phagocytic cells to mount a respiratory burst [139]. Treatment of CGD patients with subcutaneous IFN-γ decreased the incidence of infections by 67% [140], although the exact mechanism by which IFN-γ restores host defense mechanisms in these patients has not been fully elucidated [141, 142]. In a study performed in parallel with the multicenter randomized double-blind study of CGD patients [140], PMN obtained from patients of the IFN-γ-treated group showed an increased capacity to damage *Aspergillus* hyphae *in vitro* compared to PMN from placebo-treated subjects [143]. Moreover, in a related observation of patients with CGD followed at the NIH between 1988 and 1990, 9 of 37 patients (24%) who did not receive IFN-γ developed fungal infections, whereas only one fungal infection was noted among 23 patients (4%) receiving IFN-γ [144]. The capacity of murine IFN-γ to activate macrophages *in vitro* to display enhanced fungicidal activity has been described for various other organisms, such as *Blastomyces dermatitidis* [23, 24, 145], *Coccidioides immitis* [122, 146, 147], *Paracoccidioides brasiliensis* [148], *Histoplasma capsulatum* [149, 150], and *Cryptococcus neoformans* [151, 152].

Several authors have studied the effects of IFN-γ on *C. albicans* infection using *in vitro* models, but the results are somewhat divergent. The reports that human alveolar macrophages and peripheral blood monocytes can be activated by IFN-γ [93] or IFN-γ plus LPS [153] to enhanced candidastatic activity are difficult to interpret because no controls have been included to distinguish real intracellular killing of microorganisms from subtle variations in the rate of outgrowth. Brummer and coworkers have reported that overnight incubation of murine peritoneal macrophages with IFN-γ *in vitro* enabled these cells to kill 40% of the phagocytized *C. albicans* in 2 hours [24, 154, 155], whereas unactivated macrophages do not kill *C. albicans*. In contrast, murine alveolar macrophages could not be activated to exhibit candidacidal mechanisms by IFN-γ [23]. It has been suggested that the candidacidal mechanism of IFN-γ-incubated macrophages is oxygen-independent, since the inhibitory effect on *Candida* had already disappeared before IFN-γ-induced oxygen metabolites had been formed [58]. IFN-γ-activated macrophages contain phagolysosomes with a low pH (< 4.0), and increasing the lysosomal pH reduces candidacidal activity, suggesting that acidification of the phagolysosomes is an essential step in the killing of phagocytized *C. albicans* [58]. In contrast, we have not been able to confirm reports on activation of murine peritoneal macrophages *in vitro* by rIFN-γ or crude lymphokines to kill *C. albicans* under comparable conditions (unpublished data).

The ability of IFN-γ to activate PMN to enhanced killing of *C. albicans* has been studied mainly with human peripheral blood PMN [156]. Djeu *et al.* [28] have reported that incubation with human rIFN-γ for 2 hours was sufficient to augment the capacity of PMN to kill *C. albicans*, and synergy was observed during incubation with the combination of IFN-γ and TNF-α for 2 hours in amounts that were too low to activate PMN alone. However, these results are difficult to compare with other data because the uptake of [^{3}H]glucose was used as an indirect measure of growth inhibition, and the outcome was assessed after 24 h of incubation of PMN with *C. albicans* instead of the 2 or 4 hours usually studied [28]. It may be asked whether these results are in part attributable to extracellular killing of *C. albicans* hyphae, a process which is also slightly but significantly enhanced by IFN-γ *in vitro* [124]. Using a microbiological assay, we found that human peripheral blood PMN killed 41% of phagocytized *C. albicans* in 4 hours, whereas overnight incubation with 50 U/ml of human rIFN-γ increased killing to 65% ($P < 0.001$; unpublished data). Although earlier reports indicate that multiple intramuscular injections of rIFN-γ worsen the course of experimental candidiasis in mice [157, 158], we have shown that administration of a single intravenous dose of rIFN-γ reduces the outgrowth of *C. albicans* in the kidneys, liver and spleen of mice with an experimental *C. albicans* infection [159]. In mice with impaired host defense due to hydrocortisone pretreatment, rIFN-γ reduced the outgrowth of *C. albicans* in the organs only when a small number of *C. albicans* was injected. The beneficial effect of rIFN-γ on the outgrowth of *C. albicans* in the various organs could be abolished by pretreatment of mice with cyclophosphamide [159]. Since the main effect of cyclophosphamide is to reduce the number of peripheral blood PMN, these data suggest that the observed effect of rIFN-γ on disseminated candidiasis is mediated by activation of PMN. This is also supported by the observation of enhanced killing of *C. albicans* by peritoneal and peripheral blood PMN from rIFN-γ-treated mice [159]. The observation that treatment with rIFN-γ is effective even when given as late as 3 days after the onset of infection warrants further investigation of rIFN-γ as a therapeutic agent for disseminated candidiasis.

Colony-stimulating factors

The colony-stimulating factors (CSFs) are a family of polypeptides that regulate proliferation and maturation of hematopoietic precursor cells and affect the function of mature progeny [160]. Four major types of hematopoietic growth factors have been described: granulocyte (G)-CSF, monocyte (M)-CSF, granulocyte-monocyte (GM)-CSF, and multi-CSF (interleukin-3) [110, 160, 161]. The production and activities of CSFs are regulated by a variety of factors, such as IL-1, IL-6 and TNF-α. For instance, IL-1 induces the production of CSFs and acts synergistically with IL-3 and CSFs on hematopoiesis [162–164]. Apart from their effects on the proliferation and differentiation of neutrophil, monocyte and eosinophil lineages in the bone marrow, a wide range of effects of CSFs on mature cells has been described both *in vitro* and during *in vivo* administration and may contribute to the host defense against infections. Administration of CSFs during neutropenia leads to faster recovery of PMN numbers and thereby protects against infections in experimental models [165–168]. Likewise, shortening the duration of neutropenia in patients receiving cytotoxic chemotherapy should decrease the frequency of invasive fungal infections. However, randomized trials of hematopoietic growth factors have not shown a clear beneficial effect on the incidence of infections [169, 170].

Various animal studies suggest a beneficial effect of G-CSF on experimental infection with *C. albicans* [171], *A. fumigatus* [39, 171] or *C. neoformans* [171]. However, the design of these experiments may imply that CSF-treated mice had already recovered from neutropenia before or early during the fungal infection, whereas control mice were still neutropenic [171]. Thus, although of importance from a clinical point of view, these reports merely reconfirm the increased sensitivity to fungal infections in neutropenic animals as compared to animals with higher numbers of neutrophils. In contrast, it is more difficult to investigate *in vivo* whether CSFs enhance cell function independently of their effect on cell numbers.

Most evidence on the role of CSFs in the regulation of host defense has therefore been obtained from *in vitro* studies. Incubation of human PMN with GM-CSF *in vitro* increases the chemotaxis to bacterial chemoattractants, reduces random migration, and enhances the expression of cellular adhesion molecules, cytotoxicity and production of O_2^- [110, 172–174]. Human PMN exhibit enhanced phagocytosis of *S. aureus* after exposure to GM-CSF *in vitro* [175] or *in vivo* [172], but the intracellular killing of staphylococci was unaffected. Incubation of human PMN for 2 hours with rGM-CSF led to enhanced intracellular killing of *C. albicans* [176, 177]. In contrast, incubation of human PMN with rG-CSF *in vitro* enhances both the phagocytosis and killing of *S. aureus* but not *C. albicans* [178], although rG-CSF does enhance the oxidative burst of PMN in response to both blastoconidia and pseudohyphae of *C. albicans* [179] and to hyphae of *A. fumigatus* [37].

Additional evidence for the capacity of CSFs to modulate host defense has been obtained from studies with mononuclear phagocytes. Human PBMC produce increased amounts of IL-1, TNF-α and O_2^- and other ROI after incubation with rhGM-CSF [174, 180, 181] but not rhG-CSF [181], and these GM-CSF-activated cells inhibit the outgrowth of *Cryptococcus neoformans* [182]. Incubation of monocytes or macrophages with purified or recombinant GM-CSF inhibits the intracellular replication of *Trypanosoma cruzi* [183] and *Mycobacterium avium* [184]. Overnight incubation with purified murine M-CSF inhibits the outgrowth of *C. albicans* in murine peritoneal exudate macrophages [185, 186] but not in resident peritoneal macrophages [186].

Incubation with M-CSF did not prime these cells to exhibit augmented O_2^- production upon stimulation with PMA or either live or heat-killed yeasts, suggesting that the effect on *C. albicans* was oxygen-independent [186]. From animal experiments, it has been reported that repeated i. p. injections of 5×10^5 U of purified M-CSF before a lethal *C. albicans* challenge improved the survival time and reduced the outgrowth of *C. albicans* in the kidneys of mice with disseminated candidiasis [185], but others found that administration of rhM-CSF either before infection or commencing at the moment of infection aggravated the course of experimental candidemia in mice [187]. It is not clear whether the differences between these studies are due to the mouse strains used, the source of M-CSF, or the *C. albicans* strains used. Nevertheless, the beneficial effect of M-CSF has recently been validated *in vivo*, since infusion of a single dose of rhM-CSF into humans led to an enhanced respiratory burst in peripheral blood monocytes and increased phagocytosis of *Candida guillermondii* [188]. Randomized trials of rhM-CSF for hematologic patients with invasive fungal infections are now being performed [189]. Administration of GM-CSF as adjunctive therapy in patients with documented fungal infections has only been reported from uncontrolled series [190], that do not permit evaluation of the potential antifungal properties of CSFs as compared to optimal antifungal therapy alone.

Interleukin-2

IL-2, a 15. 5-kDa protein produced by activated T_{H1}-type lymphocytes, has profound effects on the immune response. The main functions of IL-2 are triggering proliferation of antigen-activated T-cells and enhancing NK-cell function, but *in vivo* experiments have indicated that IL-2 may also play a role in the non-specific host defense against infections. Administration of recombinant IL-2 enhances the survival of mice in infection models with various microorganisms [191–195]. Whereas these data indicate that IL-2 cooperates with other cytokines in the activation of macrophages or other mechanisms of host defense, administration of IL-2 to patients with cancer or AIDS has brought about an increased incidence of septicemia [196, 197], probably due to an IL-2-induced impairment of the chemotaxis of peripheral blood neutrophils [198].

Incubation of PBMC with recombinant IL-2 activates these cells to inhibit and probably kill *C. neoformans* [182]. Recent data show that two distinct IL-2-activated lymphocyte populations are responsible for this anticryptococcal effect [199]. Not only NK-cells but also T-cells are able to surround and bind to *C. neoformans in vitro*, subsequently inhibiting fungal growth. These data suggest that IL-2-activated T-cells not only mediate antifungal activity by releasing cytokines that activate macrophages or by lysis of infected cells, but also directly attack *C. neoformans* [199].

Divergent effects of IL-2 have been found in models of *C. albicans* infection. Murine spleen lymphocytes cultured in the presence of IL-2 for several days were recently shown to inhibit the outgrowth of *C. albicans* hyphae *in vitro* in the absence of macrophages [200]. Others have failed to demonstrate NK-cell-mediated activity against *C. albicans*, when either freshly isolated lymphocytes or lymphocytes activated for short periods of time with IL-2 were used [176, 201]. In contrast, Wei *et al.* [202] have shown that rhIL-2-induced lymphokine-activated killer (LAK) cells have the capacity to lyse monocytes and may impair the functional activity of monocytes against intracellular pathogens. Co-culture of IL-2-induced LAK cells with human monocytes that had phagocytized *C. albicans* led to increased outgrowth of intracellular *C. albicans* [202]. These IL-2/LAK-treated monocytes were unable to present candidal antigen to T-cells after incubation with intact *C. albicans* or soluble candidal cell wall mannoprotein and were unable to produce IL-1 [203]. These results indicate that IL-2 may suppress the host defense against *C. albicans* infection at the level of antigen presentation or activation of phagocytic cells. Interestingly, when monocytes were incubated with IFN-γ their antigen presenting function remained intact despite subsequent exposure to LAK cells [203]. *In vivo*, lymphokine-activated lymphocytes can be isolated from mice after injection of *C. albicans* [204], suggesting that these phenomena, whether beneficial or adverse, may indeed occur *in vivo* as part of the host defense against candidal infections.

Interleukin-3

IL-3, also called multi-colony-stimulating factor, is distinct among the hematopoietic colony-stimulating factors in that it stimulates the clonal proliferation of bone marrow pluripotent stem cells, leading to the production of all major blood cell types [161]. In addition to its effect on early progenitor cells, studies have shown that IL-3 exhibits biological activities on more mature cells: it prolongs the survival and enhances the functional activity of eosinophils and has a number of effects on mononuclear phagocytes: IL-3 stimulates the proliferation of peripheral blood monocytes and tissue macrophages [205, 206], enhances the expression of surface receptors, and stimulates the oxidative killing mechanisms of macrophages [207]. In addition, IL-3 induces production of IL-1, IL-6 and TNF-α [208] by macrophages, which may represent an amplification loop in the case of infection, since IL-1 in turn induces production of IL-3 [73].

Several investigators have studied the effect of IL-3 on the phagocytosis and killing of *C. albicans*. Incubation of human peripheral blood monocytes with human rIL-3 for 18 hours led to inhibition of the intracellular outgrowth of *C. albicans* [29]. Incubation of murine resident peritoneal macrophages with purified murine IL-3 *in vitro* for 15 minutes was sufficient to enhance the phagocytosis of opsonized *C. albicans* or *C. pseudotropicalis* [207]. In the same study, IL-3 enhanced the overall killing of *C. pseudotropicalis*, whereas *C. albicans* was not killed by these macrophages, whether stimulated with IL-3 or not. Since superoxide dismutase, a scavenger of superoxide anion (O_2^-), antagonizes the effect of IL-3 on the killing of *C. pseudotropicalis*, it has been suggested that IL-3 activates macrophages to express oxidative microbicidal mechanisms. The fact that IL-3 was unable to induce killing of *C. albicans* by peritoneal macrophages lends support to the observations that the killing of *C. albicans* appears to require both oxygen-dependent and oxygen-independent mechanisms, whereas *C. parapsilosis* and *C. pseudotropicalis* can be killed after stimulation of oxidative mechanisms only [25, 30, 209].

Interleukin-8

IL-8 is a polypeptide of approximately 8 kDa, originally known as neutrophil-activating factor (NAF) or monocyte-derived neutrophil chemotactic factor (MDN-CF) [210]. The effects of IL-8 on PMN include chemotaxis as well as activation, leading to the expression of surface adhesion molecules, respiratory burst, and degranulation [211, 212]. IL-1, TNF-α and LPS are able to induce production of IL-8 in monocytes, macrophages, endothelial cells and other cells [210, 213]. Thus, IL-1 and TNF-α contribute in various ways to the inflammatory event, both via direct effects and via IL-8 which is chemotactic and activates PMN.

Vogels *et al.* have recently shown that injection of recombinant human IL-8 (rhIL-8) provided some protection against a lethal infection with *K. pneumoniae* in normal but not in granulocytopenic mice [214]. The balance between the beneficial and detrimental effects of IL-8 appears to be very delicate, since in some experiments the survival was negatively affected by injection of rhIL-8 [214, 215]. Indeed, high levels of circulating IL-8 have recently been found in patients with sepsis, and IL-8 levels correlated with the presence of shock and mortality [216].

Djeu *et al.* [217] have shown that rhIL-8 is able to activate human peripheral blood PMN, but not monocytes, to kill *C. albicans* more efficiently *in vitro*. Incubation of PMN with rhIL-8 for 30 minutes did not lead to enhanced O_2^- production [217], but others have reported that rhIL-8 enhanced the respiratory burst in human PMN [212, 218]. Although, to our knowledge, it is not known whether inhibitors of the respiratory burst affect the IL-8-induced killing of *C. albicans*, it has been suggested that non-oxidative mechanisms, i. e. lysosomal enzymes, are involved in the IL-8-induced candidacidal activity [217, 219]. Limited data suggest that recombinant IL-8 also enables PMN to inhibit the outgrowth of *C. neoformans* [100]. Taken together, these observations suggest that IL-8 may play an important role in the elimination of invasive fungal infections, either after induction by IL-1 or by other mechanisms.

Conclusion

The increasing incidence of fungal infections in constitutes an important problem in the immunocompromized host. Optimal antifungal therapy, even with the recently developed new classes of agents, often fails to cure the infection, especially in patients with persistently insufficient host defense mechanisms. It is therefore rational to focus on the modulation of host defense in addition to antifungal therapy in order to cure systemic fungal infections in these patient groups. Treatment with cytokines and growth factors is beginning to find its way to therapy of infection in humans. Trials with G-CSF and M-CSF in patients with proven fungal infections are being performed. Other agents that have shown to be effective in animal models of disseminated fungal infection, such as IL-1 and IFN-γ, deserve further study both in experimental models and in selected patient groups.

References

1. Bodey GP. Candidiasis in cancer patients. Am J Med 1984; 77: 13–19.
2. Meunier-Carpentier F, Kiehn TE, Armstrong D. Fungemia in the immunocompromised host. Changing patterns, antigenemia, high mortality. Am J Med 1981; 71: 363–370.
3. Pizzo PA, Robichaud KJ, Gill FA, Witebski FG. Empiric antibiotic and antifungal therapy for cancer patients with prolonged fever and granulocytopenia. Am J Med 1982; 72: 101–111.
4. Odds FC. *Candida* and candidosis (2nd ed.). London: Ballière Tindall, 1988.
5. Bodey G, Bueltmann B, Duguid W, *et al.* Fungal infections in cancer patients: an international autopsy survey. Eur J Clin Microbiol Infect Dis 1992; 11: 99–109.
6. Beck-Sagué CM, Jarvis WR. Secular trends in the epidemiology of nosocomial fungal infections in the United States, 1980–1990. J Infect Dis 1993; 167: 1247 - 1251.
7. Edwards JE. Invasive *Candida* infections - evolution of a fungal pathogen. N Engl J Med 1991; 324: 1060–1062.
8. Pfaller MA. Infection control: opportunistic fungal infections – the increasing importance of *Candida* species. Infect Control Hosp Epidemiol 1989; 10: 270–273.
9. Van 't Wout JW, Van der Woude FJ. Fungal infections in solid organ transplant recipients. In: Powderly WB, Van 't Wout JW, ed. Fluconazole. Carnforth (UK): Marius Press, 1992; 82–91.
10. Denning DW, Stevens DA. Antifungal and surgical treatment of invasive aspergillosis: review of 2121 published cases. Rev Infect Dis 1990; 12: 1147–1201.
11. Cohen MS, Isturiz RE, Malech HL, *et al.* Fungal infection in chronic granulomatous disease. The importance of the phagocyte in defense against fungi. Am J Med 1981; 71: 59–66.
12. Denning DW, Follansbee SE, Scolaro M, Norris S, Edelstein H, Stevens DA. Pulmonary aspergillosis in the acquired immunodeficiency syndrome. N Engl J Med 1991; 324: 654–662.
13. Chuck SL, Sande MA. Infections with *Cryptococcus neoformans* in the acquired immunodeficiency syndrome. N Engl J Med 1989; 321: 794–800.
14. Lazzarin A, Umberti Foppa C, Galli M, *et al.* Impairment of polymorphonuclear leucocyte function in patients with acquired immunodeficiency syndrome and with lymphadenopathy syndrome. Clin Exp Imunol 1986; 65: 105–111.
15. Umberti Foppa C, Franzetti F, Negri C, *et al.* Role of PMN's candidacidal activity in the pathogenesis of AIDS-related systemic candidiasis. Boll Ist Sieroter Milan 1987; 66: 471–478.
16. Gutiérrez J, Maroto M, Piédrola G. Granulocyte abnormalities in parenteral drug addicts. The influence of HIV-infection. Allergol Immunopathol 1989; 17: 251–255.
17. Pos O, Stevenhagen A, Meenhorst PL, Kroon FP, Van Furth R. Impaired phagocytosis of *Staphylococcus aureus* by granulocytes and monocytes of AIDS patients. Clin Exp Immunol 1992; 88: 23–28.
18. Brummer E, McEwen JG, Stevens DA. Fungicidal activity of murine inflammatory polymorphonuclear neutrophils: comparison with murine peripheral blood PMN. Clin Exp Immunol 1986; 66: 681–690.
19. Leijh PCJ, Van den Barselaar MT, Van Furth R. Kinetics of phagocytosis and intracellular killing of *Candida albicans* by human granulocytes and monocytes. Infect Immun 1977; 17: 313–318.
20. Moser SA, Domer JE. Effects of cyclophosphamide on murine candidiasis. Infect Immun 1980; 27: 376–386.
21. Van 't Wout JW, Linde I, Leijh PCJ, Van Furth R. Contribution of granulocytes and monocytes to resistance against experimental disseminated *Candida albicans* infections. Eur J Clin Microbiol Infect Dis 1988; 7: 736–741.
22. Kullberg BJ, Van 't Wout JW, Van Furth R. Role of granulocytes in enhanced host resistance to *Candida albicans* induced by recombinant interleukin-1. Infect Immun 1990; 58: 3319–3324.
23. Brummer E, Stevens DA. Activation of pulmonary macrophages for fungicidal activity by gamma-interferon or lymphokines. Clin Exp Immunol 1987; 70: 520–528.
24. Brummer E, Morrison CJ, Stevens DA. Recombinant and natural gamma-interferon activation of macrophages *in vitro*: different dosage requirements for induction of killing activity against phagocytizable and nonphagocytizable fungi. Infect Immun 1985; 49: 724–730.
25. Sasada M, Johnston RB Jr. Macrophage microbicidal activity. Correlation between phagocytosis-associated oxidative metabolism and the killing of *Candida* by macrophages. J Exp Med 1980; 152: 85–98.
26. Sasada M, Kubo A, Nishimura T, *et al.* Candidacidal activity of monocyte-derived human macrophages: relationship between *Candida* killing and oxygen radical generation by human macrophages. J Leukocyte Biol 1987; 41: 289–294.
27. Van 't Wout JW, Poell R, Van Furth R. The role of BCG-PPD-activated macrophages in resistance against systemic candidiasis in mice. Scand J Immunol 1992; 36: 713–719.
28. Djeu JY, Blanchard DK, Halkias D, Friedman H. Growth inhibition of *Candida albicans* by human polymorphonuclear neutrophils: activation by interferon-γ and tumor necrosis factor. J Immunol 1986; 137: 2980–2984.
29. Wang M, Friedman H, Djeu JY. Enhancement of human monocyte function against *Candida albicans* by the colony-stimulating factors (CSF): IL-3, granulocyte-macrophage CSF, and macrophage CSF. J Immunol 1989; 143: 671–677.
30. Lehrer RI. The fungicidal mechanisms of human monocytes. I. Evidence for myeloperoxidase-linked and myeloperoxidase-independent candidacidal mechanisms. J Clin Invest 1975; 55: 338–346.

31. Lehrer RI, Szklarek D, Ganz T, Selsted ME. Modulation of the *in vitro* candidacidal activity of human neutrophil defensins by target cell metabolism and divalent cations. J Clin Invest 1988; 81: 1829–1835.
32. Diamond RD. Immune response to fungal infection. Rev Infect Dis 1989; 11: S1600–S1604.
33. Diamond RD, Krzesicki R, Jao W. Damage to pseudohyphal forms of *Candida albicans* by neutrophils in the absence of serum *in vitro*. J Clin Invest 1978; 61: 349–359.
34. McNamara MP, Wiessner JH, Collins-Lech C, Hahn BL, Sohnle PG. Neutrophil death as a defence mechanism against *Candida albicans* infections. Lancet 1988; 2: 1163–1165.
35. Sohnle PG, Collins-Lech C. Comparison of candidacidal and candidastatic activities of human neutrophils. Infect Immun 1990; 58: 2696–2698.
36. Schaffner A, Douglas H, Braude A. Selective protection against conidia by mononuclear and against mycelia by polymorphonuclear phagocytes in resistance to *Aspergillus*. J Clin Invest 1982; 69: 617–631.
37. Roilides E, Uhlig K, Venzon D, Pizzo PA, Walsh TJ. Enhancement of oxidative response and damage caused by human neutrophils to *Aspergillus fumigatus* hyphae by granulocyte colony-stimulating factor and gamma interferon. Infect Immun 1993; 61: 1185–1193.
38. Diamond RD, Krzesicki R, Epstein B, Jao W. Damage to hyphal forms of fungi by human leukocytes *in vitro*: a possible host defense mechanism in aspergillosis and mucormycosis. Am J Pathol 1978; 91: 313–328.
39. Polak-Wyss A. Protective effect of human granulocyte colony-stimulating factor (hG-CSF) on *Cryptococcus* and *Aspergillus* infections in normal and immunosuppressed mice. Mycoses 1991; 34: 205–215.
40. Levitz SM. The ecology of *Cryptococcus neoformans* and the epidemiology of cryptococcosis. Rev Infect Dis 1991; 13: 1163–1169.
41. Huffnagle GB, Yates JL, Lipscomb MF. Immunity to a pulmonary *Cryptococcus neoformans* infection requires both $CD4^{+}$ and $CD8^{+}$ T cells. J Exp Med 1991; 173: 793–800.
42. Lipscomb MF, Alvarellos T, Toews GB, *et al.* Role of natural killer cells in resistance to *Cryptococcus neoformans* infections in mice. Am J Pathol 1987; 128: 354–361.
43. Salkowski CA, Balish E. Role of natural killer cells in resistance to systemic cryptococcosis. J Leukoc Biol 1991; 50: 151–159.
44. Weinberg PB, Becker S, Granger DL, Koren HS. Growth inhibition of *Cryptococcus neoformans* by human alveolar macrophages. Am Rev Respir Dis 1987; 136: 1242–1247.
45. Dubos RJ, Schaedler RW. Effects of cellular constituents of mycobacteria on the resistance of mice to heterologous infections. J Exp Med 1957; 106: 703–717.
46. Sher NA, Chaparas SD, Greenberg LE, Bernard S. Effects of BCG, *Corynebacterium parvum*, and methanol-extraction residu in the reduction of mortality from *Staphylococcus aureus* and *Candida albicans* infections in immunosuppressed mice. Infect Immun 1975; 12: 1325–1330.
47. Van Dissel JT, Stikkelbroeck JJM, Van den Barselaar MT, Sluiter W, Leijh PCJ, Van Furth R. Divergent changes in antimicrobial activity after immunologic activation of mouse peritoneal macrophages. J Immunol 1987; 139: 1665–1672.
48. Langermans JAM, Van der Hulst MB, Nibbering PH, Van Furth R. Activation of mouse peritoneal macrophages during infection with *Salmonella typhimurium* does not result in enhanced intracellular killing. J Immunol 1990; 144: 4340–4346.
49. Vecchiarelli A, Cenci E, Puliti M, *et al.* Protective immunity induced by low-virulence *Candida albicans*: Cytokine production in the development of the anti-infectious state. Cell Immunol 1989; 124: 334–344.
50. Bistoni F, Vecchiarelli A, Cenci E, Puccetti P, Marconi P, Cassone A. Evidence for macrophage-mediated protection against lethal *Candida albicans* infection. Infect Immun 1986; 51: 668–674.
51. Cenci E, Romani L, Vecchiarelli A, Puccetti P, Bistoni F. Role of $L3T4^{+}$ lymphocytes in protective immunity to systemic *Candida albicans* infection in mice. Infect Immun 1989; 57: 3581–3587.
52. Cluff LE. Effects of endotoxins on susceptibility to infections. J Infect Dis 1970; 122: 205–216.
53. Parant M, Riveau G, Parant F, Dinarello CA, Wolff SM, Chedid L. Effect of indomethacin on increased resistance to bacterial infection and on febrile responses induced by muramyl dipeptide. J Infect Dis 1980; 142: 708–715.
54. Phillips NC, Chedid L. Anti-infectious activity of liposomal muramyl dipeptides in immunodeficient CBA/N mice. Infect Immun 1987; 55: 1426–1430.
55. Oppenheim JJ, Togawa A, Chedid L, Mizel S. Components of mycobacteria and muramyl dipeptide with adjuvant activity induce lymphocyte activating factor. Cell Immunol 1980; 50: 71–81.
56. Mackaness GB. Resistance to intracellular infection. J Infect Dis 1971; 123: 439–445.
57. Hashimoto T. *In vitro* study of contact-mediated killing of *Candida albicans* hyphae by activated murine peritoneal macrophages in a serum-free medium. Infect Immun 1991; 59: 3555–3561.
58. Watanabe K, Kagaya K, Yamada T, Fukazawa Y. Mechanism for candidacidal activity in macrophages activated by recombinant gamma-interferon. Infect Immun 1991; 59: 521–528.
59. Rogers TJ, Balish E. The role of activated macrophages in resistance to experimental renal candidiasis. J Reticuloendothel Soc 1977; 22: 309–318.
60. Baghian A, Lee KW. Role of activated macrophaghes in resistance to systemic candidosis. J Leucocyte Biol 1988; 44: 166–171.
61. Kampschmidt RF, Pulliam LA. Stimulation of antimicrobial activity in the rat with leukocyte endogenous mediator. J Reticuloendothel Soc 1975; 17: 162–169.
62. Dinarello CA. Interleukin-1. Rev Infect Dis 1984; 6: 51–95.
63. Dinarello CA, Cannon JG, Mier JW, Bernheim HA, LoPreste G. Multiple biological activities of human recombinant interleukin-1. J Clin Invest 1986; 77: 1734–1739.
64. Ellouz F, Adam A, Ciorbaru R, Lederer E. Minimal structural requirements for adjuvant activity of bacterial peptidoglycan derivatives. Biochem Biophys Res Commun 1974; 59: 1317–1325.
65. Parant M, Chedid L. Stimulation of non-specific resistance to infections by synthetic immunoregulatory agents. Infection 1985; 13: S251–255.
66. Cummings NP, Pabst MJ, Johnston RB Jr. Activation of macrophages for enhanced release of superoxide anion and greater killing of *Candida albicans* by injection of muramyl dipeptide. J Exp Med 1980; 152: 1659–1669.
67. Fraser-Smith EB, Matthews TR. Protective effect of muramyl dipeptide analogs against infections of *Pseu-*

domonas aeruginosa or *Candida albicans* in mice. Infect Immun 1981; 34: 676–683.
68. Fraser-Smith EB, Waters RV, Matthews TR. Correlation between *in vivo* anti-*Pseudomonas* and anti-*Candida* activities and clearance of carbon by the reticuloendothelial system for various muramyl dipeptide analogs, using normal and immunosuppressed mice. Infect Immun 1982; 35: 105–110.
69. Dinarello CA, Krueger JM. Induction of interleukin-1 by synthetic and naturally occurring muramyl peptides. FASEB J 1986; 45: 2545–2548.
70. Sanceau J, Falcoff R, Beranger F, Carter DB, Wietzerbin J. Secretion of interleukin-6 (IL-6) by human monocytes stimulated by muramyl dipeptide and tumor necrosis factor alpha. Immunol 1990; 69: 52–56.
71. Broudy VC, Kaushansky K, Shoemaker SG, Aggarwal BB, Adamson JW. Muramyl dipeptide induces production of hemopoietic growth factors *in vivo* by a mechanism independent of tumor necrosis factor. J Immunol 1990; 144: 3789–3794.
72. Vogels MTE, Van der Meer JWM. Use of immune modulators in nonspecific therapy of bacterial infections. Antimicrob Agents Chemother 1992; 36: 1–5.
73. Dinarello CA. Interleukin-1 and interleukin-1 antagonism. Blood 1991; 77: 1627–1652.
74. Oppenheim JJ, Kovacs EJ, Matsushima K, Durum SK. There is more than one interleukin-1. Immunol Today 1986; 7: 45–56.
75. Dinarello CA, Cannon JG, Wolff SM. New concepts on the pathogenesis of fever. Rev Infect Dis 1988; 10: 168–189.
76. Atkins E. Pathogenesis of fever. Physiol Rev 1960; 40: 580–646.
77. Atkins E. Fever – new perspectives on an old phenomenon. N Engl J Med 1983; 308: 958–959.
78. Kaiser HK, Wood WB Jr. Sudies on the pathogenesis of fever. IX. The production of endogenous pyrogen by polymorphonuclear leukocytes. J Exp Med 1962; 115: 27–36.
79. Platanias LC, Vogelzang NJ. Interleukin-1 – biology, pathophysiology, and clinical prospects. Am J Med 1990; 89: 621–629.
80. Di Giovine FS, Duff GW. Interleukin 1: the first interleukin. Immunol Today 1990; 11: 13–20.
81. Van der Meer JWM, Vogels MTE, Kullberg BJ. Interleukin-1 and related pro-inflammatory cytokines in the treatment bacterial infections in neutropenic and non-neutropenic animals. Biotherapy 1994; 7: 161–167.
82. Van 't Wout JW, Van der Meer JWM, Barza M, Dinarello CA. Protection of neutropenic mice from lethal *Candida albicans* infection by recombinant interleukin 1. Eur J Immunol 1988; 18: 1143–1146.
83. Kullberg BJ, Van 't Wout JW, Poell RJM, Van Furth R. Combined effect of fluconazole and recombinant human interleukin-1 on systemic candidiasis in mice. Antimicrob Agents Chemother 1992; 36: 1225–1229.
84. Czuprynski CJ, Brown JF. Purified human and recombinant murine interleukin-1 induced accumulation of inflammatory peritoneal neutrophils and mononuclear phagocytes: possible contributions to antibacterial resistance. Microb Pathogen 1987; 3: 377–386.
85. Czuprynski CJ, Brown JF, Young KM, Cooley AJ, Kurtz RS. Effects of murine recombinant interleukin 1 alpha on the host response to bacterial infection. J Immunol 1988; 140: 962–968.
86. McIntyre KW, Unowsky J, DeLorenzo W, Benjamin W. Enhancement of antibacterial resistance of neutropenic bone marrow-suppressed mice by interleukin-1α. Infect Immun 1989; 57: 48–54.
87. Stork LC, Peterson VM, Rundus CH, Robinson WA. Interleukin-1 enhances murine granulopoiesis *in vivo*. Exp Hematol 1988; 16: 163–167.
88. Fibbe WE, Daha MR, Hiemstra PS, *et al.* Interleukin 1 and poly(rI). poly(rC) induce production of granulocyte CSF, macrophage CSF, and granulocyte-macrophage CSF by human endothelial cells. Exp Hematol 1989; 17: 229–234.
89. Vogel SN, Douches SD, Kaufman EN, Neta R. Induction of colony stimulating factor *in vivo* by recombinant interleukin 1 alpha and recombinant tumor necrosis factor alpha. J Immunol 1987; 138: 2143–2148.
90. Fibbe WE, Van der Meer JWM, Falkenburg JHF, Hamilton MS, Kluin PM, Dinarello CA. A single low dose of human recombinant interleukin 1 accelerates the recovery of neutrophils in mice with cyclophosphamide-induced neutropenia. Exp Hematol 1989; 17: 805–808.
91. Kullberg BJ, Van 't Wout JW, Van Furth R. No effect of recombinant human interleukin-1 on the numbers of peripheral blood and peritoneal leukocytes during an acute inflammation. Inflammation 1991; 15: 457–470.
92. Blasi E, Farinelli S, Varesio L, Bistoni F. Augmentation of GG2EE macrophage cell line-mediated anti-*Candida* activity by gamma-interferon, tumor necrosis factor, and interleukin-1. Infect Immun 1990; 58: 1073–1077.
93. Vecchiarelli A, Todisco T, Puliti M, Dottorini M, Bistoni F. Modulation of anti-*Candida* activity of human alveolar macrophages by interferon-gamma or interleukin-1-alpha. Am J Respir Cell Mol Biol 1989; 1: 49–55.
94. Van der Meer JWM, Barza M, Wolff SM, Dinarello CA. A low dose of recombinant interleukin 1 protects granulocytopenic mice from lethal Gram-negative infection. Proc Natl Acad Sci USA 1988; 85: 1620–1623.
95. Langermans JAM, Van der Hulst MEB, Nibbering PH, Hiemstra PS, Fransen L, Van Furth R. IFN-γ-induced L-arginine-dependent toxoplasmastatic activity in murine peritoneal macrophages is mediated by endogenous tumor necrosis factor-α. J Immunol 1992; 148: 568–574.
96. Holtmann H, Wallach D. Down regulation of the receptors for tumor necrosis factor by interleukin-1 and 4β-phorbol-12-myristate-13-acetate. J Immunol 1987; 139: 1161–1167.
97. Kullberg BJ, Vogels MTE, Van der Meer JWM. Immunomodulators in bacterial and fungal infections. A review of their therapeutic potential. Clin Immunother 1994; 1: 43–55.
98. Beekhuizen H, Corsel-van Tilburg AJ, Blokland I, Van Furth R. Characterization of the adherence of human monocytes to cytokine-stimulated human macrovascular endothelial cells. Immunology 1991; 74: 661–669.
99. Pettipher R, Henderson B. Inflammatory activities of locally or systemically administered interleukin-1. In: Bomford R, Henderson B, ed. Interleukin-1, inflammation and disease. Amsterdam: Elsevier, 1989;218–228.
100. Roseff SA, Levitz SM. Effect of endothelial cells on phagocyte-mediated anticryptococcal activity. Infect Immun 1993. A. 61: 3818–3824.
101. Gresser IA and Chekhov MD, Coley's toxins. N Engl J Med 1987; 317: 457.

102. Beutler B, Cerami A. Cachectin/tumor necrosis factor: an endogenous mediator of shock and inflammation. Immunol Res 1986; 5: 281–293.
103. Dinarello CA, Cannon JG, Wolff SM. Tumor necrosis factor (cachectin) is an endogenous pyrogen and induces production of interleukin-1. J Exp Med 1986; 163: 1433–1450.
104. Cerami A, Beutler B. The role of cachectin/TNF in endotoxic shock and cachexia. Immunol Today 1988; 9: 28–31.
105. Girardin E, Grau GE, Dayer JM, Roux-Lombard P, The J5 study group, Lambert PH. Tumor necrosis factor and interleukin-1 in the serum of children with severe infectious purpura. N Engl J Med 1988; 319: 397–400.
106. Tracey KJ, Beutler B, Lowry SF. Shock and tissue injury induced by recombinant human cachectin. Science 1986; 234: 470–474.
107. Waage A, Espevik T, Lamvik J. Detection of tumor necrosis factor-like cytotoxicity in serum from patients with septicaemia, but not from untreated cancer patients. Scand J Immunol 1986; 24: 739–743.
108. Figari IS, Mori NA, Palladino MA Jr. Regulation of neutrophil migration and superoxide production by recombinant tumor necrosis factors-α and -β: comparison to recombinant interferon-γ and interleukin-1α. Blood 1987; 70: 979–984.
109. Seow WK, Thong YH, Ferrante A. Macrophage-neutrophil interactions: contrasting effects of the monokines interleukin-1 and tumour necrosis factor (cachectin) on human neutrophil adherence. Immunology 1987; 62: 357–361.
110. Steinbeck MA, Roth JA. Neutrophil activation by recombinant cytokines. Rev Infect Dis 1989; 11: 549–568.
111. Nakane A, Minagawa T, Kohanawa M, *et al.* Interactions between endogenous gamma interferon and tumor necrosis factor in host resistance and primary and secondary *Listeria monocytogenes* infections. Infect Immun 1989; 57: 3331–3337.
112. Green SJ, Crawford RM, Hockmeyer JT, Meltzer MS, Nacy CA. *Leishmania major* amastigotes initiate the L-arginine dependent killing mechanism in IFN-γ-stimulated macrophages by induction of TNF-α. J Immunol 1990; 145: 4290–4297.
113. Liew FY, Li Y, Millott S. Tumor necrosis factor-α synergizes with IFN-γ in mediating killing of *Leishmania major* through the induction of nitric oxide. J Immunol 1990; 145: 4306–4310.
114. Alexander HR, Doherty GM, Block MI, *et al.* Single dose tumor necrosis factor protection against endotoxin-induced shock and tissue injury in rats. Infect Immun 1991; 59: 3889–3894.
115. Alexander HR, Sheppard BC, Jensen JC, *et al.* Treatment with recombinant human tumor necrosis factor-alpha protects rats against the lethality, hypotension, and hypothermia of Gram-negative sepsis. J Clin Invest 1991; 88: 34–39.
116. Van der Meer JWM. The effects of recombinant interleukin-1 and recombinant tumor necrosis factor on non-specific resistance to infection. Biotherapy 1988; 1: 19–25.
117. Collins HL, Bancroft GJ. Cytokine enhancement of complement-dependent phagocytosis by macrophages: synergy of tumor necrosis factor-α and granulocyte-macrophage colony-stimulating factor for phagocytosis of *Cryptococcus neoformans*. Eur J Immunol 1992; 22: 1447–1454.
118. Cameron M, Granger D, Kozumbo W, Weinberg B, Koren H, Durack D. Human alveolar macrophage mediated fungistasis occurs independently of L-arginine oxidation. Clin Res 1989; 37: 425A.
119. Granger DL, Hibbs JB Jr, Perfect JR, Durack DT. Specific amino acid (L-arginine) requirement for the microbiostatic activity of murine macrophages. J Clin Invest 1988; 81: 1129–1136.
120. Steinshamn S, Waage A. Tumor necrosis factor and interleukin-6 in *Candida albicans* infection in normal and granulocytopenic mice. Infect Immun 1992; 60: 4003–4008.
121. Netea MG, Blok WL, Francot G, Buurman WA, Van der Meer JWM. Pentoxifylline-induced decrease in circulating TNF-concentrations is not associated with improved outcome of candidal infection in mice. Eur Cytokine Netw 1992; 3: 223.
122. Beaman L. Effects of recombinant gamma interferon and tumor necrosis factor on *in vitro* interactions of human mononuclear phagocytes with *Coccidioides immitis*. Infect Immun 1991; 59: 4227–4229.
123. Ferrante A. Tumor necrosis factor alpha potentiates neutrophil antimicrobial activity: Increased fungal activity against *Torulopsis glabrata* and *Candida albicans* and associated increases in oxigen radical production and lysosomal enzyme release. Infect Immun 1989; 57: 2115–2122.
124. Diamond RD, Lyman CA, Wysong DR. Disparate effects of interferon-γ and tumor necrosis factor-α on early neutrophil respiratory burst and fungicidal responses to *Candida albicans* hyphae *in vitro*. J Clin Invest 1991; 87: 711–720.
125. Wherry J, Wenzel R, Wunderingk R, *et al.* Monoclonal antibody to human tumor necrosis factor (TNF MAb): multi-center efficacy and safety study in patients with the sepsis syndrome. Interscience Conference on Antimicrobial Agents and Chemotherapy. New Orleans, LA, 1993: Abstr. 696, p. 246.
126. Nathan CF, Murray HW, Wiebe ME, Rubin BY. Identification of interferon-γ as the lymphokine that activates human macrophage oxidative metabolism and antimicrobial activity. J Exp Med 1983; 158: 670–689.
127. Buchmeier NA, Schreiber RD. Requirement of endogenous interferon-γ production for resolution of *Listeria monocytogenes* infection. Proc Natl Acad Sci USA 1985; 82: 7404–7408.
128. Ribeiro RA, Cunha FQ, Ferreira SH. Recombinant gamma interferon causes neutrophil migration mediated by the release of a macrophage neutrophil chemotactic factor. Int J Exp Path 1990; 71: 717–725.
129. Shalaby MR, Aggarwal BB, Rinderknecht E, Svedersky LP, Finkle BS, Palladino MA Jr. Activation of human polymorphonuclear neutrophil functions by interferon-γ and tumor necrosis factors. J Immunol 1985; 135: 2069–2073.
130. Berton G, Zeni L, Cassatella MA, Rossi F. Gamma interferon is able to enhance the oxidative metabolism of human neutrophils. Biochem Biophys Res Commun 1986; 138: 1276–1282.
131. Billiau A. Gamma-interferon: the match that lights the fire? Immunol Today 1988; 9: 37–40.
132. Doherty GM, Lange JR, Langstein HN, Alexander HR, Buresh CM, Norton JA. Evidence for IFN-γ as a mediator for the lethality of endotoxin and tumor necrosis factor-α. J Immunol 1992; 149: 1666–1670.
133. Nacy CA, Fortier AH, Meltzer MS, Buchmeier NA, Schreiber RD. Macrophage activation to kill *Leishmania major*: activation of macrophages for intracellular destruction of amastigotes can be induced by both recombinant

interferon-γ and non-interferon lymphokines. J Immunol 1985; 144: 3505–3511.
134. Nauciel C, Espinasse-Maes F. Role of gamma-interferon and tumor necrosis factor alpha in resistance to *Salmonella typhimurium* infection. Infect Immun 1992; 60: 450–454.
135. Kurtz RS, Young KM, Czuprynski CJ. Separate and combined effects of recombinant interleukin-1α and gamma interferon on antibacterial resistance. Infect Immun 1989; 57: 553–558.
136. Langermans JAM, Van der Hulst MEB, Nibbering PH, Van der Meide PH, Van Furth R. Intravenous injection of IFN-γ inhibits the proliferation of *Listeria monocytogenes* in the liver but not in the spleen and peritoneal cavity. Immunol 1992; 77: 354-361.
137. Murray HW. Interferon-γ, the activated macrophage, and host defense against microbial challenge. Ann Intern Med 1988; 108: 595–608.
138. Geertsma MF, Nibbering PH, Pos O, Van Furth R. Interferon-γ-activated human granulocytes kill ingested *Mycobacterium fortuitum* more efficiently than normal granulocytes. Eur J Immun 1990; 20: 869–873.
139. Dinauer MC, Ezekowitz RAB. Interferon-γ and chronic granulomatous disease. Curr Opin Immunol 1991; 3: 61–64.
140. Gallin JI, Malech HL, Melnick DA, The international chronic granulomatous disease cooperative study group. A controlled trial of interferon gamma to prevent infection in chronic granulomatous disease. N Engl J Med 1991; 324: 509–516.
141. Ezekowitz RAB, Sieff CA, Dinauer MC, Nathan DG, Orkin SH, Newburger PE. Restoration of phagocyte function by interferon-γ in X-linked chronic granulomatous disease occurs at the level of a progenitor cell. Blood 1990; 76: 2443–2448.
142. Ezekowitz RAB, Dinauer MC, Jaffe HS, Orkin SH, Newburger PE. Partial correction of the phagocyte defect in patients with X-linked chronic granulomatous disease by subcutaneous interferon gamma. N Engl J Med 1988; 319: 146–151.
143. Rex JH, Bennett JE, Gallin JI, Malech HL, Decarlo ES, Melnick DA.*in vivo* interferon-γ therapy augments the *in vitro* ability of chronic granulomatous disease neutrophils to damage *Aspergillus* hyphae. J Infect Dis 1991; 163: 849–852.
144. Gallin JI. Interferon-gamma in the management of chronic granulomatous disease. Rev Infect Dis 1991; 13: 973–978.
145. Brummer E, Hanson LH, Restrepo A, Stevens DA.*in vivo* and *in vitro* activation of pulmonary macrophages by IFN-γ for enhanced killing of *Paracoccidioides brasiliensis* or *Blastomyces dermatitidis*. J Immunol 1988; 140: 2786–2789.
146. Beaman L.*in vitro* response of alveolar macrophages to infection with *Coccidioides immitis*. Infect Immun 1980; 28: 594–600.
147. Beaman L. Fungicidal activation of murine macrophages by recombinant gamma interferon. Infect Immun 1987; 55: 2951–2955.
148. Brummer E, Hanson LH, Stevens DA. Gamma-interferon activation of macrophages for killing of *Paracoccidioides brasiliensis* and evidence for nonoxidative mechanisms. Int J Immunopharmacol 1988; 10: 945–952.
149. Fleischmann J, Wu-Hsieh B, Howard DH. The intracellular fate of *Histoplasma capsulatum* in human macrophages is unaffected by recombinant interferon-γ. J Infect Dis 1990; 161: 143–145.
150. Wu-Hsieh BA, Howard DH. Intracellular growth inhibition of *Histoplasma capsulatum* induced in murine macrophages by recombinant gamma interferon is not due to a limitation of the supply of methionine or cysteine to the fungus. Infect Immun 1992; 60: 698–700.
151. Perfect JR, Granger DL, Durack DT. Effects of antifungal agents and gamma interferon on macrophage cytotoxicity for fungi and tumor cells. J Infect Dis 1987; 156: 316–323.
152. Flesch IEA, Schwamberger G, Kaufmann SHE. Fungicidal activity of IFN-γ-activated macrophages: extracellular killing of *Cryptococcus neoformans*. J Immunol 1989; 142: 3219–3224.
153. Vecchiarelli A, Dottorini M, Puliti M, Todisco T, Cenci E, Bistoni F. Defective candidacidal activity of alveolar macrophages and peripheral blood monocytes from patients with chronic obstructive pulmonary disease. Am Rev Respir Dis 1992; 143: 1049–1054.
154. Brummer E, Stevens DA. Candidacidal mechanisms of peritoneal macrophages activated with lymphokines or g-interferon. J Med Microbiol 1989; 28: 173–181.
155. Brummer E, Hanson LH, Stevens DA. Kinetics and requirements for activation of macrophages for fungicidal activity – effect of protein synthesis inhibitors and immunosuppressants on activation and fungicidal mechanism. Cell Immunol 1991; 132: 236–245.
156. Perrusia B, Kobayashi M, Rossi ME, Anegon I, Trinchieri G. Immune interferon enhances functional properties of human granulocytes: role of Fc receptors and effect of lymphotoxin, tumor necrosis factor, and granulocyte-macrophage colony-stimulating factor. J Immunol 1987; 138: 765–774.
157. Garner RE, Kuruganti U, Czarniecki CW, Chiu HH, Domer JE.*in vivo* immune responses to *Candida albicans* modified by treatment with recombinant murine gamma interferon. Infect Immun 1989; 57: 1800–1808.
158. Garner RE, Kuruganti U, Al-Hussaini LA, Czarniecki CW, Domer JE. Effect of *in vivo* administration of recombinant murine gamma interferon on *in vitro* lymphoproliferative responses following immunization with *Candida albicans*. Infect Immun 1992; 60: 1927–1935.
159. Kullberg BJ, Van 't Wout JW, Hoogstraten C, Van Furth R. Recombinant interferon-γ enhances resistance to acute disseminated *Candida albicans* infection in mice. J Infect Dis 1993; 168: 436–443.
160. Metcalf D. The granulocyte-macrophage colony–stimulating factors. Science 1985; 229: 16–22.
161. Metcalf D, Begley CG, Nicola NA, Johnson GR. Quantitative responsiveness of murine hemopoietic population *in vitro* and *in vivo* to recombinant multi-CSF (IL-3). Exp Hematol 1987; 15: 288–295.
162. Mochizuki DY, Eisenman JR, Conlon PJ, Larsen AD, Tushinski RJ. Interleukin 1 regulates hematopoietic activity, a role previously ascribed to hemopoietin 1. Proc Natl Acad Sci USA 1987; 84: 5267–5271.
163. Fibbe WE, Van Damme J, Billiau A, *et al.* Interleukin-1 (22-k factor) induces release of granulocyte-macrophage colony-stimulating activity from human mononuclear phagocytes. Blood 1986; 68: 1316–1321.
164. Fibbe WE, Van Damme J, Billiau A, *et al.* Interleukin 1 induces human marrow stromal cells in long-term culture to produce granulocyte-macrophage colony-stimulating factor

and macrophage colony-stimulating factor. Blood 1988; 71: 430–435.
165. Matsumoto M, Matsubara S, Matsuno T, *et al.* Protective effect of human granulocyte colony-stimulating factor on microbial infection in neutropenic mice. Infect Immun 1987; 55: 2715–2720.
166. Matsumoto M, Tamura M, Matsubara S, Matsuno T, Ono M, Yokota T. Mechanism of protective effect of recombinant human granulocyte colony-stimulating factor (rG-CSF) on *Pseudomonas* infection. Microbiol Immunol 1991; 35: 461–474.
167. Tanaka T, Okamura S, Okada K, *et al.* Protective effect of recombinant murine granulocyte-macrophage colony-stimulating factor against *Pseudomonas aeruginosa* infection in leukocytopenic mice. Infect Immun 1989; 57: 1792–1799.
168. Vadas MA, Lopez AF, Gamble JR, Elliot MJ. Role of colony-stimulating factors in leucocyte responses to inflammation and infection. Curr Opin Immunol 1991; 3: 97–104.
169. Nemunaitis J, Rabinowe SN, Singer JW, *et al.* Recombinant granulocyte-macrophage colony-stimulating factor after autologous bone marrow transplantation for lymphoid cancer. N Engl J Med 1991; 324: 1773–1778.
170. Gorin NC, Coiffier B, Hayat M, *et al.* Recombinant human granulocyte-macrophage colony-stimulating factor after high-dose chemotherapy and autologous bone marrow transplantation with unpurged and purged marrow in Non-Hodgkin's lymphoma: a double-blind placebo-controlled trial. Blood 1992; 80: 1149–1157.
171. Uchida K, Yamamoto Y, Klein TW, Friedman H, Yamaguchi H. Granulocyte-colony stimulating factor facilitates the restoration of resistance to opportunistic fungi in leukopenic mice. J Med Vet Mycol 1992; 30: 293–300.
172. Baldwin GC, Gasson JC, Quan SG, *et al.* Granulocyte-macrophage colony-stimulating factor enhances neutrophil function in acquired immunodeficiency syndrome patients. Proc Natl Acad Sci USA 1988; 85: 2763–2766.
173. Weisbart RH, Kwan L, Golde DW, Gasson JC. Human GM-CSF primes neutrophils for enhanced oxidative metabolism in response to major physiological chemoattractants. Blood 1987; 69: 18–21.
174. Weisbart RH. Colony-stimulating factors and neutrophils. In: Weisbart RH, ed. Colony-stimulating factors and host defense. 1989: 297–303.
175. Fleischmann J, Golde DW, Weisbart RH, Gasson JC. Granulocyte-macrophage colony-stimulating factor enhances phagocytosis of bacteria by human neutrophils. Blood 1986; 68: 708–711.
176. Djeu JY. Role of tumor necrosis factor and colony-stimulating factors in phagocyte function against *Candida albicans*. Diagn Microbiol Infect Dis 1990; 13: 383–386.
177. Blanchard DK, Michelini-Norris B, Djeu JY. Production of granulocyte-macrophage colony-stimulating factor by large granular lymphocytes stimulated with *Candida albicans*: Role in activation of human neutrophil function. Blood 1991; 77: 2259–2265.
178. Roilides E, Walsh TJ, Pizzo PA, Rubin M. Granulocyte colony-stimulating factor enhances the phagocytic and bactericidal activity of normal and defective human neutrophils. J Infect Dis 1991; 163: 579–583.
179. Roilides E, Uhlig K, Venzon D, Pizzo PA, Walsh TJ. Neutrophil oxidative burst in response to blastoconidia and pseudohyphae of *Candida albicans*: augmentation by granulocyte colony-stimulating factor and interferon-γ. J Infect Dis 1992; 166: 668–673.
180. Sisson SD, Dinarello CA. Production of interleukin-1 alpha, interleukin-1 beta and tumor necrosis factor by human mononuclear cells stimulated with granulocyte-macrophage colony–stimulating factor. Blood 1988; 72: 1368-1374.
181. Smith PD, Lamerson CL, Banks SM, *et al.* GM-CSF augments human monocyte fungicidal activity for *Candida albicans*. J Infect Dis 1990; 161: 999–1005.
182. Levitz SM. Activation of human peripheral blood mononuclear cells by interleukin-2 and granulocyte-macrophage colony-stimulating factor to inhibit *Cryptococcus neoformans*. Infect Immun 1991; 59: 3393–3397.
183. Reed SG, Nathan CF, Pihl DL, *et al.* Recombinant granulocyte/macrophage colony-stimulating factor activates macrophages to inhibit *Trypanosoma cruzi* and release hydrogen peroxide. Comparison with interferon-γ. J Exp Med 1987; 166: 1734–1746.
184. Denis M. Tumor necrosis factor and granulocyte macrophage-colony stimulating factor stimulate human macrophages to restrict growth of virulent *Mycobacterium avium* and to kill avirulent *M. avium*: killing effector mechanism depends on the generation of reactive nitrogen intermediates. J Leukocyte Biol 1991; 49: 380–387.
185. Cenci E, Bartocci A, Puccetti P, Mocci S, Stanley ER, Bistoni F. Macrophage colony-stimulating factor in murine candidiasis – serum and tissue levels during infection and protective effect of exogenous administration. Infect Immun 1991; 59: 868–872.
186. Karbassi A, Backer JM, Foster JS, Moore RN. Enhanced killing of *Candida albicans* by murine macrophages treated with macrophage colony-stimulating factor: evidence for augmented expression of mannose receptors. J Immunol 1987; 139: 417–421.
187. Hume DA, Denkins Y. The deleterious effect of macrophage colony-stimulating factor (CSF-1) on the pathology of experimental candidiasis in mice. Lymphokine Cytokine Res 1992; 11: 95–98.
188. Khwaja A, Johnson B, Addison IE, *et al. In vivo* effects on macrophage colony-stimulating factor on human monocyte function. Br J Haematol 1991; 77: 25–31.
189. Nemunaitis J, Meyers JD, Buckner CD, *et al.* Phase-I trial of recombinant human macrophage colony-stimulating factor in patients with invasive fungal infections. Blood 1991; 78: 907–913.
190. Anaissie E, Wong E, Bodey GP, Obrien S, Gutterman J, Vadhan S. Granulocyte-macrophage colony-stimulating factor (GM-CSF) plus amphotericin B for disseminated mycoses in neutropenic cancer patients. Interscience Conference on Antimicrobial Agents and Chemotherapy. Houston, TX, 1989: Abstr. 73 p. 113.
191. Bermudez LEM, Young LS. Tumor necrosis factor, alone or in combination with IL-2, but not IFN-γ, is associated with macrophage killing of *Mycobacterium avium* complex. J Immunol 1988; 140: 3006–3013.
192. Bermudez LEM, Stevens P, Kolonoski P, Wu M, Young LS. Treatment of experimental disseminated *Mycobacterium avium* complex infection in mice with recombinant IL-2 and tumor necrosis factor. J Immunol 1989; 143: 2996–3000.
193. Sharma SD, Hofflin JM, Remington JS. *In vivo* recombinant interleukin 2 administration enhances survival against a lethal challenge with *Toxoplasma gondii*. J Immunol 1985; 135: 4160-4163.

194. Weyand C, Goronzy J, Fathman CG, O'Hanley P. Administration *in vivo* of recombinant interleukin-2 protects mice against septic death. J Clin Invest 1987; 79: 1756–1763.
195. Chong KT. Prophylactic administration of interleukin-2 protects mice from lethal challenge with Gram-negative bacteria. Infect Immun 1987; 55: 668–673.
196. Murphy PM, Lane HC, Gallin JI, Fauci AS. Marked disparity in incidence of bacterial infections in patients with the acquired immunodeficiency syndrome receiving interleukin-2 or interferon-γ. Ann Intern Med 1988; 108: 36–41.
197. Snydman DR, Sullivan B, Gill M, Gould JA, Parkinson DR, Atkins MB. Nosocomial sepsis associated with interleukin-2. Ann Intern Med 1990; 112: 102–107.
198. Klempner MS, Noring R, Mier JW, Atkins MB. An acquired chemotactic defect in neutrophils from patients receiving interleukin-2 immunotherapy. N Engl J Med 1990; 322: 959–966.
199. Levitz SM, Dupont MP. Phenotypic and functional characterization of human lymphocytes activated by interleukin-2 to directly inhibit growth of *Cryptococcus neoformans in vitro*. J Clin Invest 1993; 91: 1490–1498.
200. Beno DWA, Mathews HL. Growth inhibition of *Candida albicans* by interleukin-2-activated splenocytes. Infect Immun 1992; 60: 853–863.
201. Djeu JY, Blanchard DK. Regulation of human polymorphonuclear neutrophil (PMN) activity against *Candida albicans* by large granular lymphocytes via release of a PMN-activating factor. J Immunol 1987; 139: 2761–2767.
202. Wei S, Serbousek D, Mcmillen S, Blanchard DK, Djeu JY. Suppression of human monocyte function against *Candida albicans* by autologous IL-2-induced lymphokine-activated killer cells. J Immunol 1991; 146: 337–342.
203. Wei S, Blanchard DK, McMillen S, Djeu JY. Lymphokine-activated killer cell regulation of T-cell-mediated immunity to *Candida albicans*. Infect Immun 1992; 60: 3586–3595.
204. Ausiello C, Maleci A, Spagnoli GC, Antonelli G, Cassone A. Cell-mediated cytotoxicity in glioma-bearing patients: differential responses of peripheral blood mononuclear cells to stimulation with interleukin-2 and microbial antigen. J Neuro-Oncol 1988; 6: 329–338.
205. Chen BDM, Clark CR. Interleukin-3 (IL-3) regulates the *in vitro* proliferation of blood monocytes and peritoneal exudate macrophages: synergism between a macrophage specific colony-stimulating factor (CSF-1) and IL-3. J Immunol 1986; 137: 563–570.
206. Chen BDM, Mueller M, Olencki T. Interleukin-3 (IL-3) stimulates the clonal growth of pulmonary alveolar macrophage of the mouse: role of IL-3 in the regulation of macrophage production outside the bone marrow. Blood 1988; 72: 685–690.
207. Bleiberg I, Kletter Y, Riklis I, Fabian I. Induction of murine macrophage fungal killing by interleukin 3. Exp Hematol 1989; 17: 895-897.
208. Cohen L, David B, Cavaillon JM. Interleukin-3 enhances cytokine production by LPS-stimulated macrophages. Immunol Lett 1991; 28: 121–126.
209. Marodi L, Forehand JR, Johnston RB Jr. Mechanisms of host defense against *Candida* species. 2. Biochemical basis for the killing of *Candida* by mononuclear phagocytes. J Immunol 1991; 146: 2790–2794.
210. Walz A, Peveri P, Aschauer H, Baggiolini M. Purification and amino acid sequencing of NAF, a novel neutrophil-activating factor produced by monocytes. Biochem Biophys Res Comm 1987; 149: 755–761.
211. Colditz I, Zwahlen R, Dewald B, Baggiolini M. *In vivo* inflammatory activity of neutrophil-activating factor, a novel chemotactic peptide derived from human monocytes. Am J Pathol 1989; 134: 755–760.
212. Peveri P, Walz A, Dewald B, Baggiolini M. A novel neutrophil-activating factor produced by human mononuclear phagocytes. J Exp Med 1988; 167: 1547–1559.
213. Lohmann-Matthes ML. Interaction of macrophages and cytokines. Curr Opinion Immunol 1989; 2: 33–38.
214. Vogels MTE, Lindley IJD, Curfs JAHJ, Eling WMC, Van der Meer JWM. Effects of interleukin-8 on non-specific resistance to infection in neutropenic and normal mice. Antimicrob Agents Chemother 1993; 37: 276–280.
215. Vogels MTE, Lindley I, Van der Meer JWM. Interleukin-8 accelerates death of infected neutropenic mice. 30th Interscience Conference on Antimicrobial Agents and Chemotherapy. Atlanta, 1990: 140.
216. Hack CE, Hart M, Strack van Schijndel RJM, *et al.* Interleukin-8 in sepsis: relation to shock and inflammatory mediators. Infect Immun 1992; 60: 2835–2842.
217. Djeu JY, Matsushima K, Oppenheim JJ, Shiotsuki K, Blanchard DK. Functional activation of human neutrophils by recombinant monocyte-derived neutrophil chemotactic factor/IL-8. J Immunol 1990; 144: 2205–2210.
218. Nibbering PH, Pos O, Stevenhagen A, Zomerdijk TPL, Van Furth R. Interleukin-8 enhances the intracellular killing of *Mycobacterium fortuitum* by human granulocytes. Infect Immun 1993; 61: 3111–3116.
219. Ganz T, Selsted ME, Szklarek D, *et al.* Defensins: natural peptide antibiotics of human neutrophils. J Clin Invest 1986; 76: 1427–1435.

Address for correspondence: B.J. Kullberg, M.D., Ph.D., Division of General Internal Medicine, University Hospital Nijmegen, P. O. Box 9101, 6500 HB Nijmegen, The Netherlands.

Biotherapy 7: 211–221, 1994.

Cytokines in malaria, pathology and protection

Wijnand M.C. Eling[1] & Peter G. Kremsner[2]
[1]*Department of Medical Microbiology University of Nijmegen, P.O. Box 9101, 6500 HB Nijmegen, The Netherlands;*
[2]*Institut für Tropenmedizin, Engeldamm 62, 10179 Berlin, Germany*

Key words: cerebral, cytokines, malaria, *P. falciparum*, *P. berghei*

Abbreviations: IL: interleukin; GMCSF: granulocyte macrophage colony stimulating factor; CM: cerebral malaria; IFN: interferon; TNF: tumour necrosis factor; RNI: reactive nitrogen intermediates; ROI: reactive oxygen intermediates; EiA: enzyme immunoassay; ICAM-1: intercellular adhesion molecule-1; LFA-1: leucocyte function antigen-1; PMN: polymorphonuclear leucocyte; IL-1ra: interleukin-1 receptor antagonist; rH-IL-1-1ra: recombinant human-interleukin-1 receptor antagonist

Malaria

Malaria is among the most important diseases of mankind having a strong negative impact on socio-economic development. It is a threat to about one third of the world's population and particularly to people living in tropical and subtropical areas [1–4].

Malaria is caused by an unicellular parasite of the genus *Plasmodium* that completes part of its life cycle (sexual stage differentiation and development of sporozoites) in female mosquitos, which during feeding on humans (a blood meal) inject sporozoites that have matured in the salivary glands into the blood stream. The sporozoites invade liver parenchymal cells, grow and form liver schizonts. The liver cell with the mature schizont bursts and releases numerous merozoites in the blood stream that invade red blood cells. Inside the red blood cell merozoites grow out to trophozoites that develop into new schizonts that after burst release a limited number of merozoites that invade new erythrocytes establishing a cycle in itself, which takes approximately 48 hours (*Plasmodium falciparum*). This asexual erythrocytic cycle causes the disease symptoms which may vary from mild disease to a lethal cerebral malaria. Some of the merozoites that invade erythrocytes differentiate by an as yet unknown mechanism in sexual stages (gametocytes), that when taken up by a mosquito during a blood meal can establish the sexual stage differentiation in the mosquito and complete the life cycle [5].

Malaria infections occur widespread in nature, e.g., in lizards, birds, rodents, monkeys, man. Parasite species only have a limited capacity to infect several host species [5].

Man can be infected by 4 different species of malaria parasites all of which cause disease, particularly in children who have not yet developed protection of their own and people coming from areas without transmission of the parasite, e.g., tourists and migrants. Whereas in semi-immune individuals, those who have experienced malaria attacks many times, usually only a mild form of the disease is seen.

Cerebral malaria

Infection with *P. falciparum* can cause the potentially life-threatening form of the disease: cerebral malaria, particularly in children in endemic areas and people that have no recent history of repeated malaria infections [3].

Cerebral malaria may kill people within 14 days after infection and the critical phase of the disease may take only 2 days [3].

In some studies cerebral malaria is defined as unrousable coma in patients with *P. falciparum* infections (and no other cause for coma), whereas in others, cerebral involvement varies from somnolence to unrousable coma in the presence of the parasite [3].

Disturbance of brain function may be the only major organ pathology observed besides severe anemia (more common in Africa), but hypoglycemia, renal and/or hepatic failure and/or pulmonary dysfunction may further complicate the disease (more common in Asia) [3].In America, complicated malaria and death seem to be rather rare. It is not clear whether pathogenesis of acute, non-complicated and complicated cerebral malaria are based on a common principle, the differences being based on genetic differences, endemicity of malaria associated with immune reactivity or other causes.

Most studies consider sequestration, adherence of parasitized erythrocytes to the endothelial lining of capillaries and post-capillary venules in the brain, as a major factor in the pathogenesis of the cerebral complications [3, 6], while other studies of the brain show a smaller proportion of sequestration and a higher proportion of hemorrhages [7–9].

Cerebral malaria is also described in *Plasmodium berghei* infections in hamsters, rats and mice [10–18]. Sequestration of mononuclear cells that interact with and tend to migrate between the endothelium of post-capillary venules, probably causing widespread petechial hemorrhages, are a predominant characteristic of these models [11, 19]. The common denominator in cerebral malaria of man and animal seems to be the sequestration phenomenon, though the predominantly sequestered cells differ: leucocytes in murine malaria and infected erythrocytes in *P. falciparum* infections. Possibly sequestration causes stuffing of capillaries and post-capillary venules, reducing cell flow in the vascular system and permitting localized activation and release of substances that interfere with the integrity of the endothelial lining. These processes not only occur in the brain, but in the brain loss of homeostasis will be rapidly fatal.

Though, a comatose state has been described in *P. berghei*-Anka infections in CBA/Ca mice [14, 15], it is not well-established for other rodent models of cerebral malaria. It also remains to be established whether the pathogenesis of coma and hemorrhages in both human and rodent cerebral malaria are essentially the same and reflect a further evolution of ongoing pathological processes. Therefore, cerebral malaria in rodents may primarily yield information about the pathogenesis of hemorrhages.

Cells and cytokines in the pathogenesis of cerebral malaria in mice

In rodents, immunopathological reactions of the host play an important role in the development of the disease [10, 11, 15, 16]. In humans, only indirect evidence for the involvement of immunopathological reactions are available i.e. malnourished children being immunocompromised have a lower chance of developing cerebral malaria but their risk increases after refeeding [20].

More is known in the rodent and particularly in the *P. berghei*-mouse models (figure 1), but even among these models differences are observed (see below).

No cerebral malaria occurs in congenital T-cell deficient (nude) mice, or normal mice timely treated with anti-T cell antibodies particularly after depletion of $CD4^+$ T cells [11, 14–16]. Low dose irradiation of the spleen or splenectomy even when performed shortly before expected death prevents development of the syndrome, suggesting a role for T cells in the spleen [16].

The asexual blood stage life cycle of *P. berghei* is less than 24 hours and after every schizogony residual bodies are released, which are taken up by the macrophages and the Kupffer cells. This explains a strong stimulation of monocytopoiesis. Inhibition of monocytopoiesis by treatment with antibodies to IL-3 and GMCSF, as well as depletion of macrophages by treatment with liposomal-dichloromethylene diphosphonate, prevents development of the cerebral syndrome [21, 22]. The role of T-cells and macrophages was further substantiated when the role of cytokines in the pathogenesis of CM was analysed. IFNτ produced by activated $CD4^+$ T cells prime macrophages for the production of TNF and development of the cerebral syndrome was specifically associated with high levels of free TNF in the *P. berghei*-Anka mouse model [23]. Treatment with antibodies to either IFNγ [24] or TNF [23] as well as treatment with a prostacyclin analog [25] or pentoxifylline [26] which reduce TNF production, prevented CM.

Here, differences between mouse models for CM as well as between CM and non-CM models were observed.

Whereas treatment with pentoxifylline or antibodies to IFNγ prevented CM in *P. berghei*-Anka infected CBA/Ca mice, these treatments were ineffective in *P. berghei*-K173 infected C57Bl/6J mice [27] and anti-IFNγ antibodies were barely effective in K173 infected CBA/Ca mice [28]. The difference in production-capacity of IFNγ might explain the difference between

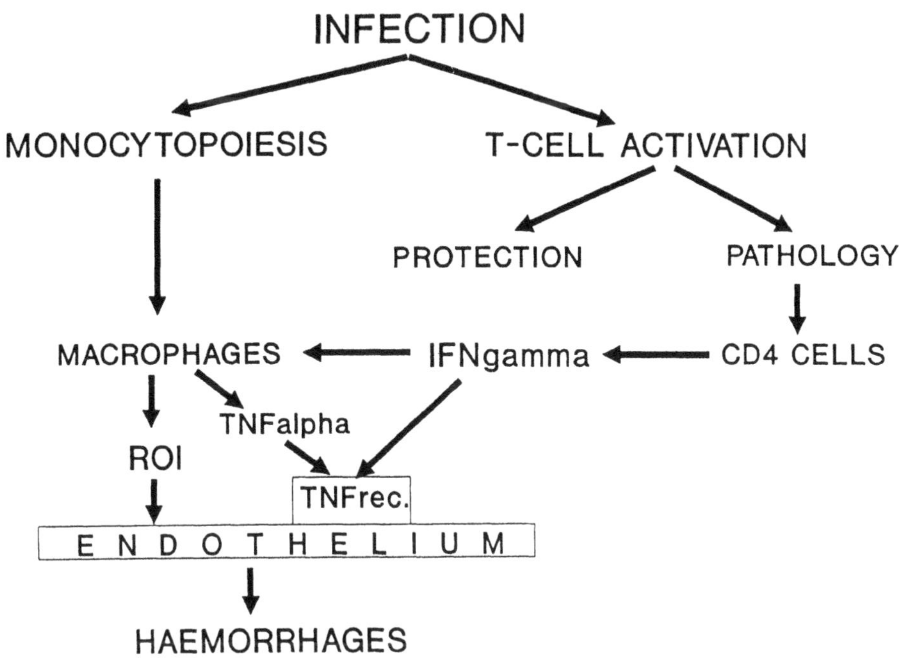

Fig. 1. Schematic representation of the possible role of T-cells and macrophages and cytokines produced by these cells in the pathogenesis of murine malaria

the CBA/Ca and C57Bl/6J mice [29], but is not sufficient to explain the difference between the parasites K-173 and Anka.

Treatment with IFNγ during infection did not enhance but delayed CM in the K173 model and inhibited parasitemia, suggesting a protective rather than an enhancing effect [28].

The protective effect of IFNγ treatment was also observed in *P. chabaudi*, *P. yoelii* and *P. vinckei*-mouse infections that do not develop CM [30–32]. Moreover, an initial burst of IFN-γ secretion occurs only in mice infected with the non-lethal variant of *P.yoelii* [32]. *P.chabaudi*-infected mice treated with neutralizing anti-IFNγ antibodies were found to develop a significantly higher degree of parasitemia than control mice [33]. Limiting dilution analysis revealed that substantial production of IFNγ by antigen specific T lymphocytes occurs early during primary non-lethal *P.chabaudi* infection [34]. Finally, early administration of IFNγ enhanced the effect of chloroquine therapy in murine *P.vinckei* malaria [35] which was at least partly due to induction of specific IgG 2a antibodies [36]. In contrast, when chloroquine and IFN-γ were combined to treat *P.vinckei* malaria in the late phase of the disease, morbidity and mortality was enhanced [37]. Pretreatment with pentoxifylline significantly decreased IFNγ-induced lethality, whereas pretreatment with an inhibitor of the production of reactive nitrogen intermediates or with neutralizing antibodies to TNF significantly increased lethality in this model [37].

In conclusion, in the experimental *Plasmodium*-mouse models IFNγ early during infection mediates an anti-parasitic activity by enhancing a non-specific immune response and possibly by helping the development of a specific immunity against malaria. In addition, IFNγ excessively produced or administered in high doses in an advanced phase of the disease in non-immune mice may have adverse effects and enhance CM and/or mortality.

In patients with *P. falciparum* malaria serum IFNγ levels were not associated with parasitemia, disease severity or complications. An increase of IFN-γ concentrations in serum of patients infected with *P.falciparum* was reported in some [38–42], but not in other studies [43–45], which may depend on different detection limits of IFN-γ in the test systems used. The levels of IFN-γ in serum of acutely infected individuals depended strongly on their immune status: non-immune individuals have a high peak of IFN-γ in serum during the malaria attack compared to semi-immune subjects who do not have significant changes in their IFN-γ serum levels [41, 42]. In addition, mononuclear leucocytes from non-immune subjects produced significantly more IFN-γ when stimulated with malarial antigen than mononuclear leucocytes from semi-immune individuals. No such difference was found when the cells were cultured with mitogen [46]. In non-immune patients during the malaria attack the delayed type hypersensitivity response to recall antigens was significantly diminished compared to semi-immune patients and control individuals [47].

TNF and the pathogenesis of cerebral malaria

There has been strong indications for a role of TNF in the pathogenesis of CM. Both in mouse and human (cerebral) malaria increased serum levels of TNF were detected, that usually correlated with parasitemia and in some studies even with CM or severity of disease [23, 26, 39, 48, 49]. In human *P. falciparum* malaria these correlations were based on the immunological detection and quantitation of TNF using a two-site EiA. In *P. berghei*-Anka CBA/Ca infections free serum TNF was found using the cell lysis assay [23]. Free, biologically active TNF in this parasite-mouse combination was only found when CM developed. It was absent in Anka infections in Balb/c mice or *P. yoelii* infections where CM does not develop.

A further indication for a role of TNF in the pathogenesis of CM came from the observation that in both the Anka and K173 model for CM, treatment with TNF during infection enhanced development of the cerebral syndrome, resulting in hemorrhages in the brain and several other organs [22, 50]. Normal mice do not show particular pathological reactions after treatment with these doses of TNF. The major difference between pathology after TNF treatment of infected mice and development of CM was the systemic (hemorrhages in several organs) rather than localized (brain only) effects observed after treatment of infected mice with TNF [22].

It was hypothesized that treatment with TNF triggered release of endogenous TNF from the pool of macrophages that was expanding considerably during infection [22]. If this were true, treatment with lower doses of TNF during infection might release TNF without approaching levels that would kill the mice. In view of the observed refractoriness of macrophages that are stimulated to release TNF for a period of approximately one week [51], this might prevent the development of CM later. Indeed, low dose TNF treatment during infection prevented CM [22].

Refractoriness to renewed stimulation of TNF production may also explain why high dose TNF treatment before or early during infection protects against infection. The injection of recombinant TNF and IFN was found to exert anti-parasitic activity *in vivo* against several *Plasmodium* infections [30, 52–54]. In addition, the early treatment with anti-TNF antibodies led to an increase of parasitemia in *P. vinckei* infected mice [55]. IFN-γ and TNF do not show a direct cytotoxic effect against murine and human malarial parasites [53, 56].

All of the above described data suggested an important role of TNF in the pathogenesis of CM and formed the basis for preliminary studies using treatment with anti-TNF antibodies in people with CM.

Meanwhile, several recent observations shed some doubt on the role of TNF in the pathogenesis of malaria and particularly CM.

No differences were found between non-immune and semi-immune patients with *P. falciparum* malaria with respect to their TNF serum levels before chemotherapy, though, TNF levels dropped significantly quicker after chemotherapy in semi-immune patients [41]. In patients suffering from *P. vivax* malaria, without signs of CM, cytokines such as TNF appeared to have extreme peak serum concentrations for only a short period [57].

In most cases, whether in experimental or human CM, TNF levels were measured by EiA that detects the molecule but does not indicate whether biologically active TNF is present. In a crucial early study, however, TNF was measured by the cell lysis assay, which measures biological activity of TNF [23].

TNF binding proteins were observed in plasma and meanwhile two different soluble TNF-receptors have been identified that are actively shed from the surface of several different cell types and block the pathological activity of free TNF when present in sufficient concentrations [58, 59].

An important further observation showed that in patients with cerebral/severe malaria, TNF could be detected by EiA but not by the cell lysis assay indicating that no free TNF was present in the plasma, while in the same plasma samples the concentrations of TNF receptors were much higher than for TNF itself [60].

These results might explain why the pilot studies using treatment with anti-TNF antibodies of patients with CM were not successful [61].

Subsequent experiments in the *P. berghei*-K173 model again showed that TNF levels as detected by EiA increased during infection, but the concentration of TNF binding proteins/soluble TNF-receptors in the plasma increased even stronger and no free TNF could be detected.

These observations may explain why treatment of *P. berghei*-K173 infected mice with anti-TNF antibody did not prevent development of CM. They may suggest the use of indirect markers of cytokine activity, such as the acute phase reactants including C-reactive protein (an easy to determine parameter) as a marker of disease severity [42, 62].

It has been shown that IL-1 and TNF are synergistic in the development of pathology [63].

Treatment of K173 infected mice with (up to 800 ng) of IL1 shortly before onset of CM did not enhance the occurrence of the CM syndrome [64]. This may be explained now by the absence of a synergistic activity because free TNF is not present in the plasma.

The picture that emerges suggests that under conditions of progressive disease, TNF production increases gradually, but so does the release of TNF receptors which prevent pathology.

Only in cases where TNF production is triggered instantaneously (e.g. treatment with lipopolysaccharide) free TNF can be found in the plasma and shedded receptor is observed later. In these cases there is pathology that could be due to free TNF and could be prevented by treatment with anti-TNF antibody [65].

A role of TNF in the pathogenesis of CM, however, is still possible. Particularly under circumstances where mononuclear cells adhere to the endothelial lining (e.g. in *P. berghei*-mouse models), activation may induce TNF release locally or even in a cell-cell contact before it is inactivated by soluble receptor or anti-TNF antibody.

Although there is substantial evidence that excessive TNF is involved in pathology, a direct lytic effect of TNF on endothelial cells has not been observed. An important question, therefore, is what causes the damage of the endothelial lining? This might be caused the local excessive production of reactive oxygen intermediates by activated macrophages [66–69], as treatment with anti-oxidants prevented murine cerebral malaria [70]. In contrast, reactive nitrogen intermediates, also produced by activated macrophages [71] and reported to kill intraerythrocytic *P. falciparum* [72], are not involved in the development of CM [73]. IFN-γ and TNF are able to induce the production of ROI and RNI by activated murine macrophages [71] and by human cells [68, 74].

Besides a possible damaging effect on endothelial lining cells, radical molecules produced by activated leucocytes are important tools of the terminal effector pathway in the killing of blood stage malarial parasites. Human and murine blood stage parasites are susceptible to destruction by ROI [66–69] and recently the intra-erythrocytic killing of *P. falciparum* by RNI was reported [72].

Local effects in the vascular system may lead to further activation of all cells present including platelets, leucocytes as well as endothelial cells, eventually leading to local damage.

The sequestration of infected erythrocytes

Sequestration of parasitized erythrocytes in the vascular sytem, particularly in the cerebral vasculature is considered a hallmark of cerebral malaria. In *post-mortem* pathology, stuffing of cerebral capillaries and post-capillary venules was used as a diagnostic character together with the presence of hemorrhages, ring hemorrhages or petecchiae.

In one study carried out on *post-mortem* material from Birma, sequestration was observed in 100% of the patients and hemorrhages in only 47% of the cases [6]. In another study on Vietnamese *post-mortem* material, only 23% of patients that died of CM exhibited the sequestration phenomenon. In these cases sequestration was not restricted to the cerebral vasculature, but was also observed in other tissues (e.g. the heart) [7, 8]. In the Vietnamese study, in approximately 75% of the cases, hemorrhages could be found. These differences in the same region of the world are remarkable. There certainly is a need for more *post-mortem* analyses [2], particularly in combination with molecular analysis of sequestration in the same patients, however, it is becoming increasingly difficult to obtain permission for *post mortem* analysis. In a recent study *post-mortem* material was obtained from 2 patients with CM both exhibiting hemorrhages in their brains. In addition, histological analysis of the brain of one patient showed a massive aggregate of peripheral blood mononuclear cells in the venous vasculature in association with coagulation of the blood (figure 2).

The significance of sequestration *in vivo* is difficult to assess. Does it block or inhibit blood flow? Does accumulation lead to a local metabolic acidosis? Are reduced flow and local metabolic acidosis the basis for coma? Such phenomena could explain why after recovery the majority of patients (85–100%) do not suffer from sequelae. On the other hand, published pictures of sequestration showing capillaries and post-capillary venules stuffed with parasitized erythrocytes

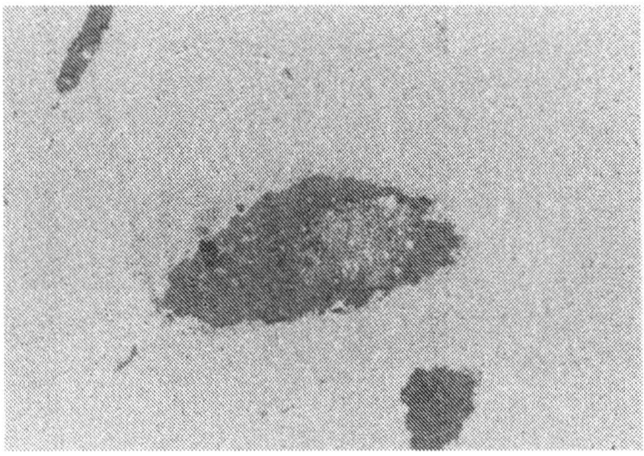

Fig. 2. Light micrograph of brain tissue from a Vietnamese patient who died with cerebral malaria. The picture shows intravascular coagulation in combination with a large aggregate of leucocytes in a vein. Goldners' trichrome stain Magn 150x

usually do not show perivascular necrosis, or even edema, despite the fact that the material is obtained from people that died of CM.

Endothelial adherence: sequestration and cerebral malaria

The molecular analysis of the phenomenon of sequestration has been extensively studied because a better understanding might help to define intervention measures.

Both light and electron microscopic studies indicated that special structures on the surface of infected erythrocytes, "the knobs", adhered to the endothelial lining of the vasculature [75]. Adherence could also be shown in *in vitro* studies using human umbilical vein endothelial cells), melanoma cells or more recently brain endothelial cells [76–78]. *In vitro* studies have helped to define five molecules present on the surface of endothelial cells, that seem to be involved in adherence of *P. falciparum*-infected erythrocytes: thrombospondin, CD36, ICAM-1, endothelial leucocyte adhesion molecule 1 (ELAM-1) and vascular cell adhesion molecule 1 (VCAM-1) [79]. The importance of each of these molecules in binding is dependent on the test system used [78], and this in turn raises the question of their relevance *in vivo* in the brain vasculature. The parasitic ligands to these molecules have not been characterized fully. Another important question is, therefore, whether all parasites express the ligands to these molecules to the same extent.

As mononuclear cells need to bind to more than one adhesion molecule for effective binding to endothelial cells, parasites may have to use more ligands too.

ICAM-1, sequestration and cytokines

Binding to endothelial ICAM-1 is interesting because it might be a common factor in human and rodent CM [80–82] (figure 3). In human CM, sequestration of parasitized erythrocytes might be mediated by ICAM-1, and sequestration of mononuclear cells in murine CM might also be mediated by ICAM-1. In both cases binding to ICAM-1 could initiate localized processes. Reduction of blood flow might allow cells to settle and/or to make contact with other cells. The presence of parasitized cells, lymphocytes and macrophages in close, or even direct contact, may result in activation of these cells and lead to the local release of all kinds of substances like cytokines, eicosanoids, reactive oxygen intermediates or reactive nitrogen intermediates. In the rodent models this apparently also leads to activation of the endothelium, as shown by increased lysosomal and even phagocytic activity [19].

In addition, in rodent CM, migration of mononuclear cells between endothelial cells is observed. This may well be a leaky process, as observed in mice with a chronic infection developing endomyocardial thrombosis [83].

The mononuclear ligand for ICAM-1 is LFA-1 and an intervention study in the *P. berghei*-Anka model has focussed on this interaction [81, 82]. Whereas treatment with recombinant ICAM-1 only delayed development of CM, treatment with antibody to ICAM-1 was deleterious causing hemorrhages in the lungs [82]. Treatment with antibody to LFA-1, however, successfully prevented CM even when given shortly before the expected death of the animal [81, 82]. Results also showed that treatment with anti-LFA-1 antibody did not change the mononuclear density in the vascular system, but only their adherence and interaction with the endothelium.

Comparable experiments in the *P. berghei*-K173 model were unsuccessful (Eling *et al.*, unpublished observation). In these experiments treatment with monoclonal antibodies to LFA-1 did not prevent development of CM for as yet unknown reasons.

ICAM-1 is constitutionally present on endothelial cells and its expression is enhanced under the influence of IFNγ or TNF [84]. The level of both these cytokines is elevated during malaria infection [38–50].

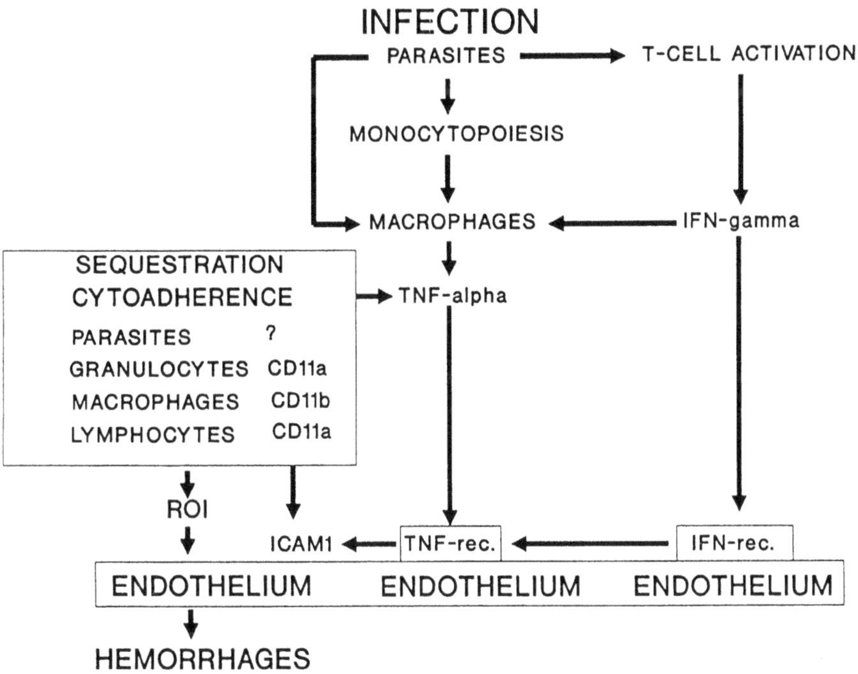

Fig. 3. Schematic representation of the possible role of adherence of leucocytes or infected red blood cells to the endothelial lining of the cerebral vasculature in the pathogenesis of cerebral malaria

Recently, it was shown that ICAM-1 is shed from the surface of cells into the plasma. Circulating ICAM-1, representing the proteolytically cleaved outer part of the molecule, can be measured [85]. Measurement of soluble ICAM-1 may reflect activation of the endothelial lining of the vasculature.

Determination of the plasma level of soluble ICAM-1 in normal uninfected controls, patients with uncomplicated *P. falciparum* malaria, patients with disturbance of brain function varying from somnolence to unrausable coma, and patients with functional disturbance in one or more organs in addition to the brain revealed a significant increase in relation to an increase in severity of the disease (Eling *et al.*, manuscript in preparation).

IL-6 and IL-8 in experimental cerebral malaria

IL-6 is probably not directly involved in the pathogenesis of CM [86] though, it is a marker of severe malaria in human *P. falciparum* infection [39]. High serum levels are found in both CM and non-lethal *P. berghei*-Anka infection. Treatment with anti-IL-6 antibody did not prevent CM [86]. Possibly IL-6 is involved in polyclonal B cell activation and stimulation of antibody production, which if timely available, may even suppress development of CM [16].

Little is known about the role of IL-8 in the pathogenesis of CM. IL-8 is a chemo-attractant for polymorphs. In the *P. berghei*-K173 model, treatment with recombinant human IL-8 had no effect on parasitemia and mortality, however, IL-8 treated and infected mice exhibited more bleedings involving other organs besides the brain, than control-treated and infected mice [87].

In human *P. falciparum* infections, IL-8 levels were elevated and remained elevated for a period of 4 weeks despite successful treatment and recovery [88].

A correlation was found between serum polymorphonuclear leucocyte elastase levels, a product of activated PMN, and severity of infection [89]. The question is whether this is only due to PMN activation or also to an (IL-8 dependent) increased PMN recruitment (see figure 2).

IL-1, IL-1 receptor antagonist and malaria

Treatment with IL-1 (α or ß) or IL-1 receptor antagonist (IL-1ra) has an effect on the parasitemia and development of CM [64, 90]. A single dose treatment, or better, multiple doses of 80 ng or more of IL-1 either per shot per mouse per day or released from an osmotic pump over 24 hours, prevented development of CM in the *P. berghei* (K173)- mouse infection. Multiple doses of 80 ng or more also progressively inhibited parasitemia, but the effect on CM was not due to the effect on parasitemia.

IL-1 treatment only excerted an effect on CM and parasitemia when given early during infection and was inactive when given shortly before the onset of CM. Whereas in shock models IL-1 and TNF have a synergistic effect on development of pathology [63], this was not observed in development of CM, which may be due to the production of large amounts of soluble TNF receptor during infection. How IL-1 treatment suppresses parasitemia and prevents CM is unclear.

P. berghei infections are sensitive to changes in erythropoietic activity and IL-1 treatment modulates erythropoiesis, however, pilot experiments did not show an inhibitory effect of IL-1 on enhanced reticulocytosis.

The IL-1 dependent inhibition of parasitemia depends on the presence of T-cells and the production of IFNγ [64]. This is in line with the observation that IL-1 stimulates IFNγ production [91], and suggests a role for CD4$^+$ T cells and possibly Th1 cells, in the IL-1 dependent inhibition of parasitemia. CD4$^+$ T cells are important for the development of CM [14], which is prevented by anti-IFNγ antibody treatment [24]. This suggests, however, that Th1 stimulation early during infection contributes to CM. On the other hand, the adjuvant effect of IL-1 on antibody production [92], as well as protection from CM and suppression of parasitemia by early treatment with specific antibody, suggest that stimulated Th2 can inhibit parasitemia and prevent CM. Thus, IL-1 treatment early during infection may interfere with the Th1-Th2 switch, either directly or through an effect on processing and presentation of parasitic antigens to these cells.

The situation is even more complicated taking into consideration the effect of IL-1 receptor antagonist on parasitemia and CM [90]. Treatment with recombinant human IL-1ra either by intraperitoneal injection during infection or through sustained release from an osmotic pump, inhibited infection and prevented development of CM, suggesting that endogenous IL-1 is involved in the development of parasitemia and CM. Since rH-IL-1ra reacts only with mouse IL-1-receptor type I (on T-cells and endothelial cells) and not type II (on monocytes and B-cells), endogenous IL-1 may contribute to CM and parasitemia by stimulating T-cells. The effect of treatment with IL-1ra on body temperature and inhibition of parasitemia during infection is weaker than for IL-1 treatment, possibly related to the inability of rH-IL-1ra to interfere with stimulation of IL-1-receptor type II. The results obtained with IL-1 and IL-1ra treatment are compatible if it is assumed that IL-1 downregulates the expression of IL-1 receptors type I and II. Exposition of cells to IL-1 *in vitro* indeed resulted in downregulation of the IL-1 receptor [93].

Dietary fish oil and the protection against malaria

The use of dietary fish oil has been shown to produce an anti-inflammatory effect in clinical and experimental situations [94, 95]. A six week fish oil diet inhibited parasitemia significantly and prevented CM compared to control-treated animals after infection with *P. berghei*-K173. How fish oil effects parasitemia and CM remains to be elucidated. The reduction of prostaglandin synthesis associated with dietary fish oil [96] could not explain the results, since indomethacin treatment did not effect parasitemia or development of CM [94]. Fish oil treated mice showed an increased level of cell-associated IL-1 and TNF production capacity. Triggering of IL-1 and/or TNF release early after infection may have the same effect as treatment with IL-1 and/or TNF which may cause temporary refractoriness of macrophages to stimulation and production of cytokin, very important for development of CM. An interesting question is whether dietary fish oil can prevent cerebral malaria in endemic areas in Africa or adults in Asia.

References

1. Clyde DF. Recent trends in the epidemiology and control of malaria. Epid Rev 1987; 9: 219–243.
2. Roman GC. Cerebral malaria: the unsolved riddle. J Neurol Sci 1991; 101: 1–6.
3. Warrell DA, Molyneux ME, Beales PF, eds. Severe and complicated malaria. Trans Roy Soc Trop Med Hyg 1990; 84 Suppl 2: 1–65.
4. Wernsdorfer G, Wernsdorfer WH. Social and economic aspects of malaria and its control. In:Wernsdorfer WH and McGregor I. editors. Malaria. Churchill Livingstone. 1992, 2. Chapter 47; 1421–1471.
5. Garnham PCC. Malaria parasites and other Haemosporidia. Blackwell Scientific Publications Oxford. 1966.
6. Oo MM, Aikawa M, Than T, Aye T, Myint PT, Igarashi I, Schoene WC. Human cerebral malaria: A pathological study. J Neuropath Exp Neurol 1987; 46: 223–231.

7. Jerusalem C, Polder T, Weijers-Rouw M, Eling W, Osonkoya BO, Trinh P. Comparative clinical and experimental study on the pathogenesis of cerebral malaria. In: Gigase PL, Mark EAE, editors. Contributions to microbiology and immunology, Vol.7 From Parasitic infection to parasitic disease. Basel, S. Karger AG. 1983: 130–138.
8. Jerusalem C, Polder T, Kubat K, Wijers-Rouw M, Trinh P. Brain edema in cerebral malaria: a comparative clinical and experimental ultrastructural and histochemical study. In:Go KG, Baethmann A, editors. Recent progress in the study and therapy of brain edema. New York, Plenum Publ. Coop. 1984: 127–135.
9. Riganti M, Ponponratn E, Tegoshi T, Loowaresuan S, Punpoowon B, Aikawa M. Human cerebral malaria in Thailand: A clinico-pathological correlation. Immunology Letters 1990; 25: 199–206.
10. Wright DH, Masemba RM, Bazira ER. The effect of antithymocyte serum on golden hamsters and rats infected with *Plasmo*dium berghei. Brit J Exp Path 1971; 52: 465–477.
11. Rest JR. Pathogenesis of cerebral malaria in golden hamsters and inbred mice. Contr Microbiol Immunol 1983; 7: 139–146.
12. Kamiyama T, Tatsumi M, Matsubara J, Yamamoto K, Rubio Z, Cortes G, Fujii H. Manifestation of cerebral malaria-like symptoms in the WM/Ms rat infected with *Plasmodium berghei* strain NK65. J Parasit 1987; 73: 1138–1145.
13. Bakker NPM, Eling WMC, de Groot AMTh, Sinkeldam EJ, Luyken R. Attenuation of malaria infection, paralysis and lesions in the central nervous system by low protein diets in rats. Acta Tropica 1992; 50: 285–293.
14. Finley RW, Mackay LJ, Lambert P-H. Virulent *P. berghei* malaria: prolonged survival and decreased cerebral pathology in T-cell nude deficient mice. J Immunol 1982; 129: 2213–2218.
15. Grau GE, Piguet P-F, Engers HD, Louis JA, Vassalli P, Lambert P-H. L3T4$^+$ T lymphocytes play a major role in the pathogenesis of murine cerebral malaria. J Immunol 1986; 137: 2348–2354.
16. Curfs JHAJ, Schetters TPM, Hermsen CC, Jerusalem CR, van Zon AAJC, Eling WMC. Immunological aspects of cerebral lesions in murine malaria. Clin Exp Immunol 1989; 75: 136–140.
17. Clark IA, Ilschner S, MacMicking JD, Cowden WB. TNF and *Plasmodium berghei*-Anka-induced cerebral malaria. Immunol Letters 1990; 25: 195–198.
18. Polder TW, Jerusalem CR, Eling WMC. Topographical distribution of the cerebral lesions in mice infected with *Plasmodium berghei*. Tropenmed Parasit 1983; 34: 235–243.
19. Polder TW, Eling WMC, Curfs JHAL, Jerusalem CR, Wijers-Rouw M. Ultrastructural changes in the blood-brain barrier of mice infected with *Plasmodium berghei*. Acta Leidensia 1992; 60: 31–46.
20. Murray MJ, Murray AB, Murray NJ, Murray MB. Diet and cerebral malaria: the effect of famine and refeeding. Am J Clin Nutr 1987; 31: 57–61.
21. Grau GE, Kindler V, Piguet P-F, Lambert P-H, Vassalli P. Prevention of experimental cerebral malaria by anticytokine antibodies. J Exp Med 1988; 168: 1499–1504.
22. Curfs JHAJ, Hermsen CC, Kremsner P, Neifer S, Meuwissen JHETh, van Rooijen N, Eling WMC. Tumor necrosis factor-α and macrophages in *Plasmodium berghei*-induced cerebral malaria. Parasitology, 1993, 107: 125–134.
23. Grau GE, Fajardo LF, Piguet P-F, Allet B, Lambert P-H, Vassalli P. Tumor necrosis factor (cachectin) as an essential mediator in murine cerebral malaria. Science 1987; 237: 1210–1212.
24. Grau GE, Heremans HJ, Piguet P-F, Pointaire P, Lambert P-H, Billiau A, Vassalli P. Monoclonal antibody against IFNτ can prevent experimental cerebral malaria and its associated overproduction of tumor necrosis factor. Proc Natl Ac Sci USA 1989; 86: 5572–5574.
25. Sliwa K, Grundmann H, Neifer S, Chaves MF, Sahlmüller G, Blitstein-Willinger E, Bienzle U, Kremsner PG. Prevention of murine cerebral malaria by a stable prostacyclin analog. Infect Immun 1991; 59: 3846–3848.
26. Kremsner PG, Grundman H, Neifer S, Sliwa K, Sahlmüller G, Hegenscheid B, Bienzle U. Pentoxifylline prevents murine cerebral malaria. J Inf Dis 1991; 164: 605–608.
27. Stoltenburg-Didinger G, Neifer S, Bienzle U, Eling W, Kremsner PG. Selective damage of hippocampal neurons in murine cerebral malaria prevented by pentoxifylline. J Neur Sci 1993; 114: 20–24.
28. Curfs JHAJ, van der Meide PH, Billiau A, Meuwissen JHETh, MCEling WMC. Recombinant interferon-τ and the development of parasitemia and cerebral lesions in *Plasmodium berghei*-infected mice. Exp Parasit. 1993; 77: 212–223.
29. Neta R. Mechanisms involved in the low responsiveness of mice in the *in vivo* release of lymphokines. In: Oppenheim JJ, Cohen S, editors. Interleukins, lymphokines and cytokines, New York: Academic Press, Inc, 711–721.
30. Clark IA, Hunt NG, Butcher GA, Cowden WB. Inhibition of murine malaria (*Plasmodium chabaudi*) *in vivo* by recombinant interferon τ or tumor necrosis factor, and its enhancement by butylated hydroxyanisole. J Immunol 1987; 13: 3493–3496.
31. Bienzle U, Fritsch KG, Hoth G, Rozdzinski E, Köhler K, Kalinowski M, Kremsner P, Rosenkaimer F, Feldmeier H. Inhibition of *Plasmodium vinckei*-malaria in mice by recombinant murine interferonτ. Acta Tropica 1988; 45: 289–290.
32. Shear L, Srinivasan R, Nolan T, Ng C. Role of IFN-τ in lethal and non-lethal malaria in susceptible and resistant murine hosts. J Immunol 1989; 143: 2038–2044.
33. Stevenson MM, Tam MF, Belosevic M, van der Meide P, Podoba JE. Role of endogenous gamma interferon in host response to infection with blood stage *Plasmodium chabaudi* AS. Infect Immun 1990; 58: 3225–3232.
34. Slade SJ, Langhorne J. Production of interferon-τ during infection of mice with *Plasmodium chabaudi chabaudi*. Immunobiology 1989; 179: 353–365.
35. Kremsner PG, Neifer S, Schermuck S, Chaves MF, Sliwa K, Bienzle U. Interferon-τ enhances the effect of anti-malarial chemotherapy in murine *Plasmodium vinckei* malaria. J Infect Dis 1991; 163: 1161–1163.
36. Finnemann S, Kremsner PG, Chaves MF, Schumacher C, Neifer S, Bienzle U. Antibody response in *Plasmodium vinckei* malaria after treatment with chloroquine and adjuvant interferon-τ. Parasitol Res 1992; 78: 629–634.
37. Kremsner PG, Neifer S, Chaves MF, Rudolph R, Bienzle U. Interferon-τ induced lethality in the late phase of *Plasmodium vinckei* malaria despite effective parasite clearance by chloroquine. Eur J Immunol 1992; 22: 2873–2878.
38. Rhodes-Feuilette A, Bellosguardo M, Druilhe P, Ballet JJ, Chousterman S, Canivet M, Peries J. The interferon compartment of the immune response in malaria: II Presence of serum-interferon gamma following the acute attack. J Interferon Res 1985; 5: 167–178.
39. Kern P, Hemmer CJ, Damme JV, Gruss HJ, Dietrich M, Elevated tumor necrosis factor alpha and interleukin-6 serum levels as markers for complicated *Plasmodium falciparum* malaria. Am J Med 1989; 87: 139–143.

40. Kwiatkowski D, Hill AVS, Sambou I, Twumasi P, Castracane J, Manogue KR, Cerami A, Brewster DR, Greenwood B. TNF concentration in fatal cerebral, non-fatal cerebral, and uncomplicated *Plasmodium falciparum* malaria. Lancet 1990; 336: 1201–1204.
41. Ringwald P, Peyron F, Vuillez JP, Touze JE, Le Bras J, Deloron P. Levels of cytokines in plasma during *Plasmodium falciparum* malaria attacks. J Clin Microbiol 1991; 29: 2076–2078.
42. Harpaz R, Edelman R, Wasserman SS, Levine MM, Davies JR, Sztein MB. Serum cytokine profiles in experimental human malaria. J Clin Invest 1992; 90: 515–523.
43. Kremsner PG, Feldmeier H, Zotter GM, Jansen-Rosseck R, Graninger W, Rocha RM, Bienzle U. Immunological alterations in uncomplicated *Plasmodium falciparum* malaria Relationship between parasitaemia and indicators of macrophage activation. Acta Trop 1989; 46: 351–359.
44. Butcher GA, Garland T, Ajdukiewicz AB, Clark IA, Plasma TNF associated with malaria in patients in the Solomon Islands. Trans Roy Soc Trop Med Hyg 1990; 84: 658–661.
45. Molyneux ME, Taylor TE, Wirima JJ, Grau GE. Tumour necrosis factor, interleukin-6, and malaria. Lancet 1991; 337: 1098.
46. Chizzolini C, Grau GE, Geinoz A, Schrijvers D. T-Lymphocyte interferon-gamma production induced by *Plasmodium falciparum* antigen is high in recently infected non-immune and low in immune subjects Clin Exp Immunol 1990; 79: 95–99.
47. Kremsner PG, Zotter GM, Feldmeier H, Graninger M, Rocha RM, Rosseck RJ, Bienzle U. Immune response in patients during and after Plasmodium falciparum infection. J Inf Dis 1990; 161: 1025–1028.
48. Grau GE, Taylor TE, Molyneux ME, Wirima JJ, Vassalli P, Hommel M, Lambert P-H. Tumor necrosis factor and disease severity in children with *Plasmodium falciparum malaria*. N Engl J Med 1989; 320: 1586–1591.
49. Shaffer N, Grau GE, Hedberg K, Davachi F, Lymba B, Hightower AW, Breman JG, Nguyen-Dinh P. Tumor necrosis factor and cerebral malaria. J Inf Dis 1991; 163: 96–101.
50. Grau GE, Piguet P-F, Vassalli P, Lambert P-H. Immunol Rev Tumor-necrosis factor and other cytokines in cerebral malaria: experimental and clinical data 1989; 112: 49–70.
51. Gifford GE, Lohmann-Matthes M-L. Gamma-interferon priming of mouse and human macrophages for induction of tumor necrosis factor production by bacterial lipopolysaccharide. J Natl Cancer Inst 1987; 78: 121–124.
52. Stevenson MM, Ghadirian E. Human recombinant tumor necrosis factor alpha protects susceptible A/J mice against lethal *Plasmodium chabaudi* – AS infection. Infect Immun 1989; 57: 3936–3939.
53. Taverne J, Tavernier J, Fiers W, Playfair JHJ. Recombinant tumor necrosis factor inhibits malaria parasites *in vivo* but not *in vitro*. Clin Exp Immunol 1987; 67: 1–4.
54. Maheshawari RK, Czarniecki CW, Dutta GP, Puri SK, Dhawan BN, Friedman RM. Recombinant human gamma-interferon inhibits simian malaria. Infect Immun 1986; 53: 628–633.
55. Neifer S, Kremsner PG, Bienzle U. Application of anti-TNF to *Plasmlaedium vinckei*-infected mice is followed by an increase in parasitaemia. Acta Trop 1989; 46: 273–275.
56. Hviid L, Reimart CM, Theander TG, Jepsen S, Bendtzen K. Recombinant human tumour necrosis factor is not inhibitory to *Plasmodium falciparum in vitro*. Trans Roy Soc Trop Med Hyg 1988; 82: 48–49.
57. Karunaweera ND, Grau GE, Gamage P, Carter R, Mendis KN. Dynamics of fever and serum levels of tumor necrosis factor are closely associated during clinical paroxysms in *Plasmodium vivax* malaria. Proc Natl Acad Sci USA 1992; 89: 3200–3203.
58. Brockhaus M, Schoenfeld HJ, Schlaeger EJ, Hunzinger W, Lesslauer W, Loetscher H. Identification of two types of tumor necrosis factor receptors on human cell lines by monoclonal antibodies. Proc Natl Ac Sci USA 1990; 87: 3127–3131.
59. Tartaglia LA, Goeddel DV. Two TNF receptors. Immunol Today 1992; 13: 151–153.
60. Kern P, Hemmer CJ, Gallati H, Neifer S, Kremsner P, Dietrich M, Porzsolt F. Soluble tumor necrosis factor receptors correlate with parasitemia and disease severity in human malaria. J Inf Dis 1992; 166: 930–934.
61. Kwiatkowski D, Molyneux M, Stephens S, Curtis N, Klein N, Pointaire P, Smit M, Allen R, Brewster D, Grau GE, Greenwood B. Anti-TNF therapy inhibits fever in cerebral malaria. Quart J Medicine 1993; 86: 91–98.
62. Graninger W, Thalhammer F, Hollenstein U, Zotter GM, Kremsner PG. Serum protein concentrations in *Plasmodium falciparum* malaria. Acta Trop 1992; 52: 121–128.
63. Dinarello CA, Interleukin-1 and interleukin-1 antagonism. Blood 1991; 71: 1627–1652.
64. Curfs JHAJ, van der Meer JWM, Sauerwein RW, Eling WMC. Low dosages of interleukin-1 protect mice against lethal cerebral malaria. J Exp Med 1990; 172: 1287–1291.
65. Beutler B, Milsark TW, Cerami AC. Passive immunization against cachectin/tumor necrosis factor protects mice from lethal effect of endotoxin. Science 1985; 229: 869–871.
66. Clark IA, Hunt NH. Evidence for reactive oxygen intermediates causing hemolysis and parasite death in malaria. Infect Immun 1983; 39: 1–6.
67. Dockrell HM, Playfair JHL. Killing of blood-state murine malaria parasites by hydrogen peroxide. Infect Immun 1983; 39: 456–459.
68. Ockenhouse CF, Schulman S, Shear HL. Induction of crisis forms in the human malaria parasite *Plasmodium falciparum* by gamma-interferon activated, monocyte-derived macrophages. J Immunol 1984; 133: 1601–1608.
69. Clark IA, Hunt NH, Cowden WB, Maxwell LE, Mackie EJ. Radical mediated damage to parasites and erythrocytes in *Plasmodium vinckei* Exp infected mice after injection of t-butyl hydroperoxide. Clin Immunol 1984; 56:524–530.
70. Thumwood CM, Hunt NH, Cowden WB, Clark IA. Antioxidants can prevent cerebral malaria in *Plasmodium berghei*-infected mice. Brit J Exp Path 1989; 70: 293–303.
71. Ding AH, Nathan CF, Stuehr DJ. Release of reactive nitrogen intermediates and reactive oxygen intermediates from mouse peritoneal macrophages. J Immunol 1988; 141: 2407–2412.
72. Rockett KA, Awburn MM, Cowden WB, Clark IA. Killing of *Plasmodium falciaprum in vitro* by nitric oxide derivatives. Infect Immun 1991; 59: 2280–3203.
73. Kremsner PG, Nüssler A, Neifer S, Chaves MF, Bienzle U, Senaldi G, Grau G. Malaria antigen and cytokine-induced production of reactive nitrogen intermediates by murine macrophages: no relevance to development of experimental cerebral malaria. Immunology 1993; 78: 286–290.
74. Nüssler AK, Di Silvio M, Billiar TR, Hoffman RA, Geller DA, Selby R, Madariaga J, Simmons RL. Stimulation of the nitric oxide synthase pathway in human hepatocytes by cytokines and endotoxin. J Exp Med 1992; 176: 261–264.
75. Warrell D. Pathophysiology of severe *falciparum* malaria in man. Parasitology 1987; 94: 853–876.
76. Udeinya IJ, Schmidt J, Aikawa M, Miller L, Green I. Falciparum infected erythrocytes specifically bind to cultured human endothelial cells. Science 1981; 213: 555–557.
77. Udeinya IJ, Graves P, Carter R, Aikawa M, Miller L. *Plasmodium falciparum*: effect of time in continuous culture on

binding to endothelial cells and amelanotic melanoma cells. Exp Parasit 1985; 56: 207–214.

78. Smith J, Nelson JA, Gahmberg CG, Crandall I, Sherman E. *Plasmodium falciparum*: cytoadherence of malaria-infected erythrocytes to human brain capillary and umbilical vein endothelial cells-A comparative study of adhesive ligands. Exp Parasit 1992; 75: 269–280.
79. Ockenhouse FC, Tegoshi T, Maeno Y, Benjamin C, Ho M, Kan KE, Tway Y, Win K, Aikawa M, Loble RR. Human vascular endothelial cell adhesion receptors for*Plasmodium falciparum*-infected erythrocytes: Role for endothelial leucocyte adhesion molecule 1 and vascular cell adhesion molecule 1. J Exp Med 1992; 176: 1183–1189.
80. Ockenhouse C, Ho M, Tandon N, van Seventer G, Shaw S, White N, Jamieson G, Chulay J, Webster K. Molecular basis of sequestration in severe and uncomplicated malaria: Differential adhesion of infected erythrocytes to CD36 and ICAM-1. J Inf Dis 1991; 164: 163–169.
81. Falanga PB, Butcher EC. Late treatment with anti-LFA-1 (CD11a) antibody prevents cerebral malaria in a mouse model. Eur J Immunol 1991; 21: 2259–2263.
82. Grau GE, Pointaire P, Piguet P-F, Vesin C, Rosen H, Stamecovic I, Takei F, Vassalli P. Late administration of monoclonal antibody to leucocyte function antigen 1 abrogates incipient murine cerebral malaria. Eur J Immunol 1991; 21: 2265–2267.
83. Eling WMC, CR Jerusalem and U Heinen-Borries Role of macrophages in the pathogenesis of endomyocardial fibrosis in murine malaria. Trans Roy Soc Trop Med Hyg 1984; 78: 43–48.
84. Simmons D, Makgoba MW,Seeb B. ICAM, an adhesion ligand of LFA-1, is homologous to the neural cell adhesion molecule NCAM. Nature 1988; 331: 624–627.
85. Rothlein R, Mainolfi EA, Czajkowski M, Marlin S. A form of circulating ICAM-1 in human serum. J Immunol 1991; 147: 3788–3793.
86. Grau GE, Frei K, Piguet P-F, Fontana A, Heremans H, Billiau A, Vassalli P, Lambert P-H, Interleukin 6 production in experimental cerebral malaria: modulation by anti-cytokine antibodies and possible role in hypergammaglobulinemia. J Exp Med 1990; 172: 1505–1508.
87. Vogels MTE, Lindley IJD, Curfs JHAJ, Eling WMC, van der Meer JWM. The effects of interleukin-8 on non-specific resistance to interfection in neutropenic and normal mice, Antimicrobial Agents and Chemotherapy 1993; 37: 276–280.
88. Friedland JS, Ho M, Remick GDG, Bunnag D, White NJ, Griffin GE. Interleukin-8 and *Plasmodium falciparum* malaria in Thailand. Trans Roy Soc Trop Med Hyg 1993; 87: 54–55.
89. Pukrittayakame S, Clemens R, Pramoolsinsap C, Karges HE, Vanijanonta S, Bunnag D, White NJ. Polymorphonuclear leucocyte elastase in *Plasmodium falciparum* malaria. Trans Roy Soc Trop Med Hyg 1992; 86: 598–601.
90. Curfs JHAJ, Vogels MTE, Eling WMC, van der Meer JWM, IL-1 receptor antagonist prevents cerebral malaria in *Plasmodium berghei*-infected mice. In: Ghezzi P, Mantovani A, editors. Pathophysiology and pharmacology of cytokines. Augusta, Georgia: Biomedical Press 1992, 105–111; Progress Biomedical Research, Vol 2, Series Editor SM Reichard.
91. Le, J, Vilcek J. Biology of disease Tumor necrosis factor and Interleukin-1: cytokines with multiple overlapping biological activities. Lab Invest 1987; 56: 234–248.
92. Staruch MJ, Wood DD. The adjuvanticity of interleukin-1 *in vivo*. J Immunol 1983; 130: 2191–2194.
93. Ye K, Clark BD, Dinarello CA. Interleukin-1 downregulates gene and surface expression of Interleukin-1 receptor type I by destabilizing its mRNA, whereas Interleukin-2 increases its expression. Immunology 1992; 75: 427–434.
94. Blok WL, Vogels MTE, Curfs JHAJ, Eling WMC, Buurman WA, van der Meer JWM. Dietary fish-oil supplementation in experimental gram-negative infection and cerebral malaria in mice. J Inf Dis 1992; 165: 898–903.
95. Editorial Fish oil Lancet, 1988; 14: 1083–1091.
96. Lee TH, Hoover RL, Williams JD, Sterling RI, Ravelese J, Spur BW, Robinson DR, Corey EJ, Lewis RA, Austen KF. Effect of dietary enrichment with eicosapentaenoic and dososahexanoic acids on *in vitro* neutrophil and monocyte leukotriene generation and neutrophil function. N Engl J Med 1985; 312: 1217–1224.

Biotherapy 7: 223–235, 1994.

Cytokines in the treatment of leishmaniasis: From studies of immunopathology to patient therapy

John L. Ho, Roberto Badaro, Dimitrios Hatzigeorgiou, Steven G. Reed & Warren D. Johnson, Jr.
Division of International Medicine, Department of Medicine, Cornell University Medical College, New York, New York 10021 and Seattle Biomedical Research Institute, Seattle, WA 98109, U.S.A.

Abstract

The genus *Leishmania*, an obligate intramacrophage parasite, causes a wide spectrum of clinical diseases. It is worldwide in distribution and causes 20 million new cases annually with an at risk population of approximately 1.5 billion persons. The most severe forms are associated with high morbidity, mortality and relapses with conventional therapy. The therapeutic issues and responses to standard and alternative therapies are reviewed. Recent developments in molecular biology and immunology methods employed in the study of leishmaniasis have defined an intricate interaction of the parasite with host immune system. Perturbation of the host immune responses may be part of the survival mechanisms of *Leishmania*. In murine model, the finding of T helper cells that differ by their panel of cytokines has allowed a more precise definition of immunopathogenesis of leishmaniasis. Preliminary data from leishmaniasis patients lend support to this concept of altered immunomodulation. Furthermore, the enhancement of therapeutic response by interferon-γ has provided a new approach for treatment of patients using recombinant cytokines and for the study of the disease. Current research for early diagnosis, alternative therapies and need for vaccines are reviewed in the context of the immunopathology of leishmaniasis.

Leishmaniasis

Leishmaniasis is caused by obligate intramacrophage parasites of the genus *Leishmania*. They are distributed worldwide [1]. There are an estimated 20,000,000 new cases annually with an at risk population of approximately 1.5 billion persons [2]. In the Americas, several forms of leishmaniasis occur from the Southern United States to Northern Argentina [3–7]. The major endemic areas in Europe and Africa center around the Mediterranean basin, sub-Sahara Africa, East and West Africa. In the Middle East and the Far East, the endemic areas are Saudi Arabia, Iran, Iraq, Afghanistan, parts of Russia, India and southwest China. Infection is transmitted by the bite of a sandfly. Rodents, small mammals and dogs are the reservoirs for *Leishmania*. In endemic areas of Brazil, dogs and living near domestic animals are major risk factors for acquisition of leishmaniasis.

The clinical manifestations of leishmaniasis range from asymptomatic infection to fatal disease [6–8]. The major clinical forms are visceral leishmaniasis (VL), cutaneous leishmaniasis (CL), mucosal leishmaniasis (ML), and diffuse cutaneous leishmaniasis (DCL) [9–11]. Classic VL is characterized by fever, hepatosplenomegaly, pancytopenia and hyperglobulinemia, and is complicated by serious infections and bleeding. Mortality rates are 5–7% in VL patients who are provided optimal therapy [9]. Mortality rates of 30% are encountered under epidemic conditions, such as the 1977 VL outbreak in India and the current epidemic in Sudan in which 30,000 and 40,000 persons respectively have died [12]. All forms of leishmaniasis are found in the New World (Americas) while only CL and VL are present in the Old World (Europe, Africa, Middle and Far East).

CL is characterized by non-diagnostic ulcers at the site of primary inoculation of the *Leishmania* species by the sandfly [9]. CL heals with a disfiguring scar. ML is a late sequela, occurring in 1–3% of patients with CL. It is characterized by granulomatous lesions of the nasal septum, with occasional involvement of adjacent structures (pharynx, palate, larynx, lips) [8, 10]. ML is chronic, difficult to treat, often disfiguring, and occasionally fatal if the upper airway is compromised [8,

10]. DCL is characterized by multiple chronic nodular skin lesions containing many parasites and by anergy to *Leishmania* antigens. It is extremely refractory to all forms of therapy [11].

Classification of clinical syndromes by causative species is inaccurate. *L. amazonensis* is associated with CL, DCL and VL [13] and recently *L. tropica*, a species that usually causes CL, has been reported to cause visceral disease in US Desert Storm troops [14]. The traditional schema has grouped human leishmaniasis into five major complexes: *L. tropica* and *L. major* (Old World leishmaniasis); *L. mexicana*, *L. amazonensis* and *L. brasiliensis* (New World leishmaniasis), and *L. donovani* species (donovani, infantum, chagasi). *Leishmania donovani spp.*, are the principal agent of VL. *L. brasiliensis* causes 85% of the CL and almost all of the ML in Brazil.

The recommended therapy for VL for over 70 years is antimony. Pentavalent antimony (Sb^5) therapy is associated with initial response rates of only 70–80%, significant drug toxicity (20–30%) and relapse rates of over 20%. This is a dramatic increase from the 5% unresponsive rate of a decade ago [15–17]. The finding of *in vitro* antimony resistance being induced by intermittent drug exposure [18] and the isolation of resistant leishmanial strains from unresponsive ML or CL cases [19] lend support for Sb^5 resistance as one cause for drug failures and relapses. The alternative drugs for VL (amphotericin B and pentamidine) are also associated with significant toxicity and relapses. All three drugs must be given IV or IM for periods of 3 to 8 weeks. Treatment failures, relapses, drug toxicity, and the requirement for parenteral administration have led to a search for alternative therapy based on the understanding of the immunopathology of leishmaniasis.

Immunology of leishmaniasis The immune response to *Leishmania* can be depicted by two opposing poles: VL and DCL on the side lacking specific cell mediated immune response with CL and ML on the side with demonstrable or hyper-responsive cell mediated immune response. Patients with acute VL lack *Leishmania*-specific delayed hypersensitivity responses (DTH), and their lymphocytes and monocytes fail to proliferate and to produce IL-1 in response to parasite antigens [20–24]. They become responsive after resolution of disease. DCL is similarly characterized by an absence of T cell proliferation or DTH response to the parasite [11, 24]. The majority (80%) of active cutaneous leishmaniasis [7–9, 24–26] demonstrate a DTH and *in vitro* proliferative responses but all respond after cured/healed disease [26]. ML is characterized by hyperactive intradermal skin tests and lymphocyte proliferative responses [7–11, 25] which may explain the destructive attack on host tissue and the paucity of parasites in mucosal lesions. Major advances in leishmaniasis immunology is the separation of $CD4^+$ T cells into functional helper (h) subsets [27–30]. The immune response in the varied clinical states and by the causative *Leishmania* is illustrated in Table 1.

Th1/Th2 response: A) murine leishmaniasis. The separation of $CD4^+$ T cells into subsets based on the repertoire of cytokines generated has provided a useful tool to characterize the response patterns and to define their role in the immunopathology of leishmaniasis and other infectious diseases. Th1 cells produce IFN-γ and IL-2 and are involved in cell-mediated immunity, while Th2 cells produce IL-4, IL-5, IL-6 and IL-10 and are more involved in humoral immunity. In experimental infections a dominant Th1 cytokine response is associated with healing while a predominantly Th2 cytokine response is associated with disease progression [29–34].

Th1/Th2 response: B) human leishmaniasis. Attempts to correlate Th1 cytokines with various clinical forms of leishmaniasis have suggested that IL-2 and IFN-γ are associated with a controlled infection or healing response in CL [24, 31] and a Th2 cytokine pattern predominates in lesions of patients with diffuse CL [31]. Other studies have addressed Th1 and Th2 cytokine production by lymphoid tissue and PBMC during VL. Karp *et al.*, [35] observed increased mRNA of IL-10 and IFN-γ in bone marrow aspirates of patients with active disease, as compared with levels in treated individuals [35]. We found IL-10 mRNA in lymph nodes from patients with acute VL, but not in nodes of the same patients following successful chemotherapy [36]. Abundant mRNA for IFN-γ was present in both pre- and post-treatment samples. IL-4 mRNA was also found to be increased in most pre-treatment, but not post-treatment, samples. Thus far, IL-10 is most clearly associated with pathology in VL. These observations, based on *in situ* measurements of cytokines, provide an accurate reflection of *Leishmania*-specific responses as bone marrow and lymph nodes are sites of parasite replication.

Role of cytokines in th selection: A) murine. *In vitro* studies on the regulation of T cell responses provide support for the role of IFN-γ, IL-4, IL-10 or IL-12

Table 1. Immune response and associations with Th phenotypes in leishmaniasis

Clinical disease	*Leishmania* species	Th phenotype predominance
Acute VL	*L. donovani* complex	Th2
	L. amazonensis	Th2
DCL	*L. amazonensis*	Th2
Active CL	*L. braziliensis*	Th1/Th2
	L. amazonensis	Th1/Th2
Healed VL		Th1
Healed CL		Th1

in Th selection [26, 33, 34, 37–48]. The cytokine milieu at the time of infection may be critical in Th-cell differentiation [34–41]. For example, treatment of resistant mice with anti-IFN-γ monoclonal antibody (mAb) abrogates Th1-cell development, and promotes Th2-cell expansion [34]. Further evidence that IFN-γ may play a role in Th-cell differentiation is provided by the adoptive transfer of T cells from BALB/c mice into severe combined immunodeficiency mice rendering them resistant to *L. major* infection [34, 37]. SCID mice with adoptive T-cells produced high levels of IFN-γ and the simultaneous administration of anti-IFN-γ abrogated the resistance to infection [37].

An example of Th2 cytokine influencing Th development is provided by the studies of anti-IL-4. Treatment of susceptible mice with anti-IL-4 mAb inhibited Th2-cell expansion, leading to Th1-cell development and cure of infection [37–39]. In contrast to the studies using mAb to block IFN-γ or IL-4 action, the administration of IFN-γ did not alter resistance. Conversely, treatment of resistant mice with IL-4 induces Th2 response and causes disease [35]. IL-4 transgenic mice with a resistant genetic background became susceptible to *L. major* infection [40]. Furthermore, when a *L. major* clone transfected with IFN-γ was used to infect nude mice, the progression of disease was slower. In BALB/c mice, the transfected *L. major* clone was unable to influence the development of Th2 cells or susceptibility [41]. Therefore, the presence of IL-4 appears to directly influence Th2 predominance, suggesting IL-4 antagonists may be a useful strategy for interrupting the pathology of leishmaniasis.

Leishmania induction of IL-12 from NK, monocytes or B cells may also modulate Th-cell phenotype selection [44]. A role for IL-12 in Th1 development is suggested by the finding that murine macrophages infected with *Listeria*, can influence the differentiation of naive T cells towards Th1-cell phenotype [45]. In *L. major* infection, exogenous administration of IL-12 to BALB/c mice enhanced Th1-cell development and promoted healing of an otherwise progressive infection [46–48]. This is the first cytokine that had a therapeutic effect when administered to *Leishmania*-infected mice. Additional evidence suggests that cytokines other than IL-12 may participate in the early events of Th selection. TNFα appears to be a costimulant with IL-12 [49] for NK cell activation, while IL-1 can act independently of NK cells to drive the selection for the Th1 phenotype [50]. All three cytokines are monokines, and raise the question of the role of macrophages in Th selection [51–53].

Role of cytokines in Th selection: B) human. The reciprocal regulatory role of cytokines in Th differentiation has been demonstrated in several antigen-specific T cells. IL-4 added to bulk lymphocyte culture before cloning shifted differentiation of PPD specific T cells from Th1 to Th0, or even to Th2 phenotype [54]. IFN-γ plus anti-IL-4 mAb or IFN-α induced allergen-specific T cells or T cells specific for helminth constituents to differentiate into Th0 or even Th1 instead of Th2 clones [54, 55]. Cytokine regulation of Th cells has similarly been shown in graft infiltrating lymphocytes obtained from rejected renal grafts. Graft infiltrating lymphocytes secrete IFN-γ, IL-6 and IL-10. The addition of IL-2 to *in vitro* cultures of these cells enhanced the frequency of IFN-γ secreting cells, while IL-4 reduced the frequency of spontaneous IFN-γ producing cells and inhibited the IL-2 enhancement of IFN-γ producing cells.

The involvement of IL-12 and NK cells in human Th selection was recently demonstrated using primed cells from patients reactive to PPD or patients allergic to *Dermatophagoides pteronyssinus* (Der p I) [56]. IL-12 reduced the ability of Der p I responsive lines to produce IL-4 and increased their ability to produce IFN-γ and developed into CD4$^+$ T cell clones. The IL-12 treated CD4$^+$ T cell clones show a Th 0 or Th1 instead of Th2-like cytokine profile. The effect of IL-12 was not blocked by anti-IFN-γ mAb but by the removal of CD16$^+$ (NK) cells. Furthermore, anti-IL-12 treatment of PPD-specific T cell lines exhibited increased ability to produce IL-4 and developed into PPD-specific CD4$^+$ T cell clones showing a Th0 instead of a Th1-like profile.

In PBMC obtained from leishmaniasis patients, we recently showed that *in vitro* addition of recombinant IL-10 blocked the *Leishmania* antigen-driven proliferation of PBMC from treated patients, and neutralizing anti-IL-10 mAb restored *Leishmania*-driven response in PBMC from acute VL patients [36]. Of particular interest, acute patient PBMC "unresponsive to *Leishmania* antigens" as measured by proliferation of IL-2/IFN-γ production, were found to produce IL-10 mRNA *in vitro* [26, 36]. These findings are of antigen primed cells and do not define the interaction of the *Leishmania*, macrophages and other immune cells that leads to Th selection.

Role of antigens in T cell selection. The primary *in vivo* immunization of mice with 5 respiratory syncytial virus (RSV) proteins using recombinant vaccinia demonstrated that specific antigens can prime for functionally different T cells including selection for CD4 vs CD8 T cells, Th1 vs Th2 phenotype and cytotoxic T cells [57]. By another approach using glutaraldehyde polymerized ovalbumin (OV-POL) investigators [58] demonstrated that immunization with ovalbumin (OV) induced equivalent amounts of Th1/Th2 cells, while OV-POL increased by 20-fold the ratio of IFN-γ/IL-4 and IFN-γ/IL-10 synthesis following short-term antigen restimulation. *In vivo* administration with anti-IFN-γ mAb and OVA or OV-POL resulted in marked increase in IL-4 or IL-10 and decreased IFN-γ production. These findings are in agreement with our *in vitro* observations with several cloned antigens of *L. braziliensis* that can selectively drive cytokine production on human cells (preliminary results). The above reports suggest that macrophages and antigen presentation may play a pivotal role in Th selection.

Macrophage and leishmaniasis. *Leishmania* is an obligate intramacrophage parasite. Upon entry *Leishmania* down-modulates *in vitro* macrophage killing capacity (superoxide production) [59, preliminary results], the induction of monokines (IL-1, TNFα) [60, 61], and expression of major histocompatibility class II antigens and antigen presentation [64]. These perturbations are actively mediated by *Leishmania* at the level of intracellular signaling [62, 63] and gene regulation [65, 66, 67]. Furthermore, *in vivo* infection with low numbers of promastigotes or administration of specific antigen protects previously susceptible mice from subsequent lethal challenge [68, 69]. These findings suggest that studies to define Th selection must include an evaluation of the macrophage in driving the predominance of one type of Th cells.

TGF-β and macrophages in leishmaniasis. TGF-β is a multifunctional molecule involved in embryonic development, tumorigenesis, wound healing and fibrosis [reviewed in 70, 71]. TGF-β is constitutively secreted as an inactive form by macrophages [72]. Acid dissociation or proteolytic cleavage leads to an active form. TGF-β plays an important role in wound healing and recruitment of monocytes. However, it acts also to down-regulate the protective responses in experimental cutaneous leishmaniasis. Macrophages are a source of pro-TGF-β that is not biologically active. In contrast, *in vivo* and *in vitro Leishmania*-infected macrophages produce active TGF-β [73, 74]. Furthermore, the pathogenicity of *L. braziliensis* strains correlates with their ability to induce active TGF-β synthesis by *in vitro* infected murine macrophages.

The participation of TGF-β in the pathogenesis of murine leishmaniasis is provided by 1) the findings of high levels of active TGF-β associated with the lesion; 2) the ability to decrease intralesional IL-4, enhance IFN-γ and promote resistance to *L. amazonensis* by administration of anti-TGF-β mAb; 3) the development of lesions in BALB/c mice injected with TGF-β and *L. braziliensis*, (which normally fails to induce disease in these mice); and 4) the development of lesions in quiescent *L. braziliensis* infection by local injection of TGF-β [73, 74]. The secreted TGF-β acts as an autocrine factor which inhibits IFN-γ activation of murine and human macrophage [75 and Ho JL personal communication). Our preliminary results indicate that human macrophages infected with *L. amazonensis* produces active TGF-β. The generation of active TGF-β may also influence the Th selection. TGF-β suppresses *in vitro* IL-1 mediated T cell proliferation [70, 71], and *in vivo* infected susceptible animals or resistant animals treated with TGF-β produce high levels of IL-10 [73] which inhibits Th1 cells and IFN-γ production.

$CD8^+$ T cells and Th2/Th1 phenotype. Although Th selection has focused on $CD4^+$ T cells, recent evidence suggests that murine $CD8^+$ T cells, which have cytolytic activity and produce IFN-γ, can be switched to $CD8^-CD4^-$ non-cytolytic cells producing IL-4, IL-5 and IL-10 [76]. The switch is mediated by the combined treatment with IL-2, IL-4, PMA and ionomycin. Interestingly, treatment with TGF-β, IL-2, PMA and ionomycin results in cells that remain $CD8^+$ but become non-cytolytic, do not produce cytokines, nor help B cells to produce Ig. Therefore, early events may modulate both $CD4^+$ and $CD8^+$ T cells to a Th2 phenotype that is deleterious for control of *Leishmania*.

In vitro and murine studies defining antimicrobial activity of cytokines. The antimicrobial and antiparasitic activity of macrophages is a complex function. The generation of reactive oxygen intermediates (ROI) and at least murine cells, reactive nitrogen intermediates (RNI) is essential for antimicrobial activity. The production of ROI and RNI in response to various stimuli can be augmented by priming macrophages with cytokines, such as IFN-γ [77, 78]. Based on this observation, attempts to improve therapy have focused on enhancing macrophage antimicrobial activity [79].

Treatment of murine and human monocytes/macrophages with IFN-γ restricts growth or increased killing of intracellular microorganisms such as *Leishmania* species, mycobacteria, *Listeria monocytogenes, Trypanosoma cruzi, Salmonella typhimurium, Candida albicans* and others (Table 2) [80–103]. In most studies with human cells, this effect was paralleled with enhancement of respiratory burst [104, 105], while in murine cells with an additional activation of the inducible form of nitric oxide synthase (NOS) [106]. The enhancement of respiratory burst by IFN-γ, in human neutrophils and monocytes is possibly attributed to the increased expression of gp91-phox, one of the NADPH oxidase components [107]. Another mechanism for the IFN-γ induced antimicrobial activity, is the synthesis of indoleamine 2,3-dioxygenase, an enzyme that cleaves typtophan, resulting in amino acid starvation of the parasite [108].

TNF-α, GM-CSF, and IL-3 have similar *in vitro* antimicrobial activities (Table 3) [85, 101, 109–132]. These cytokines augment antimicrobial function by enhancing macrophage oxidative metabolism [126, 113]. IL-1 has also been shown to protect against *in vitro Leishmania* infections, but was not associated with an increased production of ROI (personal communication, Hatzigeorgiou DE, Ho JL).

In experimental murine models of infections with *Leishmania* species, *T. cruzi, L. monocytogenes, Plasmodium* species, *Pneumocystis carinii* or *Mycobacterium* species, the systemic administration of IFN-γ resulted in control of the infection [see review in: 133]. Although activated macrophages are considered the effector cells in the defense mechanisms against the above microorganisms, the involvement of activated neutrophils can not be excluded. Furthermore, since IFN-γ inhibits the *in vitro* proliferation of murine Th2 clones [134] and IL-10 production by monocytes [135] and administration of anti-IFN-γ results in a Th2 (non-protective) cytokine response in *C. albicans* infected mice [136], it is suggested that IFN-γ may alter the T-helper cytokine balance in favor of the Th1 (protective) cytokines.

Recent studies demonstrated the protective role of IL-1, TNF-α and CSFs in experimental infections from Gram-positive and Gram-negative bacteria [review in: 136]. In addition, the involvement of IL-1 in resistance against *P. carinii* was recently shown using a SCID mice model and reconstitution with immunocompetent cells [138]. Anti-IL-1 monoclonal antibodies completely inhibited clearance of the microorganism [138]. Similary, IL-1 was shown to participate in the development of anti-*Listeria* immune responses in normal and SCID mice, without an enhancement of IFN-γ production from NK cells [50]. The mechanisms of the protection effect of IL-1 in these infections were not elucidated.

Immunotherapy in human Leishmaniasis. In 1926 Montenegro advocated that the injection of killed *Leishmania* in the skin not only recalled the "cutis reaction, but helped to heal chronic lesions" [139]. Recently Convit, *et al.*, reported on an immunotherapy using heat-killed *Leishmania* promastigotes and live BCG in Venezuelan patients with localized cutaneous leishmaniasis [140]. In a randomized trial, three vaccinations over 32 weeks gave cure rates (94%) similar to that of pentavalent antimony. Preliminary results in Brazil indicate similar responses, however the length of time for healing is 2.5 times as long as with antimony (personal communication, David J).

Ifn-γ and VL IFN-γ enhances the antimicrobial capacity of macrophages toward many microbial pathogens [141, 142 and reviewed in Table 2]. We have

Table 2. Interferon-γ enhancement of macrophage antimicrobial activity

Giardia lamblia	Human Mϕ	Belocevitc M. 1992 [80]
T. gondii	Murine Mϕ	Langermans JA. 1992 [81]
	Mice	McCabe RE. 1984 [82]
	Mice	Suzuki Y. 1988 [83]
Candida albicans	Human Mϕ	Vecchiarelli A. 1991 [84]
	Mϕ cell line	Blasi E. 1990 [85]
L. pneumophila	Human Mϕ	Nash TW. 1984 [86]
	Human Mϕ	Byrd TF. 1989 [87]
S. typhimurium	Human Mϕ	Kagaya K. 1989 [88]
	Murine Mϕ	Edwards CK. 1992 [89]
M. tuberculosis	Murine Mϕ	Flesch I. 1987 [90]
	Murine Mϕ	Flesch I. 1988 [91]
M. avium-intracellulare	Mice	Edwards CK. 1986 [92]
M. leprae	Human	Nathan CF. 1986 [93]
L. monocytogenes	Mice	Buchmeier NA. 1985 [94]
	Mice	Kiderlen AF. 1984 [95]
L. donovani	Murine Mϕ	Murray HW. 1985 [96]
	Human Mϕ	Murray HW. 1983 [97]
L. major	Murine Mϕ	Wyler DJ. 1987 [98]
	Murine Mϕ	Nelson BJ. 1991 [99]
L. mexicana	Human Mo	Murray HW. 1984 [100]
L. m. amazonensis	Human Mϕ	Ho JL. 1990 [101]
T. cruzi	Mice	Reed SG. 1988 [102]
Paracoccidiodes brasiliensis	Human Mϕ	Brummer E. 1988 [103]
Blastomyces dermatitidis	Human Mϕ	Brummer E. 1988 [103]

successfully utilized recombinant human IFN-γ with pentavalent antimony in the therapy of VL patients who had failed treatment with Sb^5 alone [143] and in patients with DCL [108]. Our first use of IFN-γ was in an 8-year-old girl with severe VL [142] refractory to antimony therapy. The subsequent studies of IFN-γ and Sb^5 therapy were in patients either previously untreated (n = 17) or refractory (n = 22). The refractory patients had remained seriously ill with persistence of *Leishmania* in splenic aspirates, despite previously receiving one or more 20 day courses of Sb^5 therapy. The untreated patients also were difficult cases with symptoms for > 6 months, hemoglobin < 9 g/dl and total white blood cell counts < 4,000 mm^3. The trials were open with IFN-γ/100 $\mu g/M^2$/daily and Sb^5 20 mg/kg/day for 20 days. An overall cure rate of 94% and 59% respectively for previously untreated patients and refractory cases was defined with a minimum of 6 months' follow-up. The immediate post-therapy clinical and parasitologic response rate, as defined by absence of symptoms and negative splenic aspirates, was 94% (16/17) in previously untreated VL patients and was 82% (18/22) in refractory VL cases [144]. During a 6 month follow-up period, clinical and parasitologic relapses were confirmed in 8/18 patients from the refractory group and in 1/16 patients who had not received prior therapy. Seven of the 9 patients were retreated with the same IFN-γ and Sb^5 protocol; 4 responded and have remained asymptomatic for > 1 year. These results are the best reported for such difficult cases [144]. Comparing the clinical efficacy of IFN-γ treatment in these patients with a historical control group consisting of 87 patients treated with only Sb^5 in the same hospital as the study patients, treatment with IFN-γ improved therapeutic outcome. While 74% of patients receiving IFN-γ and Sb^5 were treated successfully with < 20 days of combined therapy, only 43% of the controls responded to antimony alone within 20 days [108].

Studies in India and in Kenya have subsequently confirmed these results in both refractory and previously untreated VL patients [145, 146]. These studies

Table 3. Cytokine enhancement of macrophage antimicrobial activity

IL-1β & -α	*Candida albicans*	Mϕ cell line	Blasi E. 1990 [85]
		Mice	Kullberg BJ. 1990 [109]
	T. gondii	Mice	Chang HR. 1990 [110]
	S. aureus	Mice	Gladue R. 1988 [111]
	B. abortus	Mice	Zhan YF. 1991 [112]
	L. amazonensis	Human Mϕ	Hatzigeorgiou D & Ho JL. 1993 [113]
TNF-α	*M. tuberculosis*	Human Mϕ	Denis M. 1990 [114]
	M. avium-intracellulare	Human Mϕ	Denis M. 1991 [115]
	L. monocytogenes	Murine Mϕ	Denis M. 1990 [116]
		Mice	Havell EA. 1987 [117]
	Candida albicans	Mϕ cell line	Blasi E. 1990 [85]
	Chlamydia trachomatis	Cell line	Holtmann H. 1990 [118]
	L. major	Murine Mϕ	Bogdan C. 1990 [119]
		Murine Mϕ	Liew FY. 1990 [120]
	L. amazonensis	Human Mϕ	Ho JL. 1992 [121]
	T. cruzi	Cell line	Munoz-Fernandez AM. 1992 [122]
GM-CSF	CSF and resistance to acute infections		Metcalf D. 1987 [123]
	L. donovani	Human Mϕ	Weiser WY. 1987 [124]
	L. major	Murine Mϕ	Handman E. 1979 [125]
	L. amazonensis	Human Mϕ	Ho JL. 1990 [101]
		Human Mϕ	Ho JL. 1992 [121]
	T. cruzi	Human Mϕ	Reed SG. 1987 [126]
	M. avium-intracellulare	Human Mϕ	Bermudez LE. 1987 [127]
		Human Mϕ	Denis M. 1991 [128]
	T. gondi	Murine Mϕ	Nathan CF. 1984 [129]
	L. pneumophila	Human Mϕ	Jensen WA. 1988 [130]
M-CSF	*L. major*	Murine Mϕ	Ralph P. 1983 [131]
	L. amazonensis	Human Mϕ	Ho JL. 1990 [132]
IL-3	*L. amazonensis*	Human Mϕ	Ho JL. 1992 [121]
		Human Mϕ	Ho JL. 1992 [132]

also demonstrated more rapid parasitologic clearance in IFN-γ treated patients compared to those receiving only Sb^5. There are also two case reports of visceral leishmaniasis in AIDS patients which responded to combination IFN-γ and Sb^5 therapy [147].

Ifn-γ and DCL. Six DCL patients showed clinical improvement while receiving IFN-γ and Sb^5. In the 1 DCL patient who has completed treatment, skin lesions resolved with the development of a positive *Leishmania* skin test. Our preliminary experience with these patients is too limited to assess its therapeutic potential [143, 144].

Gm-csf and VL. GM-CSF enhances macrophage killing of *Leishmania* [100] and is also a multipotential growth factor of marrow stem cells [123]. It reverses neutropenia in cancer patients after chemotherapy and reduces complications such as pneumonia in neutropenic patients (p70). Our preliminary studies of GM-CSF and Sb^5 in VL patients indicate that patients with severe neutropenia resulting from VL may benefit from concomitant GM-CSH therapy.

Severe VL is associated with pancytopenia and the complications of bleeding and secondary infections. In a prospective study, bacterial nosocomial infection occurred in 14 of 18 (77%) patients with neutrophils (PMN) $< 1500/mm^3$ [149] while 6 of 12 developed bacterial infections with PMN $> 1500/mm_3$. This led us to evaluate the potential benefits of recombinant GM-CSF and document safety [150]. We studied the effect of GM-CSF in combination with one-half of the usual dose of Sb^5 against full dose Sb^5 in 20 VL patients (Badaro R, Reed S, Ho JL, *et al.* [151]). All patients had < 1500 PMN/mm^3 at entry. PMN counts significantly increased in the GM-CSF group compared to the antimony alone group ($p<0.001$). In addition, viral and bacterial nosocomial infections occurred in 8/10 patients in the Sb^5 placebo group, compared with 3/10 in the GM-CSF/Sb^5 group ($p<0.05$).

The availability of reverse transcriptase-cDNA PCR technology allowed the study of Th1/Th2 cytokine predominance in splenic cells of VL patients. Three patients studied by this technique in the randomized trial of GM-CSF and antimony have demonstrated clear shift from Th2 to a Th1 profile in one patient after receiving GM-CSF/Sb^5 for 10 days compared to 2 patients receiving Sb^5 alone. The GM-CSF patient had large amounts of IFN-γ and little IL-10 while 2 patients receiving only Sb^5 had IL-10 but no IFN-γ detected. Although both patients who received Sb^5 for 20 days were cured (parasite index of 0), both relapsed within 6 months of follow-up.

Future directions in therapy of leishmaniasis

Outpatient therapy

The aim for management of leishmaniasis in endemic areas is early diagnosis and therapy. Since persons diagnosed with subclinical disease or early acute visceral leishmaniasis are more likely to respond to therapy, it is imperative that diagnostic assays to discriminate prior infection from subclinical or early acute disease be developed. Preliminary data using a newly cloned *L. donovani* antigen, K39, suggest that presence of antibodies to this antigen using an EIA assay correlates with either subclinical or acute leishmaniasis (S.G. Reed and R. Badaro, personal communications). This antigen is currently being evaluated in larger samples of persons from different geographic regions of the world.

Individuals with less advanced illness may benefit from outpatient therapy with an oral agent along with subcutaneous injections of cytokines, such as IFN-γ and GM-CSF. Ketoconazole is one such agent. Initially developed as an antifungal drug to replace amphotericin B, it has demonstrated efficacy in cutaneous leishmaniasis [152, 153] and may be useful in visceral leishmaniasis. Two recent reports described 14 Indian patients treated with ketoconazole 600 mg daily for four weeks, after failure of prior antimony and pentamidine (4 cases). Ten of 14 (71%) patients were parasitologically cured after completion of therapy. Long term follow-up information was not provided. Allopurinol may be an alternative drug since it has been used in cutaneous disease. However, the response to allopurinol in visceral patients is poor with cure rates of 26% [154–156]. From these studies, a strategy of oral with subcutaneous administration of IFN-γ or GM-CSF may be a feasible alternative to the more toxic standard regimen of parenteral antimony.

Cytokine antagonists as adjuvant in therapy of leishmaniasis. Further studies in human leishmaniasis may confirm the murine model of Th2 cytokine imbalance in leishmaniasis. The opportunities to better define the immune response is presented in treatment of persons with acute visceral leishmaniasis. Confirmation of Th2 cytokine imbalance being associated with acute leishmaniasis may lead to studies to disrupt cytokine mediated immunopathology. Molecular biology approach has allowed the cloning and expression of an array of cytokine antagonists and soluble receptors. These recombinant molecules may be tested for their theraputic efficacy in leishmaniasis. Receptor antagonists or soluble receptors may be used in conjunction with agents that either enhance macrophage antimicrobial activity or are directly active against *Leishmania*. Therapeutically, the goals are to develp sensitive and specific diagnostic assays for early disease and to improve efficacy and decrease toxicity, duration and cost of therapy. For those at risk for infection, the development of effective and affordable vaccines is a goal of current research efforts.

Acknowledgements

This work was supported in part by the Department of Medicine, CUMC and by grants from the National Institutes of Health, AI-16282, R37–22624, TW-00018 and T32-AI-07458; Dr. Hatzigeogiou was supported in part by the "Stavaros S. Niarchos" Endowment to the Division of International Medicine.

References

1. Desjeux P. Information on the epidemiology and control of the leishmaniases by country or territory. Geneva: World Health Organization 1991; WHO/LEISH/91.30.

2. Ashford RW, Desjeux P, deRaadt P. Estimation of population at risk of infection and number of cases of leishmaniasis. Parasitology Today 1992: 104–105.
3. Lainson R, Shaw JJ. Epidemiology and ecology of leishmaniasis in Latin America. Nature 1978; 273: 595–600.
4. Marsden PD. Selective primary health care: strategies for control of disease in the developing world. XIV. Leishmaniasis. Rev Inf Dis 1984; 6: 736–744.
5. Gustafson TL, Reed CM, McGreevy PB, Pappas MG, Fox JC, Lawyer PG. Human cutaneous leishmaniasis acquired in Texas. Am J Trop Med Hyg 1985; 34: 50–63.
6. Badaro R, Jones TC, Carvalho EM, Sampaio D, Reed SG, Barral A, Teixeira R, Johnson WD Jr. New perspectives on a subclinical form of visceral leishmaniasis. J Infec Dis 1986; 154(6): 1003–10.
7. Marsden PD, Jones TC. Clinical manifestations, diagnosis and treatment of leishmaniasis. In: Chang KP, Bray RS, editors. Leishmaniasis. Amsterdam: Elsevier 1986.
8. Pearson RD, de Queiroz Sousa A. Leishmaniasis species (kala-azar, cutaneous and mucocutaneous leishmaniasis). In:Mandel GL, Douglas RG, Bennett JE, editors. Principles and Practice of Infectious Diseases. New York: John Wiley & Sons, 1985: 1522–1531.
9. Jones TC, Johnson WD Jr, Baretto A, Lago E, Badaro R, Cerf B, Reed SG, Netto EM, Tada MS, Franca F, Weise K, Golightly L, Fikrig E, Costa JMM, Cuba CG, Marsden PD. Epidemiology of American cutaneous leishmaniasis due to *Leishmania* brasiliensis brasiliensis. J Infect Dis 1987; 156: 73–83.
10. Marsden PD, Sampaio RN, Gomes LF, Costa JM, Netto EM, Viega EP, Llanos-Cuentas EA. Lone laryngeal leishmaniasis. Trans R Soc Trop Med Hyg 1985; 79: 424.
11. Bryceson ADM. Diffuse cutaneous leishmaniasis in Ethiopia: II. Treatment. Trans R Soc Trop Med Hyg 1970; 64: 369–379.12.
12. World Health Organization. TDR News 1991; 37: 1–2.
13. Barral A, Pedral-Sampaio D, Grimaldi G Jr, Momen H, McMahon-Pratt D, de Jesus AR, Almeida R, Badaro R, Barral-Netto M, Carvalho EM, Johnson WD Jr. Leishmaniasis in Bahia, Brazil: Evidence that *Leishmania* amazonensis produces a wide spectrum of clinical disease. Amer J Trop Med Hyg 1991; 44: 536–546.
14. Magill AJ, Grogl M, Gassner RA, Sun W, Oster CN. Visceral infection caused by *Leishmania tropica* in veterans of operation Desert Storm. N Engl J Med 1993; 328: 1383–7.
15. Jha TK. Evaluation of diamidine compounds (pentamidine isethionate) in the treatment of resistant cases of kala-azar occuring in North Bihar, India. Trans R Soc Trop Med Hyg 1983; 77: 167–170.
16. Thakur CP, Kumar M, Pandey AK. Comparison of regimens of treatment of antimony-resistant kala-azar patients: a randomized study. Am J Trop Med Hyg 1991; 45: 435–441.
17. Bryceson ADM, Chulay JD, Mugambi M, Were JB, Gachihi G, Chunge CN, Muigai R, Bhatt SM, Ho M, Spencer HC, Meme J, Anabwani G. Visceral leishmaniasis unresponsive to antimonial drugs. II. Response to high-dosage of sodium stibogluconate or prolonged treatment with pentamidine. Trans R Soc Trop Med Hyg 1985; 79: 705–714.
18. Grogl M, Odula AMJ, Cordero LDC, Kyle DE. *Leishmania* SPP: Development of pentostam-resistant clones *in vitro* by discontinuous drug exposure. Exp Parasitol 1989; 69: 78–90.
19. Grogl M, Thomason TN, Franke ED. Drug resistance in leishmaniasis: its implication in systemic chemotherapy of cutaneous and mucocutaneous disease. Am J Trop Med Hyg 1992; 47: 117–126.
20. Carvalho EM, Badaro R, Reed SG, Johnson WD Jr, Jones TC. Absence of gamma interferon and interleukin 2 production during active visceral leishmaniasis. J Clin Invest 1985; 76: 2066–9.
21. Holaday BJ, Pompoe MML, Evans T, Braga DNM, Texeira MJ, Sousa AQ, Sadick MD, Vasconcelos AW, Abrams JS, Person RD, Locksley RM. Correlates of *Leishmania*-Specific Immunity in the clinical spectrum of Infection with *Leishmania chagasi*. J Infect Dis 1993; 167: 411–7.
22. Ho JL, Badaro R, Schwartz A, Dinarello CA, Geifand JA, Sobel J, Barral A, Barral-Netto M, Carvalho EM, Reed SG, Johnson WD Jr. Diminished *in vitro* production of interleukin-1 and tumor necrosis factor-alpha during acute visceral leishmaniasis and recovery after therapy. J Infect Dis 1992; 165: 1094–1102.
23. Carvalho EM, Barral A, Pedral-Sampaio D, Barral-Netto M, Badaro R, Rocha H, Johnson WD Jr. Immunologic markers of clinical evolution in children recently infected with *Leishmania donovani chagasi*. J Infect Dis 1992; 165: 535–40.
24. Pirmez C, Yamamura M, Uyemura K, Paes-Oliveira M, Conceicao-Silva F, Modlin RL. Cytokine Patterns in the Pathogenesis of Human Leishmaniasis. J Clin Invest 1993; 91: 1390–5.
25. Carvalho EM, Johnson WD, Barreto E, Marsden PD, Costa JLM, Reed SG, Rocha H. Cell mediated immunity in American cutaneous and mucosal leishmaniasis. J Immunol 1985; 135: 4144–8.
26. Reed SG, Scott P. T cell and cytokine responses in leishmaniasis. Cur Op Immunol(in press).
27. Sher A, Gazzineli T, Oswald IP, Clericy M, Kullberg M, Pearce J, Berzofisky JA, Mosmann TR, James SL, Morse HC, Shearer GM. Role of T-cell derived cytokines in the down-regulation of immune responses in parasitic and retroviral infection. Immunol Rev 1992; 127: 183–204.
28. Mossman TR, Coffman RL. Thl and Th2 cells: different patterns of lymphocyte secretion lead to different functional properties. Ann Rev Immunol 1989; 7: 145–73.
29. Locksley RM, Scott P. Helper T-cell subsets in mouse leishmaniasis: induction, expansion, and effector function. Immunol Today 1991; 12: A58–A61.
30. Kaye PM, Curry AJ, Blackwell JM. Differential production of Th1- and Th2-derived cytokines does not determine the genetically controlled or vaccine-induced rate of cure in murine visceral leishmaniasis. J Immunol 1991; 146: 2763–2770.
31. Caceres-Dittmar G, Tapia FJ, Sanchez MA, Yamamura M, Uyemura K, Modlin RL, Bloom BR, Convit J. Determination of the Cytokine Profile in American Cutaneous Leishmaniasis Using the Polymerase Chain Reaction. Clin Exp Immunol 1993; 91: 500–505.
32. Aponso LCC, Scott P. Immune responses associated with susceptibility of C56BL/10 mice to *Leishmania amazonensis*. Infect Immun (in press).
33. Scott P. IFN-γ Modulates the Early Development of Th1 and Th2 Responses in a Murine Model of Cutaneous Leishmaniasis. J Immunol 1991; 147: 3149–3155.
34. Varkla K, Chatelain R, Leal LMCC, Coffman RL. Reconstitution of C.B-17 SCID mice with BALB/c T cells initiates a T helper type-1 reponse and renders them capable of healing *Leishmania* major infection. Eur J Immunol 1992; 23: 262–268.
35. Karp CL, El-Saji SH, Wynn TA, Satti MMH, Kordojani HM, Hashim FA, Hag-Ali M, Neva FA, Nutman TB, Sacks DL.

In vivo cytokine profiles in patients with kala-azar: Marked elevation of both Interleukin 10 and Interferon-gamma. J Clin Invest 1993; 91: 1644–8.
36. Ghalib HG, Piuvezam MR, Skeiky YAW, Siddig M, Hashim FA, El-Hassan AM, Russo DM, Reed SG. Interleukin 10 production correlates with pathology in human *Leishmania donovani* infections. J Clin Invest (in press).
37. Morris L, Troutt AB, Handman E, Kelso A. 1992 Changes in the precursor frequencies of IL-4 and IFN-secreting CD4+ cells correlate with resolution of lesions in murine cutaneous leishmaniasis. J Immunol 149:2715–2721.
38. Chatelain R, Varkila K, Coffman RL. IL-4 Induces a Th2 response in *Leishmania* major-infected mice. J Immunol 1992; 148: 1182–1187.
39. Sadick MD, Heinzel FP, Hodaday BJ, Pu RT, Dawkins RS, Locksley RM. Cure of murine leishmaniasis with Anti-interleukin 4 monoclonal antibody: evidence for a T Cell-dependent, Interferon-c-independent mechanism. J Exp Med 1990; 171: 115–127.
40. Leal LM, Moss DW, Kuhn R, Muller W, Liew FY. Interleukin-4 transgenic mice of resistant background are susceptible to *Leishmania* major infection. Eur J Immunol 1993; 23: 566–569.
41. Tobin JF, Reiner SL, Hatam F, Zheng S, Leptak CL, Wirth DF, Locksley RM. Trangenic *Leishmania* expressing biologically active interferon-gamma. J Immunol (in press).
42. Scharton TM, Scott P. Natural Killer Cells are a Source of IFN-γ that drives differentiation of CD4+ T Cell subsets and induces early resistance to *Leishmania* major in Mice. J Exp Med (in press).
43. Kaye PM, Bancroft GJ. *Leishmania donovani* infection in SCID mice: lack of tissue response and *in vivo* macrophage activation correlates with failure to trigger natural killer cell-derived interferon production *in vitro*. Infect Immun 1992; 60: 4335–4342.
44. Trinchieri G, D'Andrea A, Rengaraju M, Valiante NM, Kubin M, Aste M, Chehimi J. Natural killer cell stimulatory factor (NKSF) or Interleukin-12: A heterodimeric cytokine produced by accessory cells and with regulatory functions on T and NK cell responses. Prog Growth Factor Res (in press).
45. Hsieh CY, Macatonia SE, Tripp CS, Wolff SF, O'Garra A, Murphy KM. Development of Thl CD4+ T cells through IL-12 produced by *Listeria*-induced macrophages. Science 1993; 260: 547–9.
46. Henzel FP, Rerko RM, Hatam F, Locksley RM. IL-2 is necessary for the progession of leishmaniasis in susceptible murine hosts. J Immunol 1993; 150: 3924–3931.
47. Heinzel FP, Schoenhaut DS, Rerko RM, Rosser LE, Gately MK. Recombinant Interleukin 12 cures mice infected with *Leishmania major*. J Exp Med 1993; 177: 1505.
48. Sypek JP, Chung CL, Mayor SEH, Subramanyam JM, Goldman SJ, Sieburth DS, Wolf SF, Schaub RG. Resolution of cutaneous leishmaniasis: interleukin 12 initiates a protective T helper type 1 immune response. J Exp Med 1993; 177: 1797–805.
49. Tripp CS, Wolf SF, Unanue ER. Interleukin 12 and tumor necrosis factor-α are costimulators of interferon-γ production by natural killer cells in severe combined immunodeficiency mice with listeriosis, and interleukin 10 is a physiologic antagonist. J Immunol 1993; 90: 3725–9.
50. Rogers HW, Sheehan KC, Brunt LM, Dower SK, Unanue ER, Schreiber RD. Interleukin 1 participates in the development of anti-*Listeria* response in normal and SCID mice. Proc Natl Acad Sci (USA) 1992; 89: 1011–15.
51. Scott P. IL-12: initiation cytokine for cell-mediated immunity. Science 1993; 260: 496–7.
52. Le Gros G, Ben-Sasson SZ, Seder R, Finkelman FD, Paul WE. Generation of IL-4 producing cells *in vivo* and *in vitro*: IL-2 and IL-4 are required for *in vitro* generation of IL-4-producing cells. J Exp Med 1990; 172: 921–9.
53. Conrad DH, Ben-Sasson SZ, Le Gros G, Finkelman FD, Paul WE. Infection with *Nippostrongylus braziliensis* or injection of anti-IgD antibodies markedly enhances Fc-receptor-mediated IL-4 production by non-B, non-T cells. J Exp Med 1990; 171: 1497–508.
54. Maggi E, Parronchi P, Manetti R, Simonelli C, Piccinni MP, Rugiu FS, De Carli M, Ricci M, Romagnani S. Reciprocal regulatory effect of IFN-γ and IL-4 on the *in vitro* development of human Thl and Th2 clones. J Immunol 1992; 148: 2142–7.
55. Parronchi P, DeCarli M, Manetti R, Simonelli C, Sampognaro S, Piccinni MP, Macchia D, Maggi E, Del Prete GF, Romagnani S. IL-4 and IFNs (α and γ) exerts opposite regulatory effects on the development of cytolytic potential by Thl or Th2 human T cell clones. J Immunol 1992; 149: 2977–83.
56. Manetti R, Parronchi P, Giudizi MG, Piccinni MP, Maggi E, Trinchieri G, Romagnani S. Natural killer cell stimulatory factor (IL-12) induces T helper type 1 (Th1)- specific immune responses and inhibits the development of IL-4-producing Th cells. J Exp Med 1993; 177: 1199–204.
57. Alwan WH, Record FM, Openshaw PJM. Phenotype and functional characterization of T cell lines specific for individual respiratory syncytial virus proteins. J Immunol 1993; 150: 5211–8.
58. Yang X, Gieni RS, Mosmann TR, HayGlass KT. Chemically modified antigen preferentially elicits induction of Th1-like cytokine synthesis patterns *in vivo*. J Exp Med 1993; 178: 349–53.
59. McNeely TB, Turco S. Requirements of lipophosphoglycan for intracellular survival of *Leishmania* donovani within human monocytes. J Immunol 1990; 144: 2745–50.
60. Reiner NE. Parasite accessory cell interaction in murine leishmaniasis. I. Evasion and stimulus-dependent suppression of the macrophage interleukin 1 response by *Leishmania donovani*. J Immunol 1989; 138: 1919–25.
61. Reiner NE, Winnie Ng, Wilson CB, McMaster R, Burchett SK. Modulation of *in vitro* monocyte cytokine response to *Leishmania donovani*. Interferon-γ prevents parasite-induced inhibition of interleukin-1 production and primes monocytes to respond to *leishmania* by producing both tumor necrosis factor-α and interleukin-1. J Clin Invest 1990; 85: 1914–24.
62. Olivier M, Brownsey RW, Reiner NE. Defective stimulus-response coupling in human monocytes infected with *Leishmania donovani* is associated with altered activation and translocation of protein kinase C. Proc Natl Acad Sci USA 1992; 89: 7481–5.
63. McNeely TB, Turco S. Inhibition of PKC activity by *Leishmania donovani* lipophosphoglycan. Biochem Biophys Res Comm 1987; 148: 653.
64. Fruth U, Solioz N, Louis JA. *Leishmania major* interfers with antigen presentation by infected macrophages. J Immunol 1993; 150: 1857–64.
65. Descoteaux A, Turco S, Sacks DL, Matlashewski G. *Leishmania donovani* lipophosphoglycan selectively inhibits signal transduction in macrophages. J Immunol 1991; 146: 2747–53.

66. Descoteaux A, Matlashewski G. c-fos and tumor necrosis factor gene expression in *Leishmania donovani*-infected macrophages. Molec & Cell Biol 1989; 9: 5223–7.
67. Hatzigeorgiou DH, Zhang Y, Turco S, Rom WN, Ho JL. Lipophosphoglycan from *Leishmania donovani* down-regulates IL-1β gene expression in THP-1 cells. Clin Res 1993; 322A.
68. Bretscher PA, Wei G, Menon JN, Bielefeldt-Ohmann H. Establishment of stable, cell-mediated immunity that makes "susceptible" mice resistant to *Leishmania major*. Science 1992; 257: 540–4.
69. Rachamin N, Jaffe CL. Pure protein from *Leishmania donovani* protects mice against both cutaneous and visceral leishmaniasis. J Immunol 1993; 150: 2322–31.
70. Wahl SM. Transforming growth factor beta in inflammation: a cause and a cure. J Clin Immunol 1992; 12: 61–74.
71. Roberts AB, Sporn MB. Transforming growth factor-β. Adv Can Res 1988; 51: 107–145.
72. Wahl SM, Hunt DA, Bansal G, McCartney-Francis N, Ellingsworth L, Allen JB. Bacterial cell wall-induced immunosuppression: role of transforming growth factor-β. J Exp Med 1988; 168: 1403–1417.
73. Barral-Netto M, Barral A, Brownell CE, Skeiky YAW, Ellingsworth LR, Twardzik DR, Reed SG. Transforming Growth Factor-b in Leishmanial Infection: A Parasite Escape Mechanism. Science 1992; 257: 545–548.
74. Barral A, Barral-Netto M, Yong EC, Brownell CE, Twardzik D, Reed SG. Transforming Growth Factor-b as a Virulence Mechanism for *Leishmania braziliensis*. Proc Nat Acad Sci USA 1993; 90: 3442–3446.
75. Ding A, Nathan CF, Graycar J, Derynck R, Stuehr DJ, Srimal S. Macrophage deactivating factor and transforming growth factors-b1, -b2, and -b3 inhibit induction of macrophage nitrogen oxide synthesis by IFN-gamma. J Immunol 1990; 145: 940.
76. Erard F, Wild M-T, Garcia-Sanz JA, LeGros G. Switch of CD8 T cells to noncytolytic CD8-VD4- cells that make Th2 cytokines and help B cells. Science 1993; 260: 1802–5
77. Nathan CF, Horowitz CR, de la Harp J, Vadhan-Raj S, Sherwin SA, Oettgen HF, Krown SE. Administration of recombinant interferon-γ to cancer patients enhances monocyte secretion of hydrogen peroxide. Proc Natl Acad Sci USA 1985; 82: 8686–90.
78. Nathan CF. Nitric oxide as a secretory product of mammalian cells. FASEB J 1992; 6: 3051–64.
79. Ho JL. Antimicrobial activity of macrophages. In: Klempner MS, Styrt B, Ho JL, editors. Phagocyte and Diseases. New York: Plenum Press, 1989; pp. 59–90
80. Belosevíc M, Daniels CW. Phagocytosis of *Giardia lamblia* trophozoites by cytokine-activated macrophages. Clin Exp Immunol 1992; 87: 304–9.
81. Langermans JAM, van der Hulst MEB, Nibbering PH, Hiemstra PS, Fransen L, van Furth R. IFN-γ-induced L-arginine-dependent toxoplasmastatic activity in murine peritoneal macrophages is mediated by endogenous tumor necrosis factor-γ. J Immunol 1992; 148: 568–74.
82. McCabe RE, Meagher SG, Mullins BT. Endogenous interferon-γ, macrophage activation, and murine host defense against acute infection with *Trypanosoma cruzi*. J Infect Dis 1984; 163: 912–5.
83. Suzuki Y, Orellana MA, Schreiber RD, Remington JS. Interferon-γ: the major mediator of resistance against *Toxoplasma gondii*. Science 1988; 240: 516–8.
84. Vecchiarelli A, Dottorini M, Puliti M, Todisco T, Cenci E, Bistoni F. Defective candidal activity of alveolar macrophages and peripheral blood monocytes from patients with chronic obstructive pulmonary disease. Am Rev Resp Dis 1991; 143: 1049–54.
85. Blasi E, Farinelli S, Varesio L, Bistoni F. Augmentation of GG2EE macrophage cell-line-mediated anti-*Candida* activity by γ-interferon, tumor necrosis factor, and interleukin-1. Infect Immun 1990; 58: 1073–7.
86. Nash TW, Libby DM, Horwitz MA. Interaction between the legionnaires' disease bacterium (*Legionella pneumophila*) and human alveolar macrophages. Influence of antibody, lymphokines, and hydrocortisone. J Clin Invest 1984; 74: 771–82.
87. Byrd TF, Horwitz M. Interferon-γ-activated human monocytes downregulate transferrin receptors and inhibit the intracellular multiplication of *Legionella pneumophila* by limiting the availability of iron. J Clin Invest 1989; 83: 1457–65.
88. Kagaya K, Watanabe K, Fukazawa Y. Capacity of recombinant γ-interferon to activate macrophages for *Salmonella*-killing activity. Infect Immun 1989; 57: 609–15.
89. Edwards CK, Ghiasuddin SM, Yunger LM, Lorence RM, Arkins S, Dantzer R, Kelley KW. *In vivo* administration of recombinant growth hormone or γ-interferon activates macrophages: enhanced resistance to experimental *Salmonella typhimurinum* infection is correlated with generation of reactive oxygen intermedialtes. Infect Immun 1992; 60: 2514–21.
90. Flesch I, Kaufmann SHE. Mycobacterium growth inhibition by interferon-γ-activated bone marrow macrophages and differential susceptibility among strains of *Mycobacterium tuberculosis*. J Immunol 1987; 138: 4408–13.
91. Flesch I, Kaufmann SHE. Attempts to characterize the mechanisms involved in mycobacterial growth inhibition by γ-interferon-activated bone marrow macrophages. Infect Immun 1988; 56: 1464–9.
92. Edwards CK, Hedegaard HB, Zlotnik A, Gangadharam PR, Johnson RB, Pabst MJ. Chronic infection due to *Mycobacterium intracellulare* in mice: association with macrophage release of prostaglandin E_2 and reversal by injection of indomethacin, muramyl peptide, or interferon-γ. J Immunol 1986; 136: 1820–7.
93. Nathan CF, Kaplan G, Levis WR, Nusrat A, Witmer MD, Sherwin SA, Job CK, Horowitz CR, Steinman RM, Cohn ZA. Local and systemic effects of intradermal recombinant interferon-γ in patients with lepromatous leprosy. N Engl J Med 1986; 316: 6–15.
94. Buchmeier NA, Schreiber RD. Requirement of endogenous interferon-γ production for resolution of *Listeria monocytogenes* infection. Proc Natl Acad Sci USA 1985; 82: 7404–8.
95. Kiderlen AF, Kaufmann SHE, Lohmann-Matthes M-L. Protection of mice against the intracellular bacterium *Listeria monocytogenes* by recombinant immune interferon. Eur J Immunol 1984; 14: 964–7.
96. Murray HW, Gellene RA, Libby DM, Rothermel CD, Rubin BY. Activation of tissue macrophages from AIDS patients: *in vitro* response of AIDS alveolar macrophages to lymphokines and interferon-γ. J Immunol 1985; 135: 2374–7.
97. Murray HW, Rubin BY, Rothermel CD. Killing of intracellular *Leishmania donovani* by lymphokine-stimulated human mononuclear phagocytes. Evidence that interferon-γ is the activating lymphokine. J Clin Invest 1983; 72: 1506–10.

98. Wyler DJ, Beller DI, Sypek JP. Macrophage activation for antileishmanial defense by an apparently novel mechanism. J Immunol 1987; 138: 1246–9.
99. Nelson BJ, Ralph P, Green SJ, Nacy CA. Differential susceptibility of activated macrophage cytotoxic effector reactions to the suppressive effects of transforming growth factor. J Immunol 1991; 146: 1849–57.
100. Murray HW, Rubin BY, Carriero S, Acosta AM. Reversible defect in antigen-induced lymphokine and γ-interferon generation in cutaneous leishmaniasis. J Immunol 1984; 133: 2250–54.
101. Ho JL, Reed SG, Wick E, Giordano M. Effect of granulocyte-monocyte colony stimulating factor (GM-CSF) on intramacrophage survival of *Leishmania mexicana amazonensis*. J Infect Dis 1990; 157: 925–33.
102. Reed SG. *In vivo* administration of recombinant IFN-γ induces macrophage activation, and prevents acute disease, immune suppression, and death in experimental *Trypanosoma cruzi* infections. J Immunol 1988; 140: 4342–7.
103. Brummer E, Hanson LH, Restrepo A, Stevens DA. *In vivo* and *in vitro* activation of pulmonary macrophages by IFN-γ for enhanced killing of *Paracoccidioides brasiliensis* or *Blastomyces dermatitides*. J Immunol 1988; 140: 2786–89.
104. Nathan CF, Murray HW, Wiebe ME, Rubin BY. Identification of interferon-γ as the lymphokine that activates human macrophage oxidative metabolism and antimicrobial activity. J Exp Med 1983; 158: 670–89.
105. Murray HW, Rubin BY, Rothermel C. Killing of intracellular *Leishmania donovani* by lymphokine-stimulated human mononuclear phagocytes. J Clin Invest 1983; 72: 1506–10.
106. Burmudez LE. Differential mechanisms of intracellular killing of *Mycobacterium avium* and *Listeria monocytogenes* by activated human and murine macrophages. The role of nitric oxide. Clin Exp Immunol 1993; 91: 277–81.
107. Cassatella MA, Bazzoni F, Flynn RM, Dusi S, Trinchieri G, Rossi F. Molecular basis of interferon-γ and lipopolysaccharide enhancement of phagocyte respiratory burst capacity. J Biol Chem 1990; 265: 20241–6.
108. Pfefferkorn ER. Interferon-γ blocks the growth of *Toxoplasma gondii* in human fibroblasts by inducing the host cells to degrade tryptophan. Proc Natl Acad Sci USA 1984; 81: 908–12.
109. Kullberg B-J, van't Wout JW, van Furth R. Role of granulocytes in increased host resistance to Candida albicans induced by recombinant interleukin-1. Infect Immun 1990; 58: 3319–24.
110. Chang HR, Grau GE, Pechere JC. Role of TNF and IL-1 in infections with *Toxoplasma gondii*. Immunol 1990; 69: 33–7.
111. Gladue R, Girard A, Newborg M. Enhanced antibacterial resistance in neutropenic mice treated with human recombinant interleukin-1β. Agents Actions 1988; 24: 130–6.
112. Zhan YF, Stanley ER, Cheers C. Prophylaxis or treatment of experimental Brucellosis with interleukin-1. Infect Immun 1991; 59: 1790–4.
113. Hatzigeorgiou DH, He SH, Sobel J, Hafner A, Grabstein K, Ho JL. Interleukin-6 down-modulates cytokine-enhanced antileishmanial killing. J Immunol 1993; 151: 3682–92.
114. Denis M, Gregg EO, Ghandirian E. Cytokine modulation of *Mycobacterium tuberculosis* growth in human macrophages. Int J Immunopharmac 1990; 12: 721–7.
115. Denis M. Tumor necrosis factor and granulocyte macrophage colony stimulating factor stimulate human macrophages to restrict growth of virulent *Mycobacterium avium* and to kill avirulent *M. avium*: killing effector mechanism depends on generation of reactive nitrogen intermediates. J Leukocyte Biol 1991; 49: 380–7.
116. Denis M, Gregg EO. Studies on cytokine activation of *Listerial* activity in murine macrophages. Can J Microl 1990; 36: 671–5.
117. Havell EA. Production of tumor necrosis factor during murine listeriosis. J Immunol 1987; 139: 4225–31.
118. Holtmann H, Shemer-Avni Y, Wessel K, Sarov I, Wallach D. Inhibition of growth of *Chlamydia trachomatis* by tumor necrosis factor is accompanied by increased prostaglandin synthesis. Infect Immun 1990; 58: 3168–72.
119. Bogdan C, Schroppel K, Lohoff M, Rollinghoff M, Solbach W. Immunization of susceptible host with a soluble antigen fraction from *Leishmania major* leads to aggravation of murine leishmaniasis mediated by CD4^{+} T cells. Eur J Immunol 1990; 20: 2533–40.
120. Liew FY, Li Y, Millott S. Tumor necrosis factor-α synergizes with IFN-γ in mediating killing of *Leishmania major* through the induction of nitric oxide. J Immunol 1990, 145: 4306–10.
121. Ho JL, He SH, Rios MJ, Wick EA. Interleukin-4 inhibits human macrophage activation by tumor necrosis factor-alpha, granulocyte macrophage colony stimulating factor and interleukin-3. J Infect Dis 1992; 165: 344–51.
122. Munoz-Fernandez, Fernandez MA, Fresno M. Synergism between tumor necrosis factor-α and interferon-γ on macrophage activation for the killing of intracellular *Trypanosoma cruzi* through a nitric oxide-dependent mechanism. Eur J Immunol 1992; 22: 301–7.
123. Metcalf D. The role of the colony-stimulating factors in resistance to acute infections. Immunol Cell Biol 1987; 65: 35–43.
124. Weiser WY, van Niel A, Clark SC, David JR, Remold HG. Recombinant human granulocyte/macrophage colony-stimulating factor activates intracellular killing of *Leishmania donovani* by human monocyte-derived macrophages. J Exp Med 1987; 166: 1436–46.
125. Handman E, Burgess AW. Stimulation by granulocyte-macrophage colony stimulating factor of *Leishmania tropica* killing by macrophage. J Immunol 1979; 122: 1134–7.
126. Reed SG, Nathan CF, Phil DL, Rodricks P, Shanebeck K, Conlon PJ, Grabstein KH. Recombinant granulocyte/macrophage colony-stimulating factor activates macrophages to inhibit *Trypanosoma cruzi* and release hydrogen peroxide: Comparison with interferon-γ. J Exp Med 1987; 166: 1734–46.
127. Bermudez LE, Young LS. Granulocyte-monocyte colony stimulating factor activates human macrophages to kill *Mycobacterium avium* complex. Clin Res 1987; 35: 612A.
128. Denis M, Gregg EO. Modulation of *Mycobacterium avium* growth in murine macrophages: reversal of unresponsiveness to interferon-γ by indomethacin or interleukin-4. J Leukocyte Biol 1991; 49: 65–72.
129. Nathan CF, Pendergast TJ, Wiebe ME, Stanley ER, Platzer E, Remold HG, Welte K, Rubin BY, Murray HW. Activation of human macrophages: comparison of other cytokines with interferon-γ. J Exp Med 1984; 160: 600–5.
130. Jensen WA, Rose RM, Burke RH, Anton K, Remold HG. Cytokine activation of antibacterial activity in human pulmonary macrophages: comparison of recombinant interferon-γ and granulocyte-macrophage colony-stimulating factor. Cell Immunol 1988; 117: 369–77.
131. Ralph P, Nacy CA, Meltzer MS, Williams N, Nakoinz I, Leonard EJ. Colony-stimulating factors and regulation of macrophage tumoricidal and microbicidal activities. Cell Immunol 1983; 76: 10–21.

132. Ho JL, Reed SG, Sobel J, Arruda S, He SH, Wick EA, Grabstein KH. Interleukin-3 augments human macrophage antimicrobial activity against *Leishmania amazonensis* and *Trypanosoma cruzi* and tumoricidal activity. Infect Immun 1992; 60: 1984–93.
133. Kullberg B-J, van't Wout JW, Hoogstraten C, van Furth R. Recombinant interferon-γ enhances resistance to acute disseminated *Candida albicans* infection in mice. J Infect Dis 1993; 168: 436–43.
134. Gajewski TF, Fitch FW. Anti-proliferative effect of IFN-γ in immune regulation. IFN-γ inhibits the proliferation of Th2 but not Th1 murine helper T lymphocyte clones. J Immunol 1988; 140: 4245–52.
135. Chomarat P, Rissoan M-C, Banchereau J, Miossec P. Interferon-γ inhibits interleukin 10 production by monocytes. J Exp Med 1993; 177: 523–7.
136. Romani L, Cenci E, Mencacci A, Spaccapelo R, Grohmann U, Puccetti P, Bistoni F. 1992 γ-Interferon modifies $CD4^+$ subset expression in murine candidiasis. Infect Immun 60: 4950–2.
137. Vogels HW, van der Meer JM. Use of immune modulators in non-specific therapy of bacterial infections. Antimicrob Agent Chemother 1992; 36: 1–5.
138. Chen W, Havell EA, Moldawer LL, McIntyre KW, Chizzonite RA, Harmsen AG. Interleukin-1: an important mediator of host resistance against *Pneumocytis carinii*. J Exp Med 1992; 176: 713–8.
139. Montenegro J. A cutireaco na leishmaniase. Ann Fac Med, Sao Paulo 1926; 1: 1-29.
140. Convit J, Castellanos PL, Rondon A, Pinardi ME, Ulrich M, Castes M, Bloom B, Garcia L. Immunothrapy vs. chemotherapy in localized cutaneous leishmaniasis. Lancet 1987; 1: 401-405.
141. Nathan CF, Kaplan G, Levis WR, Nusrat A, Witmer MD, Sherwin SA, Job CK, Horowitz CR, Steinman RM, Cohn ZA. Local and systemic effects of intradermal recombinant interferon gamma in patients with lepromatous leprosy. N Engl J Med 1986; 324: 509-516.
142. International Chronic Granulomatous Disease Cooperative Study Group. A controlled trial of interferon gamma to prevent infection in chronic granulomatous disease. N Engl J Med 1991; 324: 509-516.
143. Badaro R, Falcoff E, Badaro FS, Carvalho EM, Pedral-Sampiao D, Barral A, Carvalho JS, Barrel-Netto M, Brandely M, Silva L, Bina JC, Teixeira R, Falcoff R, Rocha H, Ho JL, Johnson WD Jr. N Engl J Med 1990; 322: 16–21.
144. Badaro R, Johnson WD Jr. The role of interferon-gamma in the treatment of visceral and diffuse cutaneous leishmaniasis. J Infect Dis 1993; 167(Suppl 1): S13-17.
145. Sundar S, Thakur A, Mishra A, Rosenkeimer F, Murray H. Immunochemotherapy for visceral leishmaniasis in India. Clin Res 1993; 41: 381.
146. Squires KE, Rosenkeimer F, Sherwood J, Forni AL, Were ZBO, Murray HW. Immunochemical therapy for visceral leishmaniasis: A controlled pilot trial of antimony vs. antimony plus interferon-gamma. J Infect Dis (in press).
147. de Gorgolas M, Casrillo JM, Guerrero JMF. Visceral leishmaniasis in patients with AIDS: report of three cases treated with pentavalent and IFN-γ. Clin Infect Dis 1993; 17: 56–9.
148. Lieske GJ, Burgess AW. Granulocyte colony stimulating factor and granulocyte-macrophage- colony stimulating factor. N Engl J Med 1992; 327: 99–106.
149. Andrade TM, Carvalho EM, Rocha H. Bacterial infections in patients with visceral leishmaniasis. J Infect Dis 1990; 162: 1354–9.
150. Badaro R, Carvalho JS, Badaro F, Nascimento C, Sobel J, Saito Y, Johnson WD Jr, Jones TJ. Cytokines in the management of leishmaniasis. In: van Furth R, editor. Hemopoietic Growth Factors and Mononuclear Phagocytes. Basel: S Karger, 1993, pp 111–122.
151. Badaro R, Nascimento C, Carvalho JS, Badaro F, Russo D, Ho JL, Reed SG, Johnson WD Jr, Jones TC. rhGM-CSF reverses neutropenia and reduces secondary infections in visceral leishmaniasis. (submitted)
152. Berman JD, Goad LJ, Beach DH, Holz GG Jr. Effects of ketoconazole on sterol biosynthesis by *Leishmania mexicana mexicana* amastigotes in murine macrophage tumor cells. Mol Biochem Parasitol 1986; 20: 85–92.
153. Saenz RE, Paz H, Berman JD. Efficacy of ketoconazole against *Leishmaniasis braziliensis paramensis* cutaneous leishmaniasis. Am J Med 1990; 89: 147–155.
154. Martinez S, Marr JJ. Allopurinol in the treatment of American cutaneous leishmaniasis. N Engl J Med 1992; 326: 741–744.
155. Jha TK. Evaluation of allopurinol in the treatment of kala-azar occuring in North Bihar, India. Trans R Soc Trop Med Hyg 1983; 77: 204–207.
156. Kager PA, Rees PH, Wellder BT, Hockmeyer WT, Lyerly WH. Allopurinol in the treatment of visceral leishmaniasis. Trans R Soc Trop Med Hyg 1981; 75: 556–559.

Address for correspondence: John L. Ho, M.D., Division of International Medicine, Room A431, Department of Medicine, Cornell University Medical College, 1300 York Avenue, New York, NY 10021, USA

Biotherapy 7: 237–247, 1994.

The role of cytokines in toxoplasmosis

Christopher A. Hunter, Carlos S. Subauste & Jack S. Remington
Division of Infectious Diseases and Geographic Medicine, Department of Medicine, Stanford University School of Medicine and Department of Immunology and Infectious Diseases, Palo Alto Medical Foundation, Research Institute, Palo Alto, California 94301, U.S.A.

Key words: Encephalitis, immunotherapy, interferon, interleukin, *Toxoplasma gondii*, tumor necrosis factor

Abstract

Infection with *Toxoplasma gondii* is normally asymptomatic, but as a consequence of the AIDS epidemic the incidence of symptomatic disease and especially toxoplasmic encephalitis (TE) has grown in frequency. The high frequency of adverse reactions to conventional therapeutic regimens for toxoplasmosis highlight the need to develop new strategies for the management of this disease. The importance of cytokines in resistance against *T. gondii* has been shown primarily in murine models of toxoplasmosis and a number of cytokines (e.g., IFN-γ, TNF-α, IL-2 and IL-12) have been proposed for trials in patients with TE. One mechanism by which these cytokines produce their effects is through stimulation of macrophages and/or NK cells. However, there are problems with immunological intervention in immunocompromised patients with TE since the infection is present primarily in the central nervous system (CNS), an immunoprivileged site, and because certain cytokines may down regulate the immune response. While much valuable information has been obtained from studies conducted in immunocompetent strains of mice their relevance to an immunocompromised host is unknown. The development of genetically altered mice with immune deficiencies offers promising new models that may allow for more rational development of new treatment regimens.

Abbreviations: AIDS: Acquired Immunodeficiency Syndrome; CNS: Central Nervous System; GM-CSF: Granulo cyte-macrophage colony stimulating factor; HIV: Human Immunodeficiency Virus; IL: Interleukin; IFN: Interferon; LAK: Lymphokine Activated Killer; LPS: Lipopolysacharide; MIP: Macrophage Inflammatory Protein; NK: Natural Killer; PCR: Polymerase chain reaction; SCID: Severe Combined Immunodeficiency; TG: Toxoplasmic encephalitis; TGF: Transforming Growth Factor; TNF: Tumor Necrosis Factor.

Introduction

In immunocompetent individuals, infection with the obligate intracellular parasite *Toxoplasma gondii* is most often asymptomatic. The organism, which is ubiquitous in nature, is the cause of one of the most common latent infections of humans throughout the world. In terms of public health, it has long been important as a causative agent of ocular and neurological sequelae in congenitally infected infants and children whose mothers acquired the infection during pregnancy [1]. More recently it has emerged as one of the most important opportunistic pathogens in patients with the acquired immunodeficiency syndrome (AIDS) [2].

Infection is normally acquired through ingestion of tissue cysts, found in undercooked meat, or oocysts present in the feces of members of the cat family, the definitive hosts for *T. gondii* [1, 3]. The prevalence of the infection varies considerably in different geographical areas and even among different ethnic groups within the same area. As low as 3% and as high as 75% of different populations in the United States have serologic evidence of prior infection [4]. The overall prevalence in Western Europe is higher and is approximately 50–75% in many areas [5]. Thus there is a very significant population of individuals who, should they become immunocompromised, are at risk of recrudescence of the latent infection and the potentially fatal disease it can cause.

Once within its host, the tachyzoite form of *T. gondii* is capable of infecting all cell types [3]. The normal immune response is associated with disappearance of tachyzoites and thereafter the parasite is found solely within cysts as the bradyzoite form which may persist for the entire life of the individual. *T. gondii* cysts are most commonly found in the CNS, skeletal and cardiac muscles.

The increasing use of immunosuppressive drug regimens for the treatment of cancer and transplant patients has heightened awareness of this pathogen since these regimens predispose to recrudescence of the latent infection, which has persisted in the cyst stage [6]. This has become a more urgent problem due to increasing numbers of patients with AIDS. *T.gondii* is the major opportunistic pathogen to cause focal lesions in the CNS of AIDS patients [2]. This appears to result from reactivation of a pre-existing infection since approximately 95% of cases of TE in AIDS patients have serological evidence of having been exposed to toxoplasma before the onset of their TE [7]. It has been proposed that bradyzoites escape from cysts but fail to result in TE in immunocompetent hosts whereas in a setting of impaired host immunity active infection can result. Thus, it seems likely that there is immune regulation of toxoplasma throughout the body including within the immunoprivileged site of the CNS during the latent stage of the infection. Interestingly, not all AIDS patients with pre-existing antibodies to *T. gondii* develop TE. Reactivation of the infection occurs in approximately 30% of such individuals who are seropositive for *T. gondii* [7]. Whether a genetic predisposition to development of TE exists and whether a much higher percentage will develop TE if they survive longer with their AIDS is unclear. It has been reported that in France although TE is the AIDS defining diagnosis in 16% of patients, 37% of AIDS patients had histological evidence of TE at autopsy [8]. The evidence for a direct interaction between the human immunodeficiency virus (HIV) and *T. gondii* is contradictory. Whereas Kalter *et al.* [9] reported that HIV infection of macrophages increased the percentage of cells infected with *T. gondii* and led to increased multiplication rates of the intracellular parasite Welker *et al.* found no such effect [10]. It has been suggested that the neurological involvement of HIV leads to cytokine disregulation in the CNS. This in turn alters the balance of the immune response within the CNS and, as a consequence, reactivation of the latent infection occurs. *T. gondii* may also act as a co-factor that enhances the immunodeficiency induced by HIV [11].

Clinically, toxoplasmosis may be protean in its manifestations. In the majority of immunocompetent individuals there are no recognizable clinical signs of the infection. In immunocompromised patients however, toxoplasmosis manifests very differently; from the classic ring enhancing lesions found in the CNS of AIDS patients with TE and associated neuropsychiatric manifestations to chorioretinitis and complications associated with the presence of the active infection in the lungs and heart [7] as well as septic shock [12]. The lesions of TE have a central necrotic area, with inflammatory cells and tachyzoites at the periphery of the lesion [13]. Occasionally there is diffuse involvement of the brain in which abscesses are not present [14].

The most widely used therapeutic regimens for TE in AIDS patients are pyrimethamine in combination with sulfonamides or clindamycin [15]. Neither regimen results in eradication of Toxoplasma cysts which remain as individual niduses that predispose patients to relapse. While the majority of patients are responsive to antimicrobial therapy, in 20–60% of cases therapy proves inadequate or is poorly tolerated [15]. Even in treated cases, mortality may be as high as 25% or more [16]. As a consequence of these statistics, the search for new therapeutic strategies has intensified and attention has increasingly focused on the potential for intervention at the level of the immune response, in particular with immunomodulatory cytokines.

If biological response modifiers are to be used rationally to intervene in toxoplasmosis, there are a number of considerations that must be addressed. So that we will be better able to identify candidates for immune intervention in toxoplasmosis, we must gain a better understanding of those arms of the immune system and their modulators that are essential for resistance against acute infection with *T. gondii*, those that prevent relapse of the latent infection and the immunological defects that predispose to its recrudescence in the immunocompromised patient.

Immune response to T. gondii

Use of murine models of toxoplasmosis has demonstrated that macrophages from mice acutely infected with *T. gondii* inhibit parasite multiplication more efficiently than those from uninfected animals [17]. In humans it has been reported that macrophages from different anatomical sites do not require prior activation in order to inhibit parasite replication [18]. While these results indicate the importance of cells of the mononuclear phagocytic system in the anti-parasite response they also illustrate the suitability of macrophages as host cells for *T.gondii,* providing they are not activated. The mechanisms that lead to macrophage activation and subsequent parasite inhibition and killing *in vivo* include a number of antimicrobial mechanisms such as the respiratory burst and a hostile lysosomal system capable of killing parasites. Recent work has highlighted reactive nitrogen free radicals as being of primary importance in preventing replication of *T. gondii* within activated murine macrophages [19, 20]. Macrophages are also intimately involved in the regulation of cellular immunity through their production of immunological mediators, such as prostaglandins and cytokines. Thus, the role of macrophages in the immune response is not solely as effector cells but also to regulate the immune response to *T. gondii.*

Both $CD4^+$ and $CD8^+$ T lymphocytes are involved in mediating protective immunity [21–24]. It appears that while $CD8^+$ T cells are crucial to this immunity, they are most effective when working in conjunction with $CD4^+$ T cells. Although the results obtained in different murine models differ, perhaps the most striking evidence for the importance of the $CD4^+$ and $CD8^+$ T-cell populations in regulating clinical disease is found in AIDS patients who, almost invariably, have $CD4^+$ T-cell counts that have fallen to less than $100/mm^3$ with a corresponding reduction in $CD8^+$ T-cells at the time they present with clinical TE [7].

Cytotoxic cells have been associated with a role in anti-tumour or anti-viral activity and their role as effector cells in toxoplasmosis in the intact host is uncertain. Recent work has demonstrated that $CD8^+$ T-cells and lymphokine activated killer (LAK) cells are capable of lysing *T. gondii* infected cells [25–27]. Increased natural killer (NK) cell activity has also been reported during the course of *T. gondii* infection in mice [28]. In addition to their roles as cytotoxic effector cells, these cells mediate their protective effects via production of cytokines, such as IFN-γ.

Infection with *T. gondii* induces an antibody response that is associated with protective immunity [3]. Specific anti-toxoplasma antibodies bind to the parasite surface and activate the complement pathway thereby resulting in lysis of the parasite [29] or phagocytosis by macrophages via Fc receptors which results in killing of the parasite [30]. This highly efficient protective mechanism is dependant upon the access of antibody to the parasite. However, *T. gondii* is frequently protected from antibodies by its intracellular location and its location within the CNS.

Cytokines in toxoplasmosis

Several approaches have been used in attempts to understand the role of cytokines in the immune response to *T. gondii.* Detection of elevated cytokine levels in infected humans and in murine models of the infection suggest they play an important role in the immune response and immunopathology associated with toxoplasmosis. Their importance has also been demonstrated *in vitro* and *in vivo* in experiments in which the cytokines or antibodies against these same cytokines were administered. In the following section, we present a summary of certain data on the role of various cytokines in toxoplasmosis.

Interferon-γ. This cytokine is produced in both resistant and susceptible strains of mice during the course of infection [31] and has also been detected in acutely infected humans and congenitally infected newborns [32]. The importance of endogenous IFN-γ in mediating resistance to *T. gondii* was first demonstrated by Suzuki *et al.* [33]. Mice infected with an avirulent strain survived the infection whereas those treated with an antibody against IFN-γ all died of toxoplasmosis. Administration of IFN-γ has been demonstrated to protect against acute *T. gondii* infection in mice [34] and to decrease the pathology associated with TE [35] whereas administration of anti-IFN-γ increased the severity of the encephalitis [36]. The finding that peripheral blood lymphocytes obtained from AIDS patients who were seropositive for toxoplasma antibodies could not secrete IFN-γ in response to stimulation with Toxoplasma lysate antigen [37], suggests that deficient production of IFN-γ may be one of the underlying reasons why this infection has become so important in AIDS.

There are three sources of IFN-γ, $CD4^+$ and $CD8^+$ T-cells and NK cells. Gazzinelli *et al.* demonstrated that $CD4^+$ T cells were the major source of this cytokine in mice immunized with *T. gondii*, although $CD8^+$ T cells also contributed to production of this cytokine [38]. The role of NK cells in mediating resistance to this infection by production of IFN-γ has received much attention recently. In mice that lack $CD8^+$ T cells, NK cells have been found to produce increased levels of IFN-γ [39]. In this regard, we have recently demonstrated an *in vivo* mechanism of resistance to *T. gondii* in SCID mice that relies on endogenous IFN-γ, and since these mice lack functional $CD4^+$ and $CD8^+$ T cells, we have implicated NK cells as a source of this cytokine [40]. Sharma *et al.* reported that the stimulation with Toxoplasma antigen of human, nylon wool non-adherent peripheral blood lymphocytes (containing NK cells) from uninfected donors resulted in production IFN-γ [41]. Similarly, NK cells from uninfected SCID mice will produce IFN-γ in response to Toxoplasma antigen preparations as well as exposure to live parasites; this response requires the presence of macrophages [42, 43]. *In vivo*, infection of SCID mice with *T. gondii* results in increased NK cell activity; this correlates with the increased ability of spleen cells from infected mice to produce IFN-γ when stimulated with *T. gondii* [43]. IFN-γ is involved in regulation of this NK cell activity since administration of anti-IFN-γ to *T. gondii* infected SCID mice ablates the increase in NK cell activity associated with *T. gondii* infection [43].

When parasite killing by macrophages was used as an assay of macrophage activation, peritoneal and alveolar macrophages from mice treated with IFN-γ were found to effect increased parasite killing while in those from mice treated with anti-IFN-γ, the level of infection was comparable to that observed in macrophages obtained from uninfected controls [44]. This antimicrobial activity of IFN-γ activated macrophages has been reported to be mediated by reactive nitrogen intermediates [19, 20]. The relevance of this IFN-γ dependant, antimicrobial mechanism against infection of other host cells is unclear. IFN-γ also induces indoleamine 2,3 dioxygenase, an enzyme involved in tryptophan catabolism [45]. This effect of IFN-γ leads to depletion of tryptophan, an amino acid necessary for the parasites intracellular growth and survival. It will be important to clarify the role of this mechanism in resistance against *T. gondii in vivo*.

Tumor necrosis factor-α. The initial results with TNF-α in murine models of toxoplasmosis presented conflicting results. Treatment of infected animals with TNF-α resulted in increased survival [46] while in other studies it resulted in increased mortality [47]. The reason for these different results remain unexplained. Serum levels were found to be elevated during the course of acute and chronic Toxoplasma infection in mice [46, 48]. Administration of neutralizing antibodies to TNF-α increased mortality rates in infected mice [49]. This indicates a role for endogenous TNF-α as a mediator of protection against *T. gondii*. Our data also demonstrate a similar role for endogenous TNF-α in SCID mice infected with *T. gondii* [40].

In vitro, TNF-α alone failed to activate macrophages to inhibit or kill *T. gondii*, but did so when combined with IFN-γ [50]. Indeed, recent experiments have shown that under stringent endotoxin free conditions, IFN-γ alone was unable to activate macrophages to kill Toxoplasma but addition of small amounts of TNF-α or LPS could restore this inhibition of parasite growth [50].

Recent work in which the genetic basis of resistance to development of TE was examined revealed that differences in the genes within the H-2D region correlated with resistance or susceptibility to development of TE in a murine model [51]. The genes for TNF-α and lymphotoxin (TNF-β) lie within this region. Freund *et al.* [52] reported that differences between susceptible and resistant strains of mice could be correlated with specific RFLP and microsatellite variants in the TNF-α gene. These data suggest that differences in regulation of TNF-α production may contribute to differences in susceptibility to disease following *T. gondii* infection.

Interferon α/β. Interferon-α and interferon-β, when used alone, fail to activate macrophages to inhibit Toxoplasma growth *in vitro* [53]. However, the combination of IFN-β and LPS markedly inhibited parasite replication within human macrophages [54]. The activity of this combination appears to be mediated, at least in part, through tryptophan starvation. The *in vivo* activity of IFN-β has also been demonstrated in a murine model of toxoplasmosis in which treatment with IFN-β increased survival times in infected mice [55].

Interleukin-1. IL-1α and IL-1β are important in the induction and propagation of the inflammatory response and are intimately involved in the regulation of the acute phase response. Treatment of acutely infected mice with either of these cytokines led to significant protection against death due to *T. gondii* [46]. However, *in vitro*, IL-1α or IL-1β had no effect on the antimicrobial activity of macrophages infected with *T. gondii* [56].

Interleukin-2. This product of $CD4^+$ lymphocytes is associated with the T helper 1 subset that is considered important in mediating resistance against a variety of different intracellular parasites and viruses [57]. Sharma *et al.* [58] reported that administration of IL-2 to mice resulted in significant survival after a lethal challenge with *T. gondii.* In addition, *in vivo* administration of IL-2 to mice infected with *T. gondii* resulted in a decrease in the number of Toxoplasma cysts in the brains of the mice. These effects did not appear to be mediated by increased antibody production or enhanced killing of *T. gondii* by macrophages. The authors proposed that the protective effects of IL-2 might be associated with the *in vivo* augmentation of NK cell activity observed in animals treated with this cytokine. Since NK cells produce IFN-γ when stimulated with IL-2 [59], an IL-2 mediated increase in production of IFN-γ may account for the observed protective effect. An alternative explanation may be found in the work of Kelly *et al.* [60] who described the IL-2 dependant production of IFN-γ by human $CD4^+$ T lymphocytes from a seropositive donor when they were stimulated *in vitro* with Toxoplasma antigen.

Lymphokine activated killer (LAK) cells are effector cells that upon culture with IL-2 become cytotoxic for NK resistant targets, including fresh autologous and allogenic tumor cells and tumor cell lines. Purified NK and T cells from healthy seronegative donors do not exhibit significant cytotoxic activity against *T. gondii*-infected cells [27]. However, Subauste *et al.* [27] have demonstrated that the use of IL-2 to produce standard LAK cell preparations induced in them a remarkable cytotoxic activity against *T. gondii*-infected cells. Both cells with NK cell phenotype and cells with a T cell phenotype were precursors of the effector cells that displayed cytolytic activity against *T. gondii*-infected targets. This effect of IL-2 may represent a mechanism of defense against *T. gondii in vivo.*

Interleukin-6. IL-6 has been detected in serum of both resistant and susceptible strains of mice infected with *T. gondii* [61]. IL-6 levels may be intimately involved in the pathogenesis of this infection or may simply reflect the severity of the disease since it is closely associated with an acute phase response. Recent work from our laboratory has demonstrated that pretreatment of macrophages *in vitro* with IL-6 leads to increased intracellular replication of the parasite and that IL-6 antagonizes the ability of IFN-γ to activate macrophages to inhibit parasite replication [62]. These studies have been extended to *in vivo* models in which the use of a monoclonal antibody that neutralizes IL-6 led to increased survival of *T. gondii* infected immunocompetent [61] as well as SCID mice [40]. These latter results may reflect *in vivo* inhibition by IL-6 of IFN-γ mediated activation of macrophages. Alternatively, neutralization of IL-6 during acute toxoplasmosis may have abrogated the pathological effects of high levels of this cytokine.

Interleukin-10. IL-10 was initially characterized by its production by the Th2 subset of $CD4^+$ T cells and its immunosuppressive effect on the Th1 type subset [63]. It is now recognized that this cytokine may be produced by other T cell subsets as well as by B cells and macrophages and exert a number of immunosuppressive and immunostimulatory effects [63]. Gazzinelli *et al.* [64] demonstrated that IL-10 inhibits the ability of IFN-γ to activate macrophages to inhibit multiplication of intracellular Toxoplasma. This activity appears to be through inhibition of the production of reactive nitrogen intermediates. IL-10 has also been reported to down regulate IFN-γ production by NK and $CD4^+$ T cells through its inhibitory effect on production of cytokines, including TNF-α, and IL-1α by macrophages [65–66]. The broad immunosuppressive activities of IL-10 on production of cytokines involved in resistance to *T. gondii* strongly implicate this cytokine in down regulation of the protective immune response to this parasite. Certainly, IL-10 is a potent inhibitor of production of IFN-γ by spleen cells from uninfected SCID mice or SCID mice infected with *T. gondii* [42, 43] furthermore, neutralization of endogenous IL-10 in SCID mice infected with *T. gondii* delays time to death [40]. Sher and colleagues have proposed that parasite induced production of IL-10 may be an important strategy for a variety of different parasites to avoid the consequences of cell mediated immune killing [67].

Interleukin 12. This cytokine was initially identified by its ability to enhance spontaneous NK cell mediated cytotoxicity. It has subsequently been shown to stimulate IFN-γ production by $CD4^+$ and $CD8^+$ T cells and NK cells [68]. Gazzinelli *et al.* have reported that macrophages produced IL-12 following their incubation with Toxoplasma lysate and that administration of IL-12 to SCID mice infected with *T. gondii* prolonged their survival times [69]. They propose that macrophages are activated by *T. gondii* infection to produce IL-12. The latter would then stimulate NK cells to produce IFN-γ and mediate resistance to *T. gondii* [42].

The CNS and Toxoplasma

Because the CNS is the organ most frequently affected in clinical toxoplasmosis and one of the main sites for persistence of the cyst stage of the parasite, the interaction of the CNS, the immune system and *T. gondii* will be considered separately from the interaction of the parasite with the systemic immune system. The CNS was, until quite recently, regarded as essentially immunologically isolated since it has little interaction with the systemic immune system. The presence of the blood brain barrier serves to restrict access to the CNS of immune effector cells and molecules such as cytokines and antibodies. In addition, the lack of a lymphatic system and low levels of basal MHC expression add to this immunologically pristine state of the CNS. However, glial cells are now known to be capable of interacting with the immune system and that limited trafficking of lymphocytes through the CNS may occur [70–71].

The critical importance of T cells as mediators of protective immunity against latent *T. gondii* infection within the CNS is evidenced by the close correlation of fall in peripheral T cell numbers with the development of TE in AIDS patients. Depletion of T cell populations also results in reactivation of *T. gondii* in chronically infected mice [22]. Although the mechanism of T cell mediated protection within the CNS remains to be defined, these cells may interact directly with the parasite, parasite infected cells, or both, within the CNS and also stimulate glial cells to control the infection. In addition, cytotoxic cells may exert their activity directly within the CNS against infected glial and neuronal cells.

The severity of toxoplasmic encephalitis has been altered by systemic administration of cytokines or cytokine neutralizing antibodies [22, 33, 35, 36]. It is difficult to dissociate the effect of these treatment forms on the systemic immune and inflammatory responses versus that which may be unique to the CNS itself. Recent studies have characterized cytokine mRNA levels within the CNS of mice with TE [72–74]. These have employed the sensitive technique of PCR assisted amplification of mRNA to detect the presence of RNA transcripts for TNF-α, MIP-1, GM-CSF, IL-1α, IL-1β, IL-6, IL-2, IL-4, IL-10, TGF-β, and IFN-γ. Levels of transcripts vary depending on the susceptibility of the strains of mice investigated and the severity of the encephalitis [73, 74]. In resistant mice, there was an early peak of IFN-γ production whereas in susceptible mice, transcripts for IFN-γ were present throughout the course of the encephalitis [73–74]. The finding that the encephalitis progressed despite the presence of high levels of IFN-γ transcripts may have been due to the increased levels of IL-10 we have observed in the CNS of susceptible mice with TE (Hunter *et al.*, unpublished observations).

The difficulty with these types of studies is that they do not readily distinguish the roles of the cytokines in either immunopathology or in mediation of protective immunity. Indeed, the presence of cytokine transcripts within the CNS is no guarantee that they are translated to produce biologically active proteins. While there are many possible sources of the transcripts detected, in particular the inflammatory cells or resident microglia, the intense astrocyte activation observed in mice with TE highlights these cells as possible candidates for production of cytokines within the CNS [72–73]. In particular, microglia and astrocytes may produce TNF-α, IL-6 and IL-1 *in vitro* [75–76].

Although production of cytokines within the CNS may be beneficial in terms of an anti-parasite response, it also may have adverse effects. TNF-α, IL-1α and MIP-1 have each been shown to directly initiate meningeal inflammation [77–78] and it has been proposed that local production of these cytokines contribute to the pathogenesis of TE [72–73]. Although IFN-γ can stimulate microglia to kill intracellular *T. gondii* [79] it can also induce production of nitrogen free radicals which are cytotoxic for neurons [80]. TNF-α has also been reported to be cytotoxic for oligodendrocytes [81].

Immunotherapy of toxoplasmosis

Since seropositivity may be used to distinguish patients at risk of developing TE, this information can potentially be used as an opportunity to initiate immunotherapeutic measures to prevent development of clinical TE. However, the patients who initially would most likely be targeted for immunotherapy would be those who have failed to respond to what would be accepted as optimal anti-toxoplasma therapy and as such would have active TE. Although there will be problems associated with attempting to stimulate specifically an adequate anti-parasite immune response to control the parasite within the CNS in immunocompromised patients, the promising results observed in murine models of the disease would suggest that studies of such an approach are warranted. When considering this approach, the possible deleterious consequences of attempting to manipulate the immune system must be considered. In addition to its potential for a beneficial effect, the enhancement of the immune response to parasites within the CNS could lead to more severe immunopathology when there is increased numbers of immune effector cells entering the brain parenchyma. In addition, use of regimens designed to decrease the extent of the inflammatory response may remove the protective immune response within the CNS. In the absence of this immune surveillance, unrestricted multiplication of the parasite might occur.

There are other considerations that must be recognized if cytokine therapy is to be used to treat AIDS patients with TE. The use of biological response modifiers in HIV infected patients with toxoplasmosis may have an effect on the viral load and HIV disease status in these patients. TNF-α has been shown to increase expression of the HIV reverse transcriptase and could also be involved in the activation and resulting differentiation of infected macrophages into mature macrophages, a step necessary for efficient production of viral progeny in HIV infected macrophages [82]. TNF-α and IL-1α have both been shown to be capable of reactivating HIV in infected fetal glial cell cultures [82]. Thus, immunotherapy that results in increased levels of these cytokines in the CNS has the potential to increase the severity of the underlying HIV infection.

Based on the results reviewed above, it appears that there are several strategies that may prove useful in stimulating cell mediated immunity to kill parasitized cells and perhaps the parasites themselves. IFN-γ in particular is a strong candidate for use in AIDS patients with TE, especially since administration of IFN-γ restores depressed immune function in immunocompromised individuals with impaired production of IFN-γ [83]. At present only a single clinical trial is underway for the immunotherapy of toxoplasmosis (Henry Murray, personal communication). There is also a potential role for other cytokines, eg. IL-10 and IL-6. But before they can be used, it will be advisable to further characterize their role in down regulating the anti-parasite response. Neutralization of the effects of these cytokines by antibodies or receptor antagonists may lead to the enhancement of an existing or therapeutically enhanced immune response,

Adoptive immunotherapy using LAK cells and $CD8^+$ T cells has been suggested for patients with TE and has proven useful in conferring protection to humans and animals against certain types of cancer and infections with other intracellular pathogens [84, 85]. Our results *in vitro* suggest that administration of $CD8^+$ T cells or LAK cells might prove of therapeutic use in immunocompromised patients with toxoplasmosis.

The most likely use of immune response modifiers would be in conjunction with chemotherapy. There is already experimental evidence supporting this strategy since IFN-γ has been shown to act synergistically with roxithromycin in a murine model of toxoplasmosis [86]. These results raise the possibility that cytokines and antimicrobial agents when used together may act synergistically, thereby allowing the dose of the antimicrobial or cytokine, or both, to be lowered. This then would be useful to reduce the toxic side effects of either of these agents.

The future

Most of the *in vivo* studies described above have employed immunocompetent mice, with different genetic susceptibilities to toxoplasmosis. Although they do not take into consideration the immunodeficiency that underlies the majority of patients that present with TE, they have proven to be extremely useful for study of the immunopathogenesis of the infection and to define promising antimicrobial agents and biological response modifiers. With the increasing availability of genetically manipulated mouse strains that display different immunodeficiencies it becomes increasingly possible to investigate this infection against an immune background which is perhaps more relevant to clinical presentation of opportunistic infections. The availability of mouse strains that lack certain effector arms of the immune system, such as the nude or SCID mouse, or more specifically which lack the ability to produce certain cytokines such as IFN-γ [87] or the ability to respond to IFN-γ [88] or TNF-α [89] should allow for a better understanding of the actual role of cytokines in the immune response to this and other infectious diseases.

We, and others, have developed a new murine model of reactivation, using SCID mice, that leads to development of brain lesions similar to those observed in AIDS patients with TE [90–92]. Thus the CNS pathology and underlying immunocompromised of the SCID mouse model, when compared to most immunocompetent mouse models, appears to more closely resemble the situation in AIDS patients. Since the effects of different cytokines or cytokine neutralizing antibodies is likely to differ in immunodeficient and immunocompetent patients, use of SCID mice will be helpful in determining whether use of immunotherapy might be suitable for study in AIDS patients with TE. The same is also true for conventional drug regimens used for treatment of TE since recent work has shown that the efficacy of anti-toxoplasma drug regimens is dependant on an intact immune system [93–94].

Conclusions

Despite the possible difficulties associated with immunotherapy of this disease, there is at least a basis on which to approach this problem, i.e. this infection normally induces a strong protective immune response. Therefore, the aim of any form of immunotherapy of this disease must be to boost the immune response in an attempt to achieve its previous anti-toxoplasma activity. Whether this is achievable in the presence of the underlying HIV infection is not yet clear. Based on results of previous studies and with the availability of new and improved models of TE and of new biological response modifiers, including recombinant cytokines, humanized antibodies and receptor antagonists, rapid progress is being made in our understanding of the potential for immunotherapy in toxoplasmosis.

Acknowledgements

This work was supported by the U. S. Public Health Service Grants AI04717 and AI30320 from the National Institutes of Health and a MacArthur Foundation Grant in Molecular Parasitology. C.S. is the recipient of a grant from the American Foundation for AIDS Research and from the University of California Universitywide AIDS Research Program.

References

1. Remington JS, Desmonts G. Infectious diseases of the fetus and the newborn infant. In: Remington JS, Klein JO, eds. Toxoplasmosis. Philadelphia: W.B. Saunders & Co., 1990: 89–95.
2. McCabe R, Remington JS. Toxoplasmosis: The time has come., N Engl J Med 1988; 318: 313–315
3. Krahenbuhl JL, Remington JS. The immunology of Toxoplasma and toxoplasmosis. In: Cohen S, Warren KS, eds. Immunology of Parasitic Infections. London: Blackwell Scientific Publications 1982: 356–421.
4. Porter SB, Sande M. Toxoplasmosis of the central nervous system in the acquired immunodeficiency syndrome. N Engl J Med 1992; 327: 1643–1648.
5. Clumeck N. Some aspects of the epidemiology of toxoplasmosis and pneumocystosis in AIDS in Europe. Eur J Clin Microbiol Infect Dis 1991; 10: 177–178.
6. Derouin F, Devergie A, Auber P, Gluckman E, Beauvais B, Garin YJF, Lariviere M. Toxoplasmosis in bone marrow-transplant recipients: Report of seven cases and review. Clin Infect Dis 1992; 15: 267–270.
7. Israelski DM, Remington JS. AIDS associated toxoplasmosis. In: Sande MA, Volberding PA, eds. The Medical Management of AIDS, Third Edition, Philadelphia: W.B. Saunders Company 1992: 319–345.
8. Khuong MA, Matheron S, Marche C, De Truchis C, Coulaud JP, Saimot AG. Diffuse toxoplasmic encephalitis (DTE) without abscesses in AIDS patients 1990. Abstr 1157, In: 30th Interscience Conferen Antimicrob Agents Chemotherapy, Atlanta, Georgia, October 21–24.
9. Kalter DC, Gendelman H, Orenstein J, Meltzer MS, Reed S. HIV-infection alters the interaction of macrophages with *Toxoplasma* and *Leishmania*. 1989. Abstr W.C.P. 63. V Inter Conferen on AIDS, The Scientific and Social Challenge, Montreal, Quebec, Canada, June 4 – 9.
10. Welker Y, Molina JM, Poirot C, Ferchal F, Decazes JM, Lagrange P, Deouin F. Interactions between human immunodeficiency virus and *Toxoplasma gondii* replication in dually infected monocytoid cells. Infect Immun 1993; 61: 1596–1598.
11. Lin D-S, Bowman DD. *Toxoplasma gondii*: An AIDS enhancing cofactor. Med Hypotheses 1992: 39; 140–142.
12. Lucet JC, Bailly MP, Bedos JP, Gachot B, Casalino E, Wolff M, Vachon F. Septic shock due to *Toxoplasma gondii* in AIDS patients. Abstr 32nd Interscience Conf. on Antimicros Agents and Chemo Oct. 11–14 Anaheim CA 1992; 1212.
13. Post MJ, Chan JC, Nensley GT, Hoffman TA, Moskowitz LB, Lippmann S. Toxoplasma encephalitis in Haitian adults with acquired immunodeficiency syndrome: a clinical-pathologic-CT correlation. Am Neuro Radio 10 1983 4: 155-162.
14. Gray F, Gherardi R, Wingate E, Wingate J, Fenelon G, Gaston A, Sobel A, Poirier J. Diffuse "encephalitic" cerebral toxoplasmosis in AIDS. J Neurol 1989: 236: 273-277.
15. Beaman MH, Luft BJ, Remington JS. Assessment of therapy for toxoplasmic encephalitis. Ann Intern Med 1992: 117: 163-164.
16. Haverkos HW. Prophylaxis for toxoplasmosis in AIDS. Am J Med 1987: 83: 907–914.
17. Jones TC, Len L, Hirsch JG. Assessment *in vitro* of immunity against *Toxoplasma gondii*. J Exp Med 1975: 141: 466–482.
18. Catterall JR, Black CM, Leventhal JP, Rizk NW, Wachtel JS Remington JS. Nonoxidative microbicidal activity in normal human alveolar and peritoneal macrophages. Infect Immun 1987: 55: 1635–1640.
19. Adams LB, Hibbs JB, Taintor RR, Krahenbuhl JL. Microbiostatic effect of murine-activated macrophages for *Toxoplasma gondii*. J Immunol 1990: 144: 2725–2729.
20. Langermans JAM, van der Hust MEB, Nibbering PH, Hiemstra PS, Fransen L, van Furth R. IFN-γ induced L-arginine dependant toxoplasmastatic activity in murine peritoneal macrophages is mediated by endogenous tumor necrosis factor-alpha. J Immunol 1992: 148: 568–574.
21. Araujo F G. Depletion of L3T4^{+} (CD4^{+}) T lymphocytes prevents development of resistance to *Toxoplasma gondii* in mice. Infect Immun 1991: 59: 1614–1619.

22. Gazzinelli R, Xu Y, Hieny S, Cheever A, Sher A. Simultaneous depletion of $CD4^+$ and $CD8^+$ T lymphocytes is required to reactivate chronic infection with *Toxoplasma gondii*. J Immunol 1992: 149: 175–180.
23. Parker SJ, Robert CW, Alexander J. $CD8^+$ T cells are the major lymphocyte population involved in the protective immune response to *Toxoplasma gondii* in mice. Clin Exp Immunol 1991: 84: 207–212.
24. Suzuki Y, Remington JS. Dual regulation of resistance against *Toxoplasma gondii* by Lyt-2^+ immune T cells against toxoplasmosis in mice. J Immunol 1988: 140: 3943–3946.
25. Hakim FT, Gazzinelli RT, Denkers E, Hieny S, Shearer GM, Sher A. $CD8^+$ T cells from mice vaccinated against *Toxoplasma gondii* are cytotoxic for parasite-infected or antigen-pulsed host cells. J Immunol 1991: 147: 2310–2316.
26. Subauste CS, Koniaris AH, Remington JS. Murine $CD8^+$ cytotoxic T lymphocytes lyse *Toxoplasma gondii*-infected cells. J Immunol 1991: 147: 3955–3959.
27. Subauste CS, Dawson L, Remington JS. Human lymphokine-activated killer cells are cytotoxic against cells infected with *Toxoplasma gondii*. J Exp Med 1992: 176: 1511–1519.
28. Hauser WE, Sharma SD, Remington JS. Natural killer cells induced by acute and chronic *Toxoplasma* infection. Cell Immunol 1982: 69: 330–346.
29. Fuhrman SA, Joiner KA. *Toxoplasma gondii*: mechanism of resistance to complement-mediated killing. J Immunol 1989: 142: 940–947.
30. Sibley DL, Weidner E, Krahenbuhl JL. Phagosome acidification is blocked by intracellular *Toxoplasma gondii*. Nature 1985: 315: 416–419.
31. Suzuki Y, Orellana MA, Wong SY, Conley FK, Remington JS. Susceptibility to chronic infection with *Toxoplasma gondii* does not correlate with susceptibility to acute infection in mice. Infect Immun 1993; 61: 2284–2288.
32. Raymond J, Poissonnier MH, Thulliez PH, Forestier F, Daffos F, Lebon P. Presence of gamma interferon in human acute and congenital toxoplasmosis J Clin Microbiol 1990; 28: 1434–1437.
33. Suzuki Y, Orellana MA, Schreiber RD, Remington JS. Interferon-γ: The major mediator of resistance against *Toxoplasma gondii*. Science 1988; 240: 516–518.
34. McCabe RE, Luft BJ, Remington JS. Effect of murine interferon gamma on murine toxoplasmosis. J Infect Dis 1984; 150: 961–962.
35. Suzuki Y, Conley FK, Remington JS. Treatment of toxoplasmic encephalitis in mice with recombinant gamma interferon. Infect Immun 1990; 58: 3050–3055.
36. Suzuki Y, Conley FK, Remington JS. Importance of endogenus IFN-γ for prevention of toxoplasmic encephalitis in mice. J Immunol 1989; 143: 2045–2050.
37. Murray HW, Rubin BY, Masur H, and Roberts RB. Impaired production of lymphokines and immune (gamma) interferon in the acquired immunodeficiency syndrome. N Eng J Med. 1984; 310: 883–889.
38. Gazzinelli RT, Hakim FT, Hieny S, Shearer GM, Sher A. Synergistic role of $CD4^+$ and $CD8^+$ T lymphocytes in IFN-γ production and protective immunity induced by an attenuated *Toxoplasma gondii* vaccine. J Immunol 1991; 146: 286–292.
39. Denkers E, Gazzinelli RT, Sher A. Natural killer cells replace $CD8^+$ lymphocytes as effectors of immunity to *Toxoplasma gondii* in vaccinated β2-microglobulin negative mice. Progr Abstr 41st Ann Meet Amer Soc Trop Med Hyg, Seattle, Washington. 1992; 47: 4, Abstr 195.
40. Hunter CA, Abrams JS, Beaman MH, Remington JS. Cytokine mRNA in the CNS of SCID mice with *Toxoplasma gondii*: Importance of T-cell independant regulation of resistance to *T. gondii*. 1993 Infect Immun. 1993 61: 4038–4044.
41. Sharma SD, Verhoef J, Remington JS. Enhancement of human natural killer cell activity by sub-cellular components of *Toxoplasma gondii*. Cell Immunol 1984; 86: 317–326.
42. Sher A, Oswald IP, Hieny S, Gazzinelli RT. *Toxoplasma gondii* induces a T-independant IFN-γ response in natural killer cells that requires both adherent accessory cells and tumor necrosis factor-α. J Immunol 1993; 150: 3982–3989.
43. Hunter CA, Subauste C, Remington JS. Production of IFN-γ by NK cells from *Toxoplasma gondii* infected SCID mice: regulation by IL-10, IL-12 and TNF-α. 1994 .Infect Immun. 62: 2818–2824.
44. Black CM, Catteral JR, Remington JS. *in vivo* and *in vitro* activation of alveolar macrophages by recombinant interferon-γ. J Immunol 1987; 138: 491–495.
45. Pfefferkon ER, Guyre PM. Inhibition of growth of *Toxoplasma gondii* in cultured fibroblasts by human recombinant gamma interferon. Infect Immun 1984; 44: 211–216.
46. Chang HR, Grau GE, Pechere JC. Role of TNF and IL-1 in infection with *Toxoplasma gondii*. Immunol 1990; 69: 33–37.
47. Black CM, Israelski DM, Suzuki Y, Remington JS. Effect of recombinant tumor necrosis factor on acute infection in mice with *Toxoplasma gondii* or *Trypanosoma cruzi*. Immunol 1989; 68: 570–574.
48. Beaman MH, Pearce MK, Abrams JS, Remington JS. Serum cytokine profile in lethal murine toxoplasmosis. Proceed First Inter Congr Biological Response Modifiers, Quebec City, Abstr 61. 1991.
49. Johnson LJ. A protective role for endogenous tumor necrosis factor in *Toxoplasma gondii* infection. Infect Immun 1992; 60: 1979–1983.
50. Sibley LD, Adams L, Fukutomi Y, Krahenbuhl JL. Tumor necrosis factor-α triggers antitoxoplasmal activity of IFN-γ primed macrophages. J Immunol 1991; 147: 2340–2345.
51. Suzuki Y, Joh K, Orellana MA, Conley FK, Remington JS. A gene(s) within the H-2D region determine development of toxoplasmic encephalitis in mice. Immunol 1991; 74: 732-739.
52. Freund YR, Sgarlato G, Jacob CO, Suzuki, Remington JS. Polymorphisms in the tumor necrosis factor-α (TNF-α) gene correlate with murine resistance to development of toxoplasmic encephalitis and with levels of TNF-α mRNA in infected brain tissue. J Exp Med 1992; 172: 683–688.
53. Nathan CF, Prendergast TJ, Wiebe ME, Rubin BY. Activation of human macrophages. Comparison of other cytokines with IFN-γ. J Exp Med 1984; 160: 600–605.
54. Schmitz JL, Carlin JM, Borden EC, Byrne GI. Beta interferon inhibits *Toxoplasma gondii* growth in human monocyte-derived macrophages. Infect Immun 1989; 57: 3254–3256.
55. Orellana MA, Suzuki Y, Araujo F, Remington JS. Role of beta interferon in resistance to *Toxoplasma gondii* infection. 1991. Infect Immun 1991; 59: 3287–3290.
56. Hughes HPA, Speer CA, Kyle JE, Dubey JP. Activation of murine macrophages and a bovine monocyte cell line by bovine lymphokines to kill the intracellular pathogens *Eimeria bovis* and *Toxoplasma gondii*. Infect Immun 1987; 55: 784–791.
57. Cox FEG, Liew FY. T-cell subsets and cytokines in parasitic infections. Immunol Today 1992; 13: 445–448.
58. Sharma SD, Hofflin JM, Remington JS. *In vivo* recombinant interleukin-2 administration enhances survival against a lethal challenge with *Toxoplasma gondii*. J Imunol 1985; 135: 4160–4163.

59. Perussia, B. Lymphokine-activated killer cells, natural killer cells and cytokines. Curr Op Immunol 1991; 3: 49–55.
60. Kelley CD, Welte H, Murray HW. Antigen-induced human interferon-γ production. Differential dependence on interleukin-2 and its receptor. J Immunol 1987; 139: 2325–2328.
61. Beaman MH, Abrams JS, Remington JS. Serum cytokine profile in acute and chronic Toxoplasma infections of mice: Evidence for the role of interleukin-6 in pathogenesis. 1994 (submitted).
62. Beaman MH, Hunter CA, Remington JS. Enhancement of intracellular replication of *Toxoplasma gondii* by interleukin-6: interactions with interferon-γ and tumor necrosis factor-α 1994. (submitted).
63. Howard M, O'Garra A, Ishida H, de Waal Malefyt R, de Vries, J. Biological properties of interlukin 10. J Clin Immunol 1992; 12: 239–247.
64. Gazzinelli R, Oswald IP, James SL, Sher A. IL-10 inhibits parasite killing and nitrogen oxide production by IFN-γ activated macrophages. J Immunol 1992; 148: 1792–1796.
65. Fiorentino DF, Zlotnik TR, Mosmann TR, Howard M, O'Garra A. IL-10 inhibits cytokine production by activated macrophages. J Immunol 1991; 147: 3815–3822.
66. de Wall Malefyt R, Abrams J, Bennett B, Figdor C, de Vries J. IL-10 inhibits cytokine synthesis by human monocytes: an autoregulatory role of IL-10 produced by monocytes. J Exp Med 1991; 174: 1209–1220.
67. Gazzinelli RT, Oswald IP, Hieny S, James SL, Sher A. The microbicidal activity of interferon-γ-treated macrophages against *Trypanosoma cruzi* involves an L-arginine-dependant, nitrogen oxide-mediated mechanism inhibitable by interleukin-10 and transforming growth factor-β. Eur J Immunol 1992; 22: 2501–2506.
68. Perussia B, Chan SH, D'Andrea A, Tsuji K, Santoli D, Pospisil M, Young D, Wolf SF, Trinchieri G. Natural killer (NK) cell stimulatory factor or IL-12 has differential effects on the proliferation of TCR-ab$^+$, TCR-γd$^+$ T lymphocytes and NK cells. J Immunol 1992; 149: 3495–3502.
69. Gazzinelli RT, Hieny S, Wynn T, Wolf S, Sher A. IL-12 is required for T-independant induction of IFN-γ by *Toxoplasma gondii* and mediates resistance against the parasite in SCID mice. Joint Meet Amer Assoc Immunol Clin Immunol Soc 1993; Abstr 478.
70. Benveniste EN. Lymphokines and monokines in the neuroendocrine system. Prog Allergy 1988; 43: 84–120.
71. Fontana A, Frei K, Bodmer S, Hofer E. Immune-mediated encephalitis: on the role of antigen presenting cells in brain tissue. Immunol Rev 1987; 100: 185–201.
72. Hunter CA, Roberts CW, Murray M, Alexander J. Detection of cytokine mRNA in the brains of mice with toxoplasmic encephalitis. Parasite Immunol 1992; 14: 405–413.
73. Hunter CA, Roberts CW, Alexander J. Kinetics of cytokine mRNA production in the brains of mice with progressive toxoplasmic encephalitis. Eur J Immunol 1992; 22: 2317–2322.
74. Freund Y, Wong SY, Hunter CA, Beaman MH, Remington JS. Kinetics of cytokine mRNA expression during disease development in brains of mice which differ in susceptibility to toxoplasmic encephalitis. 1994 (submitted).
75. Fontana A, Hengartner H, de Tribolet N, Weber E. Glioblastoma cells release interleukin-1 and factors inhibiting interleukin-2 mediated effects. J Immunol 1984; 132: 1837–1844.
76. Lieberman AP, Pitha PM, Shin, HS, Shin, ML. Production of tumor necrosis factor and other cytokines by astrocytes stimulated with lipopolysaccharide or a neurotropic virus. Proc Natl Acad Sci 1989; 36: 6348–6352.
77. Saukkonen K, Sande S, Cioffe C, Wolpe S, Sherry B, Cerami A, Tuomanen E. The role of cytokines in the generation of inflammation and tissue damage in experimental gram-positive meningitis. J Exp Med 1990; 171: 439–448.
78. Ramilo O, Saez-Lorens X, Mertsola H, Jafari H, Olsen KD, Hansen EJ, Yoshinaga M, Ohkawara S, Nariuchi H, McCracken GH. Tumor necrosis factor/cachectin and interleukin 1 initiate meningeal inflammation. J Exp Med 1990; 172: 497–507.
79. Chao CC, Hu S, Gekker G, Novick WJ, Remington JS, Peterson PK. Effects of cytokines on multiplication of *Toxoplasma gondii* in microglial cells. J Immunol 1993; 150: 3404–3410.
80. Piani D, Spranger M, Frei K, Schaffner A, Fontana A. Macrophage-induced cytotoxicity of N-methyl-D-aspartate receptor positive neurons involves excitatory amino acids rather than reactive oxygen intermediates and cytokines.Eur J Immunol 1992; 22: 2429–2436.
81. Selmaj KW, Raine CS. Tumor necrosis factor mediates myelin and oligodendrocyte damage *in vitro*. Ann Neurol 1988; 23: 339–346.
82. Geleziunas R, Schipper HM, Wainberg MA. Pathogenesis and therapy of HIV-1 infection of the central nervous system. AIDS 1992; 6: 1411–1426.
83. Murray HW, Scavuzzo D, Jacobs JL, Kaplan MH, Libby DM, Schindler J, Roberts RB. *in vitro* and *in vivo* activation of human mononuclear phagocytes by interferon-γ. J Immunol 1987; 138: 2457–62.
84. Rosenberg SA, Lotze MT, Muul S, Chang SE, Ettinghausen, YL, Matory JM, Skibber E, Shiloni JT, Vetto, *et al.* observations on the systemic administration of autologous lymphokine-activated killer cells and recombinant interleukin-2 to patients with metastatic cancer. N Engl J Med 1985; 313: 1485.
85. Riddell SR, Watanabe KS, Goodrich JM, Li, Cr, Agha ME Greenberg PD. Resoration of viral immunity in immunodeficient humans by the adoptive transfer of T cell clones. Science 1992; 257: 238–241.
86. Hofflin JM, Remington JS. *in vivo* synergism of roxithromycin (RU 965) and interferon against *Toxoplasma gondii*. Antimicrob Agents Chemother 1987; 31: 346–348.
87. Dalton DK, Pitts-Meek S, Keshav S, Figari IS, Bradely A, Stewart T. Multiple defects of immune cell function in mice with disrupted interferon-γ genes. Science 1993; 259: 1739–1742.
88. Huang S, Hendriks W, Althage A, Hemmi S, Bluethmann H, Kamijo R, Vilcek J, Zinkernagel RM, Aguet M. Immune response in mice that lack the interefron-γ receptor. Science 1993; 259: 1742–1745.
89. Pfeffer K, Matsuyama T, Kundig TM, Wakeham A, Kishihara K, Shahinian A, Wiegmann K, Ohashi PS, Kronke K, Mak, TW. Mice deficient for the 55 kd tumor necrosis factor receptor are resistant to endotoxic shock, yet succumb to *L.monocytogenes* infection. Cell 1993; 73: 457–467.
90. Johnson LJ. SCID mouse models of acute and relapsing chronic *Toxoplasma gondii* infections. Infect Immun 1992; 60: 3719–3724.
91. Schluter D, Deckert-Schluter M, Schwendemann G, Brunner H, Hof H. Expression of major histocompatability complex class II antigens and levels of interferon-γ, tumor necrosis factor, and interleukin-6 in cerebrospinal fluid and serum in *Toxoplasma gondii*-infected SCID and immunocompetent C.B-17 mice. Immunology 1993; 78: 430–435.

92. Beaman MH, Araujo FG, Remington JS. Protective reconstitution of the SCID mouse against reactivation of toxoplasmic encephalitis. J Infect Dis 1994 169: 375–383.
93. Araujo FG. Depletion of $CD4^+$ T cells but not inhibition of the protective activity of IFN-γ prevents cure of toxoplasmosis mediated by drug therapy in mice. J Immunol 1992; 149: 3003–3007.
94. Murray HW, Teitelbaum R, Hariprashad J. Response to treatment for an intracellular infection in a T-cell-deficient host: Toxoplasmosis in nude mice. J Infect Dis 1993; 167: 1173–1177.

Biotherapy 7: 249–259, 1994.

Cytokines in the treatment of primary immunodeficiency

Benjamin A. Kruskal[1,3] & R. Alan B. Ezekowitz[1,2,3]
Divisions of [1] Infectious Diseases and [2] Hematology/Oncology, The Children's Hospital, 300 Longwood Av., Boston, MA 02115, USA and [3] Department of Pediatrics, Harvard Medical School

Key words: Colony-stimulating factor, cytokine, immunodeficiency, interferon, interleukin

Abstract

Cytokines have great potential in the treatment of primary immunodeficiencies, which is just beginning to be realized. We discuss some general considerations in the use of cytokines in this setting, and review the clinical use of a number of cytokines. The best proven example to date is the use of interferon-γ in chronic granulomatous disease, which significantly reduces infectious complications of this disease. We also discuss the potential use of interferon-γ in the hyperimmunoglobulin E syndrome and in newborns. Granulocyte-colony stimulating factor usage in congenital neutropenias is reviewed. The use of IL-2, thymic hormones, and interferon-α are briefly discussed. Strategies for the design of clinical trials of cytokines in these uncommon illnesses are proposed.

Abbreviations: ANC: absolute neutrophil count; CGD: chronic granulomatous disease; CSF: colony-stimulating factor; CVID: common variable immune deficiency; G-CSF: granulocyte colony-stimulating factor; GM-CSF: granulocyte-macrophage colony-stimulating factor; HIE: hyperimmunoglobulinemia E; IL: interleukin; NBT: nitroblue tetrazolium; SCID: severe combined immune deficiency; Th1, Th2: T helper type 1 and type 2

Introduction

The last decade has yielded a plethora of information pertaining to the characterization and molecular cloning of molecules regulating the growth, differentiation, and function of cells participating in host defense. *In vitro* and *in vivo* studies have revealed activities of almost overwhelming complexity ascribed to growth factors and cytokines invididually and in combination. It is therefore not surprising that the two most successful cytokines in clinical practice appear to act predominantly by the simple mechanism of increasing the number of mature effector cells; mature red blood cells in the case of erythropoetin [66], and granulocytes in the case of granulocyte colony-stimulating factor (G-CSF) [53]. Although other cytokines, such as interferon-γ, interleukin 2 and granulocyte-macrophage colony-stimulating factor (GM-CSF) have also found their way into clinical practice, a general consensus as to their utility is yet to be reached. The challenge to the physician engaged in the care of children with primary immunodeficiencies is most commonly associated with a single genetic defect which disables a vital part of the immune system. Defects in the gene that codes for the CD40 ligand result in an X-linked disorder which is characterized by the failure to switch from immunoglobulin M to immunoglobulin G synthesis [1–5]. In other instances, similar or identical clinical phenotypes may occur as a result of defects in many independent genes. For example, severe combined immunodeficiency (SCID) is known to be caused by lymphocyte metabolic disorders (adenosine deaminase deficiency, purine nucleoside phosphorylase deficiency) as well as by defects in interleukin-2 production [6] or mutations in the interleukin-2 receptor [7]. In these instances, rational therapeutic interventions require a detailed knowledge of the underlying genetic defect that gives rise to the phenotype. In chronic granulomatous disease, the inability to convert molecular oxygen into reactive oxygen intermediates results in susceptibility to recurrent pyogenic bacterial and fungal infections.

This phenotype may result from defects in at least four independent genes, all of which play a critical role in the assembly of the superoxide generating enzyme (the NADPH oxidase) [15].

The rarity of most congenital immunodeficiencies provides another obstacle in evaluating the efficacy of therapies. It may be difficult to find enough patients to achieve statistical significance in a traditional, placebo-controlled randomized trial. One method of circumventing this difficulty is the so-called "n-of-1", individual patient trial [8]. Using this strategy, a patient is given a placebo and a treatment in a crossover trial with the patient and other evaluators blinded to crossover time and sequence, and with clearly defined objective outcome measures. This provides objective assurance that for the individual patient, at least, the therapy is effective.

Despite all of these potential hurdles, there have been notable clinical successes in the relatively safe and effective use of cytokines in primary immune deficiencies. The aim of this review is to highlight these achievements and indicate possible future directions for rational therapies in the treatment of immunodeficiencies. It is important, where possible, to quantitatively evaluate cytokine therapies with regard to both risk and benefit. The advent of gene therapy for primary immunodeficiencies [9, 10], although clearly in its infancy, suggests that a careful comparison of risks and benefits of cytokine therapy and gene therapy will be necessary to choose between these therapeutic modalities as they both mature.

Interferon-γ

Biology of interferon-γ

Interferon-γ is a small glycoprotein secreted by activated T cells and NK cells [11]. Although it was originally characterized by its antiviral activity (shared with the classical interferons, interferon-α and -β), it is a pleiotropic modulator of immune functions. Its targets are widespread; interferon-γ receptors are found on phagocytes, B- and T-lymphocytes, NK cells, and even fibroblasts and epithelial cells. Interferon-γ enhances antigen presentation by up-regulating MHC Class II expression, stimulates generation of cytotoxic T cells, stimulates NK activity, and activates PMNs. It influences B-cell differentiation and isotype and subtype switching. It is also probably the single most important macrophage activating factor, enhancing phagocytosis and microbicidal activities, and stimulating secretion of other proinflammatory cytokines such as IL-1 and TNF. Evidence in experimental animals suggests that it is an important, if not crucial, part of host defense against intracellular pathogens such as *Mycobacteria tuberculosis* and *leprae*, *Listeria*, *Chlamydia*, *Toxoplasma*, and *Leishmania* [67].

Pharmacology

Interferon-γ is a recombinant protein produced in *E. coli* and is available for parenteral use only [12]. It can be given by intravenous or intramuscular injections, but the usual route is subcutaneous, which provides the most sustained release. Pharmacokinetic data (derived from healthy volunteers) demonstrate rapid clearance after intravenous administration. Mean half-times for a dose of 100 μg/M^2 by the i.v., i.m. and s.c. routes are, respectively, 0.6, 2.9, and 5.9 hours. In a large placebo-controlled clinical trial of interferon-γ (50 μg/M^2 or 1.5 μg/kg for patients less than 0.5 M^2) for chronic granulomatous disease [13], the drug was generally well-tolerated. Adverse reactions reported significantly more frequently from treated patients included fever, headache, chills, and erythema at the site of injection. The magnitude of these reactions was usually mild, and they were effectively treated symptomatically (i.e. acetaminophen). The drug caused fewer reactions when given at bedtime, and patients younger than 10 years had fewer adverse effects than older patients. Only four of the 128 patients had to discontinue treatment because of toxicity. Patients treated with much higher doses (e.g. >100 μg/M^2) rarely had more severe reactions, e.g. cardiovascular (hypotension, syncope, tacharrhythmias, heart block, congestive heart failure and myocardial infarction), pulmonary (bronchospasm, intersitial pneumonia), CNS (confusion, seizures, Parkinsonism, transient ischemic attacks), hemostatic (deep vein thrombosis and pulmonary embolism), metabolic (hyperglycemia and hyponatremia), GI (bleeding, hepatic insufficency, pancreatitis), and reversible renal insufficiency.

Interferon-γ in chronic granulomatous disease

Chronic granulomatous disease (CGD) is an immunodeficiency characterized by recurrent pyogenic infections beginning early in life [14, 15]. Phagocytes from CGD patients fail to produce superoxide and other reactive oxygen intermediates important in bacterial killing. This results from failure of a membrane-associated NADPH oxidase which contains a unique, phagocyte-specific cytochrome b. CGD is known to be genetically heterogeneous, with a common X-linked form, and less common variant X-linked and autosomal recessive forms. Classical X-linked CGD results from mutations or deletions in the gp91*phox* gene [16], which encodes the phagocyte-specific cytochrome b [17]. The molecular defects in most of the other forms have also been elucidated [18–25].

The initial rationale for the use of interferon-γ in CGD came from *in vitro* experiments demonstrating that it could increase the magnitude of the respiratory burst [26], and increase expression of gp91*phox* in phagocytes from normal patients [27]. *In vitro* interferon-γ treatment of phagocytes from patients with X-linked CGD resulted in increased superoxide production [28, 29]. A trial of interferon-γ *in vivo* in four patients with X-linked CGD demonstrated a long-lasting improvement in oxidative metabolism, bacterial killing and cytochrome b content [30]. The longevity of the improvement (detectable weeks after two daily doses) was shown to result from an effect on myeloid progenitor cells, which resulted in circulating progeny with restored activity [31].

This set the stage for a large placebo-controlled double-blinded randomized clinical trial of interferon-γ in CGD [13]. One-hundred and twenty-eight patients with various forms of CGD were randomized to receive either interferon-γ (50 μg/M^2 s.c., 3 times weekly) or placebo. The end-point of the study was time to the first serious infection (requiring intravenous antibiotics and hospitalization). Seventy-nine percent of the patients on interferon therapy were free of serious infections after twelve months, compared to thirty percent in the placebo group. The relative risk of serious infection with interferon was one third the risk with placebo. The total number of serious infections was also significantly different (56 in the placebo group vs. 20 in the treated group). Patients in the placebo group required three times as many hospital days as those in the interferon group. Subgroup analysis revealed interferon benefit without regard to gender, mode of inheritance, or use of prophylactic antibiotics. Patients younger than 10 years derived a greater benefit than older patients.

No serious adverse effects could be attributed to the interferon-γ. Only four patients had to withdraw because of toxicity: two with constitutional symptoms (a "flu-like" sydrome), one with rash, and one with worsening of CGD-related granulomatous colitis. No abnormalities were seen with monitoring of hematologic or biochemical indices. Mild elevations of liver enzymes were equally common in both the treated and placebo groups.

Monitoring of phagocyte oxidative metabolism from a subgroup of patients in the trial revealed the surprising result that the clinical benefit of interferon-γ was unaccompanied by improvements in respiratory burst activity as assayed by superoxide production, NBT staining, or cytochrome b content [32, 33]. Several non-oxidative neutrophil antimicrobial proteins were also unaffected by treatment [33]. In some patients, a small subset of NBT$^+$ circulating monocytes were observed [32]. It is possible that this small subset provided sufficient activity to explain the observed protection.

In summary, a large controlled trial of interferon-γ in CGD revealed clear clinical benefit in reducing the number of serious infections with minimal toxicity. However, the mechanism by which this salutary effect was achieved remains unclear.

Hyperimmunoglobulinemia E/Job's syndrome

Hyperimmunoglobulinemia E (HIE), also referred to as Job's syndrome, is characterized by recurrent staphylococcal abscesses without overt signs of inflammation ("cold" abscesses), along with eczema and recurrent sinopulmonary infections [34, 35]. Immunologic abnormalities present in this disease include extreme elevations in the serum IgE, abnormal delayed-type hypersensitivity, and defective PMN chemotaxis (which is presumed to cause the "cold" nature of the abscesses). Del Prete *et al.* [36] reported that circulating T cells from patients with HIE produced much less interferon-γ in response to the non-specific T-cell mitogen phytohemagglutinin than T cells from controls. Production of TNF was also decreased, whereas IL-4 and IL-2 were unchanged. Since interferon-γ is known to decrease IgE synthesis, this suggested that interferon-γ deficiency may be part of the defect in HIE. However, Vercelli and colleagues [37] have performed similar experiments with HIE patient cells and have not found any difference in interferon-γ or IL-4 production between patient and normal cells. In addition, interferon-γ had no effect on spontaneous IgE synthesis by HIE patient cells, suggesting instead that the IgE synthesis in HIE is due to terminally differentiated B cells which are independent of cytokine stimuli. The results of Vercelli *et al.* [37] are difficult to reconcile with those of Del Prete *et al.* [36] King *et al.* [38]

demonstrated reduction of IgE synthesis *in vitro* and *in vivo* in patients with HIE.

The effect of interferon-γ on the defective neutrophil chemotaxis in HIE was studied by Jeppson and colleagues [39]. *In vitro* treatment with interferon-γ stimulated patient neutrophil chemotaxis, with stimulated patient levels reaching almost or above normal unstimulated levels. This suggests that interferon-γ might be beneficial in reducing the incidence of bacterial infections in HIE by enabling PMN to reach sites of infection.

In summary, the scientific rationale for the use of interferon-γ in HIE is controversial. Thus far there is no compelling evidence of its efficacy in this disorder. The physician treating a patient with this disorder is thus left with the hope that in the individual patient, the benefit outweighs the risks of therapy described above.

Gamma-interferon in the newborn

Human newborns have an increased susceptibility to a variety of infections, as compared with older children and adults. A number of immune functions have been shown to be depressed in the neonate, including chemotaxis, adherence and chemiluminescence of phagocytes, as well as decreased nonspecific mononuclear and T-cell cytotoxicity [40, 41]. Many, if not most, of these defects may be explained by decreased production of cytokines IL-2 production by neonatal cells appears to be normal. However, production of another crucial cytokine, interferon-γ , by newborn T cells is substantially depressed [40, 41]. Treatment of newborn PMN with interferon-γ *in vitro* can significantly stimulate chemotaxis [41].

A rational argument can be made for the use of interferon-γ as replacement therapy for low birth weight babies who are at significant risk for infections. A phase I safety study in twelve low birth weight infants (750–1500 g) has been conducted. The agent was administered three times weekly for four weeks, and the patients have been followed for one year. Our preliminary findings indicate that the cytokine can be safely administered [Ringer S, Ezekowitz RAB. Unpublished observations]. The next challenge is to define reliable endpoints by which we can determine the efficacy of interferon-γ prophylaxis in the reduction of morbiditiy and mortality associated with bacterial and fungal infections in the newborn period. The design of such a trial is underway, and it is our hope that this population may benefit most from interferon-γ adjuvant therapy.

Other primary immunodeficiencies

Surveys of peripheral blood mononuclear cells from patients with assorted congenital immunodeficiencies (common variable immunodeficiency, ataxia telangiectasia, and others) have revealed apparent deficiencies in interferon-γ production *in vitro* in some patients with each diagnosis [42]. These results presumably reflect the intrinsic heterogeneity of the clinical diagnoses. They suggest that trials of interferon-γ may be warranted in these diagnoses. Selecting patients with *in vitro* deficient interferon-γ production and with the ability to respond *in vitro* to exogenous cytokine may be desirable.

Omenn's syndrome is a rare combined immunodeficiency accompanied by hypereosinophilia [43]. One patient who was studied intensively had elevated levels of circulating IL-5 (normally undetectable in serum) [44]. The patient also had high levels of *in vitro* IL-4 and IL-5 production, with low levels of interferon-γ and IL-2, when compared to normal controls. This patient entered a compassionate-use protocol under which he was treated with interferon-γ *in vivo*, as his condition was unresponsive to conventional therapy. On interferon-γ therapy, he displayed a rapid clinical and radiologic resolution of diffuse interstitial pneumonitis (no pathogen identified), a decrease in the circulating eosinophil count, and a reversal in the pattern of cytokines produced *in vitro* from a "Th2'-like pattern (predominance of IL-4, IL-5, and IL-10) to a "Th1'-like pattern (predominance of IL-2 and interferon-γ) [44].

These anecdotal accounts indicate that a detailed knowledge of the basic defects that underly primary immunodeficiencies is an essential prerequisite to instituting cytokine therapy.

Interleukin-2

Biology of interleukin-2

IL-2 is a small glycoprotein produced by activated T cells, primarily of the CD4 ("helper") class [45, 46]. Its production is induced by antigen (or experimentally by plant mitogens) in combination with macrophage-derived interleukin-1. This combination of stimuli lead to a coordinated response leading to the synthesis of both IL-2 and its receptor. IL-2, in combination with antigen, then continues to stimulate the responding T-cells in a positive feedback loop. IL-2 is an essential part of the activation pathway of T lymphocytes for proliferation as well as the development of effector functions, e.g. cytotoxic T cells, NK cells, and possibly for B-cell immunoglobulin secretion.

Pharmacology of IL-2

Interleukin-2, like many of the other cytokines, has a very short half-life when given intravenously [45, 46]. Subcutaneous administration provides a more prolonged effect. IL-2 is most commonly used in a recombinant preparation which is not glycosylated, but which seems to have equivalent *in vitro* bioactivity to the native human molecule. Doses exceeding 10^5 U/kg (or 3–6 $\times$ 10^5 U/kg/day) typically cause significant side effects including fever, chills, tachcardia, headache, malaise, nausea and vomiting, diarrhea, and a vascular leak syndrome resulting in fluid retention, dyspnea and pulmonary edema. Less common symptoms include myalgias, arthralgias, coagulopathy, hypoglycemia, lymphopenia and thrombocytopenia. Laboratory abnormalities include increased serum creatinine, bilirubin, and cortisol, as well as anemia and eosinophilia. Some of the adverse effects (fever, chills, and myalgias) may be effectively prevented by pre-treatment with aspirin or other non-steroidal anti-inflammatory drugs. Since the half-life in the circulation is short, and toxicity may be dose-limiting, localized injection of IL-2 has been employed in various illnesses with localized lesions (e.g. tumors, leprosy) with some success, although the numbers of patients were small.

Common variable immune deficiency (CVID)

CVID is a heterogeneous group of disorders involving deficient production of immunoglobulin or of effective antibodies. Cunningham-Rundles and colleagues [47] selected a group of CVID patients with decreased T helper activity and *in vitro* proliferative response to PEG-IL-2 (the modification of IL-2 with polyethylene glycol greatly increases its *in vivo* half-life) for a trial of this cytokine *in vivo*. During 3 months of treatment and for weeks thereafter, patient B cells secreted 10–1000 fold more immunoglobulin *in vitro*. Patient T cells also had increased activity, stimulating B cells from normals 10–1000 fold better than before treatment. No change was seen in serum immunoglobulin levels during treatment, but patients continued to receive intravenous immune globulin throughout the trial. *In vitro* production of specific anti-tetanus antibody, absent before the trial, was observed during treatment. While the trial was not designed to rigorously assess clinical benefit, some observations were made. A patient with opacified nasal sinuses had radiographic clearing during PEG-IL-2 treatment without antibiotic therapy. Another patient with chronic pneumonia and bronchitis, usually maintained on chronic, rotating antibiotics, was able to stay off antibiotics for 90% of his seven-month treatment period. A third patient with mucocutaneous candidiasis had clearing of skin lesions during treatment.

Other IL-2 deficiency syndromes

Weinberg and Parkman [6] described a patient with a severe combined immunodeficiency (SCID) phenotype who had normal numbers of circulating T lymphocytes, but defective proliferation in response to non-specific stimuli (mitogen, or phorbol ester and ionophore). Direct assay of IL-2 mRNA revealed complete absence of detectable message, despite normal levels of interferon-γ mRNA. This suggests a primary IL-2 deficiency. Such a patient might benefit from treatment with IL-2, either prophylactically or as adjuvant therapy with infections.

Chatila and colleagues have described a patient with SCID with normal signal transduction but with decreased transcription of multiple cytokine genes, including those for IL-2, -3, -4, -5, and interferon-γ [48]. They treated this patient with recombinant IL-2 after failure of two bone marrow transplants [49]. She tolerated treatment well, and has been maintained on thrice-weekly IV infusions of IL-2 with no serious infections since beginning therapy.

Five patients with various primary immunodeficiencies (two with Nezelof's syndrome, three with SCID) were studied by Flomenberg *et al.* [50]. Two of the five children (both with Nezelof's syndrome) had depressed *in vitro* IL-2 production, but only one had an *in vitro* proliferative response to exogenous IL-2, suggesting that he might be a candidate for IL-2 therapy.

A patient with ataxia telangiectasia who had no *in vitro* IL-2 production, had severe, refractory pnemonia and was treated with IL-2 [51]. He had transient clinical improvement, but with continued administration he worsened, despite an increase in IL-2 dosage. Laboratory results of therapy included a selective increase in serum IgM and restoration of *in vitro* lymphocyte proliferation.

Buckley and others [52] treated a patient presenting in infancy with T lymphocytosis, decreased *in vitro* proliferation and IL-2 production, low B and NK cell numbers, and hypogammaglobulinemia. One month of IL-2 therapy resulted in marked improvement of massive pyoderma gangrenosum. However, they also treated an infant with DiGeorge syndrome who on treatment developed T cells with a normal cell-surface phenotype, but the lymphocytes did not respond to mitogen.

These experiences indicate that IL-2 can be clinically useful in individual patients. The challenge lies in identifying these patients.

Colony-stimulating factors

Biology of G- and GM-CSF

G-CSF is a small glycoprotein produced by monocyte/macrophage cells as well as nonhematopoetic cells [53]. At low concentrations, it stimulates developement of pure neutrophil colonies; at higher concentrations, macrophage colonies also arise. It also has actions on mature neutrophils, lengthening *in vitro* survival, sensitizing PMN to stimuli and enhancing their maximal response.

GM-CSF is a variably glycosylated protein, produced by endothelial cells and fibroblasts; glycosylation affects biologic activity. It stimulates formation of neutrophil, eosinophil, and monocyte/macrophage colonies, as well as stimulating various functions of mature cells of these lineages. GM-CSF increases PMN and eosinophil survival, and PMN and monocyte/macrophage phagocytosis, adhesion, and secretion, as well as secondary cytokine secretion and Class II MHC expression by mononuclear phagocytes. G-CSF, and to a lesser extent GM-CSF, has been used succcessfully to treat neutropenia induced by myelotoxic chemotherapy as well as other acquired neutropenias.

Pharmacology of G- and GM-CSF

GM-CSF and G-CSF are both produced as recombinant molecules in bacteria [53]. Despite the changes in biologic activity *in vitro* with nonglycosylated GM-CSF, *in vivo* studies have shown no difference in efficacy.

G-CSF given intravenously has a slower clearance (half-life of 1–7 hr) from the circulation than some of the other cytokines described above. In addition, its half-life was prolonged above a threshold dose, suggesting a saturable clearance mechanism. Subcutaneous administration provides a still more prolonged effect. G-CSF is usually quite well tolerated at doses required to produce a clinical effect. Doses producing a leukocytosis in excess of 20,000/μL may produce medullary bone pain. In one patient, a cutaneous necrotic vasculitis developed after 12 days of therapy, forcing a dose reduction [54].

GM-CSF has a somewhat shorter circulatory half-life, although subcutaneous administration still provides a prolonged maintenance of high levels in the serum. Toxicities of GM-CSF include lethargy, myalgia, anorexia, rash, and flushing, although these are rarely severe enough to necessitate stopping the drug. Lesions may develop at the injection site, suggesting the desirability of rotating the site. Fever may occur at moderate doses (>3 μg/kg/dose). A characteristic first–dose reaction characterized by flushing, tachycardia, hypotension, pain, nausea and vomiting, dyspnea, and decreases in arterial blood oxygen saturation may occur. This first-dose reaction appears to be related to the peak dose, occurring more commonly after intravenous than subcutaneous administration. Doses exceeding 20 μg/kg usually produce severe, dose-limiting adverse effects including fluid retention and weight gain, pleural and pericardial inflammation and effusions, and thrombotic events.

CSF's in congenital neutropenia

Congenital agranulocytosis, or Kostmann's syndrome, is characterized by a persistent severe neutropenia accompanied by maturational arrest of bone marrow myeloid progenitors. Five patients were treated with G-CSF [55] in doses ranging from 3–60 μg/kg/day in a single intravenous daily dose, with gradual titration upward of dose until a peripheral blood response was seen. In all five patients, the drug was effective, producing an increase in circulating PMN counts approximately 8 days after an effective dosage was reached. The absolute neutrophils counts rose from 0–114/μL to 1300–9500/μL on therapy. Bone marrow sampling revealed maturation of neutrophil precursors, although still at reduced levels. Clinical response included total disappearance of chronic oral ulcerations, good skin healing, and a ten-fold decrease in days of antibiotic therapy for documented infection (During the year prior to the trial, the five patients received a mean of 90 days of antibiotics; during a follow-up year on therapy, the average was 9.6 days.) Adverse effects were minimal, with medullary pain coinciding with increasing WBC counts in one patient. Two patients developed moderate increases in spleen size, and serum alkaline phosphatase levels increased. No serious toxicity was encountered. A curious feature of this study is that cycling of neutrophil counts was seen (see discussion below).

Weston and colleagues studied seven patients with congenital agranulocytosis [56]. Patients were treated with 10 μg/kg/day in two divided doses for four months. There was a marked clinical improvement in periodontitis/gingivitis, although eroded alveolar bone did not re-accumulate during the four-month treatment period. In addition, all patients had complete disappearance of oral ulcerations with no recurrence while on treatment. Similar to the observation of Bonilla *et al.* [55], one subgroup of four patients had oscillations of their ANC while on therapy, with periods ranging from 7–22 days. These patients had low superoxide production and cytochrome b content, while the other three patients, whose ANC rose and remained steadily at a normal level, had normal superoxide production and cytochrome b content. The existence of these two subgroups suggests the possibility of diverse pathophysiologic mechanisms in Kostmann's syndrome. The cycling of neutrophil counts observed in these two studies suggests that some cases of congenital neutropenia may arise from underlying defects similar to those in cyclic neutropenia.

Welte *et al.* [54] treated five patients with GM-CSF (dose, 3–30 μg/kg/day) for 6 weeks. Four out of five patients had increased peripheral blood eosinophil count; only one patient had an increase in the absolute neutrophil count (ANC). Subsequently, all five patients were treated with G-CSF; all responded with increased ANC which could be maintained by prolonged maintenance therapy. All five patients were infection-free during 3 months or more of treatment, having suffered at least one serious bacterial infection in the 6 months prior to initiation of G-CSF. One patient developed a leukocytoclastic vasculitis of both legs, necessitating a drug vacation and resumption at lower dose. This reaction recurred when dose re-escalation was attempted. The patient was able to be maintained at the lower dose without any ill effects. A single patient had an increase in serum alkaline phosphatase.

G-CSF in cyclic neutropenia

Cyclic neutropenia is a rare disease with periodic decreases in the circulating neutrophil count (usually accompanied by similar decreases in monocytes, eosinophils, lymphocytes, platelets, and reticulocytes), occurring usually at 21 day intervals. Clinical manifestations include periodic occurrence of fever and mucosal ulcerations, and occasional serious bacterial infections during periods of neutropenia. Hammond *et al.* [57] treated six patients with 3–10 μg/kg/day of G-CSF (initially intravenously, later subcutaneously). The cycling of ANC continued, but the length of the period decreased from 21 to 14 days, and the time of severe neutropenia (ANC < 200/μL) was decreased (from 12 days/month to 0.7 days/month). The mean nadir ANC increased from 17 to 1393/μL. Clinically, therapy reduced oral ulcers and febrile episodes, as well as the incidence of serious infections. The drug was well tolerated; two patients had transient bone pain during the first few days of therapy. All six patients had moderate splenomegaly and increased serum alkaline phosphatase.

A single patient treated by Hanada and colleagues [58] did well with G-CSF therapy intermittently, started at the first signs of gingivostomatitis.

Boxer and colleagues [59] report a series of 41 patients in an open-label trial of G-CSF administered to patients with various forms of severe primary neutropenias (congenital, cyclic or other chronic forms). Treatment resulted in maintenance of the ANC above 1500/μL in 40 of the 41 patients. There was complete resolution of ginigivitis and oral ulcers in 40 of the 41 patients, and no serious infections occurred. Several patients experienced transient bone pain not requiring dose modification. Other minimal adverse effects included rash, splenomegaly, and increases in serum alkaline phosphatase, lactate dehydrogenase, and uric acid. Some patients experienced thrombocytopenia necessitating drug withdrawal, but were later able to tolerate G-CSF therapy without problems.

GM-CSF and chronic granulomatous disease

A patient with variant X-linked CGD with a liver abscess refractory to standard medical treatment was treated with GM-CSF [60]. This therapy was administered in an attempt to avoid the need for surgical drainage. The patient had increased circulating granulocytes (primarily eosinophils), but no change in respiratory burst activity as measured by

NBT reduction, superoxide production or phagocyte-specific cytochrome b content. There was no clinical benefit. Thus, although this is a single patient, the data do not suggest utility of GM-CSF in variant X-linked CGD.

Summary

Studies of G-CSF therapy in both congenital and cyclic neutropenia demonstrate that it is both safe and effective. There may be rare cases of either disorder which are resistant to treatment, reflecting heterogeneity of the underlying pathophysiology. The case cited above of GM-CSF adjuvant therapy in CGD showed no benefit. However, since this was a single patient, no firm conclusion can be drawn concerning possible benefit of CSFs in CGD. They may have a role in combination with interferon-γ , but it is unlikely that a clinical trial which includes enough patients will ever be effected so as to answer this question definitively.

Interferon-α

Interferon-α, the protype antiviral interferon, has some immunomodulatory activities as well. Interferon-α *in vitro* decreases IgE synthesis by peripheral blood mononuclear cells, leading to its use in a patient with the hyperimmunoglobulin E syndrome [61]. The patient had severe eczema, which resolved rapidly on twice-weekly interferon-α therapy, and recurred after cessation of therapy. Other objective results of therapy included a dramatic decrease in serum IgE and decreased circulating $CD23^+$ cells.

Thymic hormones

Numerous thymus-derived molecules with biological activity have been characterized. Several of these have been used in uncontrolled trials in small numbers of patients with T cell immunodeficiencies. These include thymosin fraction 5, a crude fraction of thymic extract containing several polypeptides; thymostimulin, a crude calf thymic extract; and two pure polypeptides, FTS (Factor thymique serique) and thymopoietin (usually a synthetic pentapeptide, termed TP-5 is used, as this has equivalent *in vitro* bioactivity and is more easily synthesized).

Wara, Amann and colleagues have treated patients with various immunodeficiencies with thymosin. Patients with thymic hypoplasia, Wiskott-Aldrich syndrome, and chronic mucocutaneous candidiasis had clinical improvement coincident with treatment [62, 63].

Aiuti and colleagues have attempted therapy of various immunodeficiences with TP-5. Treatment of three patients with DiGeorge syndrome (congenital athymia) and three with primary T-cell defects has produced both increased immune function and apparent clinical benefit [64]. Two patients treated with TP-5 for 14 months (from birth) have had no serious infections and no obvious adverse effects of the drug [65]. Results in other immune deficiences have been less encouraging [63, 64].

Some patients with T-cell developmental abnormalities appear to benefit from thymic hormone preparations. The multitude of different preparations and the small number of patients treated make it is difficult to ascertain the magnitude of benefit under these circumstances. This situation might well benefit from a individual patient-based, "n-of-1" placebo-controlled blinded cross-over trial [8] with objective outcome measures such as number of infections, hospital admissions, days of school or work missed, etc.

Conclusions

Cytokines have an important place in the treatment of primary immunodeficiencies. In some cases, cytokines serve as replacement therapy for molecules deficient as the primary cause of an immunodeficiency or as a secondary consequence. In other cases, they may be able to activate compensatory mechanisms.

The best proven example of the benefit of cytokine therapy is in chronic granulomatous disease, in which a large, placebo-controlled trial was able to show the positive effect of interferon-γ on many clinical endpoints. This trial suggests some considerations for clinical trials of other cytokines in primary immunodeficiencies:

1. To amass enough patients with this rare disease required an international, multicenter cooperative effort. Some immunodeficiencies may not be prevalent enough to accumulate enough patients even with such massive effort. These diseases may need to be studied with individual patient-based "n-of-one" randomized crossover trials.
2. When the trial was started, the spectrum of different molecular defects underlying CGD was known, and these individual defects had been elucidated.

Attempting a trial for a disease which is defined only as a phenotype, without corresponding molecular pathophysiologic knowledge may lead to confusing results if that phenotype has many underlying causes. It may even lead to the abandonment of a therapy which would be effective for patients with a particular form of the disease (i.e. molecular defect). In some cases, *in vitro* assays of cytokine effect on patient cells may lead to more appropriate selection of patients for *in vivo* trials.

3. It is essential to develop objective endpoints for assesment of drug benefit i.e. primarily clinical endpoints. Immunologic assays may be useful as surrogate end points.

As our understanding of the molecular defects underlying these diseases increases, selection of additional candidate diseases for cytokine therapy may be possible. Clinical trials must be carefully designed to allow the recognition of situations in which cytokines are truly beneficial and to ensure the appropriate use of these powerful and costly drugs. It should be noted that the follow-up of patients on chronic prophylaxis with both interferon-γ and G-CSF is relatively short thus far, hence it is extremely important to follow these patients closely and to continue to reevaluate the benefits of cytokine therapy compared with the potential long term toxicities.

References

1. Allen RC, Armitage RJ, Conley ME, Rosenblatt H, Jenkins NA, Copeland NG, Bedell MA, Edelhoff S, Disteche CM, Simoneaux DK, *et al.* CD40 ligand gene defects responsible for X-linked hyper-IgM syndrome. Science 1993; 259: 990–3.
2. Aruffo A, Farrington M, Hollenbaugh D, Li X, Milatovich A, Nonoyama S, Bajorath J, Grosmaire LS, Stenkamp R, Neubauer M, *et al.* The CD40 ligand, gp39, is defective in activated T cells from patients with X-linked hyper-IgM syndrome. Cell 1993; 72: 291–300.
3. DiSanto JP, Bonnefoy JY, Gauchat JF, Fischer A, de Saint Basile G. CD40 ligand mutations in x-linked immunodeficiency with hyper-IgM. Nature 1993; 361: 541–3.
4. Fuleihan R, Ramesh N, Loh R, Jabara H, Rosen RS, Chatila T, Fu SM, Stamenkovic I, Geha RS. Defective expression of the CD40 ligand in X chromosome-linked immunoglobulin deficiency with normal or elevated IgM. Proc Natl Acad Sci USA 1993; 90: 2170–3.
5. Korthauer U, Graf D, Mages HW, Briere F, Padayachee M, Malcolm S, Ugazio AG, Notarangelo LD, Levinsky RJ, Kroczek RA. Defective expression of T-cell CD40 ligand causes X-linked immunodeficiency with hyper-IgM. Nature 1993; 361: 539–41.
6. Weinberg K, Parkman R. Severe combined immunodeficiency due to a specific defect in the production of interleukin-2. N Engl J Med 1990; 322: 1718–1723.
7. Noguchi M, Yi H, Rosenblatt HM, Filipovich AH, Adelstein S, Modi WS, McBride OW, Leonard WJ. Interleukin-2 receptor γ chain mutation results in X-linked severe combined immunodeficiency in humans. Cell 1993; 73: 147–157.
8. Guyatt GH, Keller JL, Jaeschke R, Rosenbloom D, Adachi JD, Newhouse MT. The n-of-1 randomized controlled trial: clinical usefulness. Ann Int Med 1990; 112: 293–299.
9. Blaese RM. Development of gene therapy for immunodeficiency: adenosine deaminase deficiency. Pediatr Res 1993; 33: S49–53; discussion S53–5.
10. Culver KW, Anderson WF, Blaese RM. Lymphocyte gene therapy. Hum Gene Ther 1991; 2: 107–9.
11. Lewis DB, Wilson CB. Gamma-interferon: an immunoregulatory lymphokine with immunotherapeutic potential. Ped Inf Dis J 1990; 9: 642–651.
12. Todd PA, Goa KL. Interferon gamma-1b. A review of its pharmacology and therapeutic potential in chronic granulomatous disease. Drugs 1992; 43: 111–22.
13. The International Chronic Granulomatous Disease Study Group. A controlled trial of interferon gamma to prevent infection in chronic granulomatous disease. N Engl J Med 1991; 324: 509–516.
14. Tauber AI, Borregaard N, Simons E, Wright J. Chronic granulomatous disease: a syndrome of phagocyte oxidase deficiencies. Medicine 1983; 62: 286–309.
15. Dinauer MC, Orkin SH. Chronic granulomatous disease. Annu Rev Med 1992; 43: 117–24.
16. Royer-Pokora B, Kunkel LM, Monaco AP, Goff SC, Newburger PE, Baehner RL, Cole FS, Curnutte JT, Orkin SH. Cloning the gene for an inherited human disorder-chronic granulomatous disease-on the basis of its chromosomal location. Nature 1986; 322: 32–38.
17. Dinauer MC, Orkin SH, Brown R, Jesaitis AJ, Parkos CA. The glycoprotein encoded by the X-linked chronic granulomatous disease locus is a component of the neutrophil cytochrome b complex. Nature 1987; 327: 717–720.
18. Curnutte JT, Berkow RL, Roberts RL, Shurin SB, Scott PJ. Chronic granulomatous disease due to a defect in the cytosolic factor required for nicotinamide adenine dinucleotide phosphate oxidase activation. J Clin Invest 1988; 81: 606–10.
19. Curnutte JT, Scott PJ, Mayo LA. Cytosolic components of the respiratory burst oxidase: resolution of four components, two of which are missing in complementing types of chronic granulomatous disease. Proc Natl Acad Sci USA 1989; 86: 825–9.
20. Volpp BD, Nauseef WM, Clark RA. Two cytosolic neutrophil oxidase components absent in autosomal chronic granulomatous disease. Science 1988; 242: 1295–7.
21. Volpp BD, Nauseef WM, Donelson JE, Moser DR, Clark RA. Cloning of the cDNA and functional expression of the 47-kilodalton cytosolic component of human neutrophil respiratory burst oxidase. Proc Natl Acad Sci USA 1989; 86: 7195–9.
22. Nunoi H, Rotrosen D, Gallin JI, Malech HL. Two forms of autosomal chronic granulomatous disease lack distinct neutrophil cytosol factors. Science 1988; 242: 1298–301.
23. Leto TL, Lomax KJ, Volpp BD, Nunoi H, Sechler JM, Nauseef WM, Clark RA, Gallin JI, Malech HL. Cloning of a 67-kD neutrophil oxidase factor with similarity to a noncatalytic region of p60c-src. Science 1990; 248: 727–30.
24. Lomax KJ, Leto TL, Nunoi H, Gallin JI, Malech HL. Recombinant 47-kilodalton cytosol factor restores NADPH oxidase in chronic granulomatous disease. Science 1989; 245: 409–12.
25. Dinauer MC, Pierce EA, Bruns GA, Curnutte JT, Orkin SH. Human neutrophil cytochrome b light chain (p22-phox).

Gene structure, chromosomal location, and mutations in cytochrome-negative autosomal recessive chronic granulomatous disease. J Clin Invest 1990; 86: 1729–37.
26. Berton G, Zeni L, Cassatella NA, Rossi F. Gamma interferon is able to enhance the oxidative metabolism of human neutrophils. Biochem Biophys Res Comm 1986; 138: 1276–1282.
27. Newburger PE, Ezekowitz RA, Whitney C, Wright J, Orkin SH. Induction of phagocyte cytochrome b heavy chain gene expression by interferon gamma. Proc Natl Acad Sci USA 1988; 85: 5215–9.
28. Sechler JM, Malech HL, White CJ, Gallin JI. Recombinant human interferon-gamma reconstitutes defective phagocyte function in patients with chronic granulomatous disease of childhood. Proc Natl Acad Sci USA 1988; 85: 4874–8.
29. Ezekowitz RAB, Orkin SH, Newburger PE. Recombinant interferon gamma augments phagocyte superoxide production and X-chronic granulomatous disease gene expression in X-linked variant chronic granulomatous disease. J Clin Invest 1987; 80: 1009–1016.
30. Ezekowitz RAB, Dinauer MC, Jaffe HS, Orkin SH, Newburger PE. Partial correction of the phagocyte defect in patients with X-linked chronic granulomatous disease by subcutaneous interferon gamma. N Engl J Med 1988; 319: 146–151.
31. Ezekowitz RAB, Sieff CA, Dinauer MC, Nathan DG, Orkin SH, Newburger PE. Restoration of phagocyte function interferon-g in X-linked chronic granulomatous disease occurs at the level of a progenitor cell. Blood 1990; 76: 2443–2448.
32. Woodman RC, Erickson RW, Rae J, Jaffe HS, Curnutte JT. Prolonged recombinant interferon-gamma therapy in chronic granulomatous disease: evidence against enhanced neutrophil oxidase activity. Blood 1992; 79: 1558–62.
33. Muhlebach TJ, Gabay J, Nathan CF, Erny C, Dopfer G, Schroten H, Wahn V, Seger RA. Treatment of patients with chronic granulomatous disease with recombinant human interferon-gamma does not improve neutrophil oxidative metabolism, cytochrome b558 content or levels of four antimicrobial proteins. Clin Exp Immunol 1992; 88: 203–6.
34. Leung DY, Geha RS. Clinical and immunologic aspects of the hyperimmunoglobulin E syndrome. Hematol Oncol Clin North Am 1988; 2: 81–100.
35. Geha RS, Leung DY. Hyper immunoglobulin E syndrome. Immunodefic Rev 1989; 1: 155–72.
36. Del Prete G, Tiri A, Maggi E, De Carli M, Macchia D, Parronchi P, Rossi ME, Pietrogrande MC, Ricci M, Romagnani S. Defective *in vitro* production of γ-interferon and tumor necrosis factor-α by circulating T cells from patients with the hyperimmunoglobulinemia E syndrome. J Clin Invest 1989; 84: 1830–1835.
37. Vercelli D, Jabara HH, Cunningham-Rundles C, Abrams JS, Lewis DB, Meyer J, Schneider LC, Leung DY, Geha RS. Regulation of immunoglobulin (Ig)E synthesis in the hyper-IgE syndrome. J Clin Invest 1990; 85: 1666–71.
38. King CL, Gallin JI, Malech HL, Abramson SL, Nutman TB. Regulation of immunoglobulin production in hyperimmunoglobulin E recurrent-infection syndrome by interferon gamma. Proc Natl Acad Sci USA 1989; 86: 10085–9.
39. Jeppson JD, Jaffe HS, Hill HR. Use of recombinant human interferon gamma to enhance neutrophil chemotactic responses in Job syndrome of hyperimmunoglobulinemia E and recurrent infections. J Peds 1991; 118: 383–387.
40. Wilson CB, Lewis DB. Basis and implications of selectively diminished cytokine production in neonatal susceptibility to infection. Rev Infect Dis 1990; [12 Suppl 4]: S410–20.
41. Hill HR. Modulation of host defenses with interferon-γ in pediatrics. J Infec Dis 1993; 167: S23–28.
42. Paganelli R, Capobianchi MR, Ensoli B, D'Offizi GP, Facchini J, Dianzani F, Aiuti F. Evidence that defective gamma interferon production in patients with primary immunodeficiencies is due to intrinsic incompetence of lymphocytes. Clin Exp Immunol 1988; 72: 124–129.
43. Omenn GS. Familial reticuloendotheliosis with eosinophilia. N Engl J Med 1965; 273: 427–432.
44. Schandene L, Ferster A, Mascart-Lemone F, Crusiaux A, Gerard C, Marchant A, Lybin M, Velu T, Sariban E, Goldman M. T helper type 2-like cells and therapeutic effects of interferon-gamma in combined immunodeficiency with hypereosinophilia (Omenn's syndrome). Eur J Immunol 1993; 23: 56–60.
45. Welte K, Mertelsmann R. Human interleukin 2: biochemistry, physiology, and possible pathogenetic role in immunodeficiency syndromes. Cancer Invest 1985; 3: 35–49.
46. Hadden JW. Recent advances in the preclinical and clinical immunopharmacology of interleukin-2: emphasis on IL-2 as an immunorestorative agent. Cancer Det Prev 1988; 12: 537–552.
47. Cunningham-Rundles C, Mayer L, Sapira E, Mendelsohn L. Restoration of immunoglobulin secretion *in vitro* in common variable immunodeficiency by *in vivo* treatment with polyethylene glycol- conjugated human recombinant interleukin-2. Clin Immunol Immunopathol 1992; 64: 46–56.
48. Chatila T, Castigli E, Pahwa R, Pahwa S, Chirmule N, Oyaizu N, Good RA, Geha RS. Primary combined immunodeficiency resulting from defective transcription of multiple T-cell lymphokine genes. Proc Natl Acad Sci USA 1990; 87: 10033–7.
49. Pahwa R, Chatila T, Pahwa S, Paradise C, Day NK, Geha R, Schwartz SA, Slade H, Oyaizu N, Good RA. Recombinant interleukin 2 therapy in severe combined immunodeficiency disease. Proc Natl Acad Sci USA 1989; 86: 5069–73.
50. Flomenberg N, Welte K, Mertelsmann R, Kernan N, Ciobanu N, Venuta S, Feldman S, Kruger G, Kirkpatrick D, Dupont B, O'Reilly R. Immunologic effects of interleukin 2 in primary immunodeficiency diseases. J Immunol 1983; 130: 2644–50.
51. Doi S, Saiki O, Hara T, Sugita T, Ha-Kawa K, Tanaka T, Hara H, Negoro S, Yabuuchi H, Kishimoto S. Administration of recombinant IL-2 augments the level of serum IgM in an IL-2 deficient patient. Eur J Peds 1989; 148: 630–633.
52. Buckley R, Schiff R, Schiff S, Markert L, Gerber P, Paradise C. Recombinant human interleukin 2 (rhIL-2) therapy in primary immunodeficiency. J Allergy Immunol 1989; 83: 296.
53. Lieschke GJ, Burgess AW. Granulocyte colony-stimulating factor and granulocyte-macrophage colony-stimulating factor. N Engl J Med 1992; 327: 28–35.
54. Welte K, Zeidler C, Reiter A, Müller W, Odenwald E, Souza L, Riehm H. Differential effects of granulocyte-macrophage colony-stimulating factor and granulocyte colony-stimulating factor. Blood 1990; 75: 1056–1063.
55. Bonilla MA, Gillio AP, Ruggeiro M, al. e. Effects of recombinant human granulocyte colony-stimulating factor on neutropenia in patients with congential agranulocytosis. N Engl J Med 1989; 320: 1574–1580.
56. Weston B, Todd R3, Axtell R, Balazovich K, Stewart J, Locey BJ, Mayo-Bond L, Loos P, Hutchinson R, Boxer LA. Severe congenital neutropenia: clinical effects and neutrophil function during treatment with granulocyte colony-stimulating factor. J Lab Clin Med 1991; 117: 282–90.
57. Hammond WP, Price TH, Souza LM, Dale DC. Treatment of cylic neutropenia with granulocyte colony-stimulating factor. N Engl J Med 1989; 320: 1306–1311.

58. Hanada T, Ono I, Nagasawa T. Childhood cyclic neutropenia treated with recombinant human granulocyte colony stimulating factor. Br J Haematol 1990; 75: 135–137.
59. Boxer LA, Hutchinson R, Emerson S. Recombinant human granulocyte-colony-stimulating factor in the treatment of patients with neutropenia. Clin Immunol Immunopathol 1992; 62: S39–46.
60. Muhlebach TJ, Feickert HJ, Welte K, Seger RA. Granulocyte-macrophage colony stimulating factor does not improve neutrophil oxidative metabolism in a patient with variant X-linked chronic granulomatous disease. Eur J Pediatr 1991; 150: 575–8.
61. Souillet G, Rousset F, De Vries JE. Alpha-interferon treatment of patient with Hyper IgE syndrome. Lancet 1989; 1: 1384.
62. Wara DW, Goldstein AL, Doyle NE, Ammann AJ. Thymosin activity in patients with cellular immunodeficiency. N Engl J Med 1975; 292: 70–4.
63. Wara DW, Ammann AJ. Thymosin treatment of children with primary immunodeficiency disease. Transplant Proc 1978; 10: 203–9.
64. Aiuti F, Businco L, Fiorilli M, Galli E, Quinti I, Rossi P, Seminara R, Goldstein G. Thymopoietin pentapeptide treatment of primary immunodeficiencies. Lancet 1983; 1: 551–4.
65. Businco L, Rubaltelli FF, Paganelli R, Galli E, Ensoli B, Betti P, Aiuti F. Results in two infants with the DiGeorge syndrome–effects of long-term TP5. Clin Immunol Immunopathol 1986; 39: 222–30.
66. Adamson JW, Eschbach JW. Treatment of the anemia of chronic renal failure with recombinant human erythropoietin. Annu Rev Med 1990; 41: 349–60.
67. Murray HW. Cytokines as antimicrobial therapy for the T cell-deficient patient: Prospects for treatment of nonviral opportunistic infections. [Review] Clin Infect Dis 17 Suppl 2: S407–13.

Biotherapy 7: 261–269, 1994.

Cytokines as potential vaccine adjuvants

Anju Nohria & Robert H. Rubin
*From the Center for Experimental Pharmacology and Therapeutics, Harvard-M.I.T. Division of Health Sciences and Technology, Cambridge, Massachusetts, 02142**

Key words: cytokines, vaccines, vaccine adjuvants

Abstract

There is a compelling clinical need for adjuvants suitable for human use to enhance the efficacy of vaccines in the prevention of life-threatening infection. Candidate populations for such vaccine-adjuvant strategies include normal individuals at the two extremes of life, as well as the ever increasing population of immunocompromised individuals. In addition, adjuvants that would increase the efficiency of vaccination with such vaccines as those directed against hepatitis B and *Streptococcus pneumoniae* would have an even greater general use. Cytokines, as natural peptides intimately involved in the normal immune response, have great appeal as potential adjuvants. An increasing body of work utilizing recombinant versions of interleukin-l, -2, -3, -6, -12, gamma-interferon, tumor necrosis factor, and granulocyte-monocyte-colony stimulating factor has shown that cytokines do have vaccine adjuvant activity. However, in order to optimize adjuvant effect and minimize systemic toxicity, strategies in which the cytokine is fused to the antigen, or the cytokine is presented within liposomes or microspheres appear to be necessary to make this a practical approach suitable for human use. There is much promise in this approach, but there is much work to be accomplished in order to optimize the pharmacokinetics of cytokine administration as well as its side effect profile.

Abbreviations: IL: interleukin; TNF: tumor necrosis factor; NK: natural killer; pIL-1: interleukin-1 peptide; LPS: lipopolysaccharide; r: recombinant; HSV-2: herpes simplex virus 2; γ: gamma

The prevention of clinical infection, rather than its treatment, is the goal of all practitioners. Although desirable for the entire population, the need for an effective preventative strategy is particularly great in those individuals whose host defenses against infection are attenuated by age, metabolic disturbance, immunosuppressing illness, or immunosuppressive therapy. At present, the most generally effective infection prevention strategy involves the use of vaccines. However, even with the currently licensed vaccines, certain problems remain: several vaccines are relatively weak antigens, and require either a series of injections over time to confer immunity or regular booster shots to maintain immunity; both neonates and the elderly, populations in particular need for vaccine protection, have attenuated responses to many vaccines; and immunocompromised patients may respond not at all, or only transiently, to conventional immmunizing programs. There is, then, a compelling need for vaccination programs that will successfully immunize those individuals with the greatest need for vaccine induced protection, preferrably with a single immunization that will provide sustained protection. Neither currently available vaccines nor those in development accomplish this, and alternative strategies are needed. Perhaps the most promising approach to this problem involves the use of immunomodulators, administered in conjunction with appropriate vaccines, to improve vaccine efficacy [1].

* Address for reprints: Dr. Robert h. Rubin, Director, HST Center for Experimental Pharmacology and Therapeutics, Massachusetts Institute of Technology, Clinical Research Center, 40 Ames Street, Building E18-435, Cambridge, Massachusetts 02142-1308.

Immunomodulators are biological or non-biological substances that "directly influence a specific immune function or modify one or more components of the immunoregulatory network to achieve an indirect effect on a specific immune function"[2]. An adjuvant is an immunomodulator that acts in a non-specific manner to augment specific immunity to an antigen [3]. Adjuvants are employed to (i) make antigens more immunogenic, (ii) increase the immune response in a situation where the antigen is limited, (iii) elicit an immune response in populations that are immunocompromised, and (iv) accentuate particular aspects of an immune response, whether it be humoral or cellular immunity. This last appears to be determined by which subset of cells, as determined by the profile of cytokines produced, is produced from previously naive CD4 positive T cells: T_H1 cells which produce interleukin-2 and γ-interferon and mediate the cellular immune response; and T_H2 cells that produce interleukins -4, -5, and -10, and stimulate the humoral immune response. An important aspect of adjuvant function is which of these two CD4 T-cell differentiation patterns is stimulated [4].

At present, only aluminum compounds are licensed for use as human adjuvants. These are prepared either by precipitating the antigen with a solution of alum or by adsorbing the antigen onto preformed aluminum compounds such as aluminum phosphate or hyroxide. Aluminum compounds accomplish their adjuvant function by two mechanisms: they may serve as an antigen depot, slowing the time of antigen absorption and elimination, thereby prolonging the time period during which antigen can interact with antigen presenting cells and lymphocytes. Alternatively, aluminum compounds may lead to an increased immune response by inducing an inflammatory response at the site of injection. Aluminum based formulations have been used successfully for diphtheria and tetanus toxoid vaccines, cholera vaccines in children under five years of age, and rabies vaccines. However, they appear to be useful only in circumstances that require augmentation of humoral immunity and are relatively ineffective with antigens that require a cell mediated response. Moreover, aluminum based formulations do not work for all antigens, cannot be lyophilized (therefore, requiring refrigeration for the vaccine), and can induce an anaphylactic response [3]. There is, thus, a continuing need for additional effective non-toxic adjuvants that will increase the immune response to different vaccines, especially for those antigens that need to induce cell mediated immunity.

Cytokines are immunomodulatory proteins that are secreted by a variety of cells, particularly those involved in the immune response. They are known to mediate the adjuvant effects of such biologic products as lipopolysaccharide (LPS), but have only recently themselves been studied as possible immune adjuvants [4,5]. Cytokines are particularly attractive as potential adjuvants for several reasons: advances in recombinant technology have made cytokines abundantly available for study; they represent natural proteins that are unlikely to elicit an allergic response; and initial studies have shown them to have potential efficacy as adjuvants for viral, bacterial, and parasitic vaccines in animal models. Furthermore, the use of cytokines may allow one to selectively enhance particular immune parameters that are needed to optimize the effects of a particular vaccine. In this review, we will review the evidence supporting the use of cytokines as vaccine adjuvants, and delineate both the problems and the opportunities inherent with this approach. In doing so, the effects of cytokines in augmenting both the cell mediated and humoral (T-cell dependent and independent) immune responses will be assessed.

Studies in animal models

Interleukin-1

Interleukin-1 (IL-1) is a primary mediator of fever and the acute phase response. Specifically, IL-1 enhances cell mediated immunity by activating T cells and increasing T cell expression of both IL-2 and the IL-2 receptor. IL-1 also acts synergistically with IL-4 to activate B cells, augmenting the humoral arm of the immune response. It also stimulates non-specific immunity through the activation of natural killer (NK) cells, in combination with IL-2 and gamma-interferon. It is likely that much of the adjuvant effect that occurs following the injection of the bacterial cell wall components LPS and muramyl. dipeptide are mediated by an IL-1 response, since both LPS and muramyl dipeptide stimulate the release of IL-1 from macrophages [6,7]. These increase T cell dependent antibody responses following antigen administration [8,9]. On the basis of these observations, IL-1 became a likely candidate as a vaccine adjuvant.

The first direct evidence that IL-1 could be used as an adjuvant came from studies by Staruch and Wood [10], which demonstrated the following: the administration of 1000-3000 lymphocyte activating factor units of a purified IL-1 preparation intraperitoneally two hours after the subcutaneous administration of bovine serum albumin (BSA) led to a 20 fold increase in anti-BSA antibody levels after a booster immunization with BSA alone. Subsequently, it was shown that recombinant human IL-1β (r-hu-IL-1β) was capable of increasing the number of plaque forming cells to sheep red blood cells (a T cell dependent B cell response) and to a T cell independent carbohydrate antigen derived from *Streptococcus pneumoniae*[11]. In this study the number of antibody producing spleen cells (the plaque forming cells) was increased with both primary and secondary exposure to sheep red blood cells, with the secondary response being increased regardless of whether the cytokine was administered at the time of primary antigen exposure or with the booster dose. The antibody response to both the sheep red blood cells and the pneumococcal antigen occurred even though the antigenic challenge was administered at a separate site from the IL-1.

Although IL-1 was found to be effective as an adjuvant, it exerted significant pyrogenic effects at the doses required for optimal adjuvant activity [11]. Nencioni, et al [11], identified an IL-1B peptide fragment corresponding to residues 163-171 (pIL-1) which lacked the pyrogenicity of IL-1 but retained the adjuvant activity of IL-1 when used at significantly higher doses (50 mg/kg of pIL-1 were equivalent to 10 mg/kg of intact IL-1). In other studies, the intraperitoneal administration of a fusion protein consisting of pIL-1 and hepatitis B surface antigen (HBsAg, residues 12–32) resulted in secondary antibody levels that were greater than those obtained with the administration of a mixture of pIL-1 and H BsAg [12].

Studies with tumor cell vaccines have demonstrated the following: McCune and Marquis [13] have reported that rIL-1a, rIL-1β, and pIL-1 act as effective vaccine adjuvants in combination with an irradiated tumor cell vaccine in BALB/c mice challenged with alveolar cell lung tumor cells. Their results showed that the daily administration of r IL-1α and -β intradermally near the site of antigen exposure or subcutaneously at a distant site, for eight consecutive days after antigen administration, rendered 7 out of 10 mice tumor free compared with 2 out of 10 animals treated with the vaccine alone. The adjuvanticity of rIL-1 was directly proportional to the dosage and the the number of doses administered. High doses of rIL-1α and -β were associated with pro-inflammatory side effects which were significantly reduced by using pIL-1. However, far higher doses of the peptide fragment were required to exert an equivalent adjuvant effect. In other studies [14], rIL-1, but not pIL-1, was effective as an adjuvant in inducing specific immunity to sialyl-Tn, a carbohydrate antigen expressed by several carcinomas.

These experiments suggest that IL-1, but not pIL-1, is an effective adjuvant against both T-cell dependent protein antigens and T-cell independent carbohydrate antigens. Therefore, the use of IL-1 as a vaccine adjuvant potentially overcomes one of the major deficiencies associated with the use of currently available aluminum adjuvants. IL-1, thus, could be useful in potentiating the effects of pneumococcal and other carbohydrate antigen vaccines. The adjuvant effects occur regardless of the site of injection relative to the site of antigen administration, emphasizing the systemic aspects of this process. It does appear that multipe doses of IL-1 are required for optimal adjuvant effect. The mechanism by which IL-1 accomplishes its adjuvant effect is presumably through its ability to activate T helper cells and B cells [15–17].

Peptide fragments of IL-1, such as pIL-1, eliminate many of the systemic side effects associated with the administration of intact IL-1. However, pIL-1 is not an effective adjuvant for carbohydrate antigens [14], and much higher doses are required than for the intact molecule [11,13]. It is conceivable that segments of the IL-1 protein other than pIL-1 (residues 163–171) either alone or in combination could overcome these defects. Alternatively, the fusion of one or another of these fragments with the antigen may be a better strategy for reducing the dosage of the IL-1 peptide fragments needed for an adjuvant effect [12].

Interleukin-2

Interleukin-2 (IL-2) is a cytokine secreted by activated T-helper cells that is capable of stimulating the growth and proliferation of antigen specific helper-, cytotoxic-, and suppressor-T cells. These activated T-cells in turn produce cytokines such as IL-4, 5, and 6 that promote the differentiation of antigen specific B-cells. IL-2 also promotes the secretion of r-interferon by activated T-cells. r-interferon induces the expression of Major Histocompatibility Complex (MHC) Class II molecules on the surfaces of antigen presenting cells (APC), thus further enhancing cellular immunity [15,18]. In view of all these actions of IL-2, it is not surprising that it has been studied extensively as a potential vaccine adjuvant, especially with antigens that elicit a cell mediated immune response.

Anderson, *et al.*, [19] demonstrated that IL-2 enhances the immune response to *H. pleuropneumoniae* vaccine in swine. In these experiments, swine were immunized with a mixture of IL-2 and bacterin from *H. pleuropneumoniae* and with IL-2 alone for 5 days thereafter. The animals received a booster dose of the antigen-IL-2 mixture on day 21 and were challenged intranasally with a virulent strain of *H. pleuropneumoniae* on day 42. The protective effect of IL-2 was measured by comparing the number of diseased lungs at necropsy between the groups of animals receiving IL-2 and those receiving bacterin alone. They found that daily treatment with IL-2 at the time of antigen presentation and for 5 days thereafter resulted in <1% infected lungs as compared with 32% in animals treated with a single dose of vaccine alone. Moreover, protection from disease was markedly enhanced with multiple injections of IL-2 (<1%) as opposed to a single additional dose of IL-2 (16%).

IL-2 has been succcessfully used as an adjuvant in conferring immunity to herpes simplex virus 2 (HSV-2) in a guinea pig model. In these studies guinea pigs were immunized subscutaneously with two or three doses of a crude extract of HSV-2 or recombinant glycoprotein D devived from HSV-2 at two week intervals. In addition, a group of animals were injected subcutaneously with 5×10^4 units of rIL-2 daily for 17 days. The animals were then challenged intravaginally with HSV-2 on day 23. Both the incidence and severity of clinical disease were significantly lower in those that had received both the vaccine and IL-2 as opposed to those who were immunized with vaccine alone. Of particular interest, rechallenge of these animals with HSV-2 two months later, resulted in continued protection in 75% of animals, suggesting that long term immunity was provided by the vaccine-IL-2 combination [20].

The daily administration of 0.03–0.1 mg/g of rIL-2 in conjuction with inactivated rabies vaccine was able to increase the potency of the vaccination at least 25 fold in mice, as measured by survival following challenge with live rabies virus. In this study, the mice were vaccinated twice intraperitoneally, on days 1 and 7, with rIL-2 administered via twice daily subcutaneous injection for five days after each antigen dose [21]. Of interest, protection was not correlated with the level of antibody achieved, an observation also noted in the swine *H. pleuropneumoniae* experiments [19]. These findings suggest the importance of an augmented cell mediated immune response in effecting protection in these systems. Further support for the belief that IL-2 has an important effect in augmenting the cytotoxic T cell response in these systems comes from the observation that T cell mediated lysis of HSV-2 infected fibroblasts was significantly higher in animals that had received both vaccine and rIL-2, as opposed to vaccine alone. This cytotoxic activity correlated with the degree of disease protection [20].

Presently available data suggest that IL-2 is only effective against T-cell dependent antigens, and is effective only when administered in multiple doses. Like IL-l, IL-2 also appears to be active as an adjuvant regardless of the site of administration relative to that of the antigen.

Interleukin-3

Interleukin-3 (IL-3) is a cytokine derived from activated T cells. It does not appear to directly stimulate the proliferation or growth of any cells of the B- or T-cell lineage, but it may have a role in the proliferation and differentiation of macrophages, and thus may modulate the immune response by affecting antigen presentation [22].

Continuous perfusion for one week with rIL-3 in mice one day before immunization with Human IgG resulted in a five fold increase in the level of antibody to the human protein as compared to the response when the protein was administered alone. Immunization with the antigen one day after the perfusion with the IL-3 resulted in no increased immunity. The IL-3 infusion did not result in any increased response against a T-cell independent polysaccharide antigen [22].

Thus, like many other cytokines, IL-3 appears to be useful only with T-cell dependent antigens. The fact that its presence is essential at the time of antigen administration for an adjuvant effect to be observed suggests that its enhancement of antigen presentation to T-helper cells is a transient phenomenon requiring its physical presence to occur.

Interleukin-6

Interleukin-6 (IL-6) is a cytokine produced by activated T-cells that is involved in the final maturation of B-cells into plasma cells. When human recombinant IL-6 is administered to mice inoculated with sheep red blood cells, both the primary and secondary antibody response are enhanced. *In vitro* experiments assessing the primary response of murine B cell-enriched spleen cells to sheep red blood cells revealed that IL-6 was capable of increasing the number of spleen cells that were responsive to sheep red blood cells. The specificity of the adjuvant effect in this case was shown by the observation that antibodies against IL-6 inhibited this response. T-cell and macrophage depleted spleen cell preparations resulted in a decreased augmentation of the immune response, suggesting that IL-6 probably requires other cytokines to optimize its adjuvant activity- a property probably true of most of the cytokines; that is, combinations may well be more potent than individual molecules [23].

Interleukin-12

Interleukin-12 (IL-12) is produced by macrophages, and stimulates α-interferon production by both NK cells and T-cells. IL-12 promotes the development of a T_H1 cellular response when administered in conjunction with a vaccine. The net result is enhanced cell mediated immunity to the antigen(s) that were administered with it. Thus, in a mouse model of leishmaniasis, a striking protective effect was shown when IL-12 was administered with vaccine, whereas the vaccine itself was ineffective [4]. It has been shown that many bacteria and their products (including *Listeria monocytogenes*, lipopolysaccharide, *Staphylococcus aureus*, *Mycobacterium tuberculosis*, and *Corynebacterium parvum*) when used as vaccine adjuvants do so by stimulating IL-12 production by macrophages [24,25]. Since IL-12 administration appears to be relatively free of many of the systemic side effects associated with bacterial adjuvant administration, it appears to be a very promising adjuvant strategy for those systems where stimulation of a cell mediated immune response appears to be important.

Tumor necrosis factor

Tumor necrosis factor (TNF) enhances the expression of MHC antigens on endothelial cells, fibroblasts, and T cells. It activates neutrophils and induces the release of colony stimulating factors. It also induces prostaglandin secretion by fibroblasts and synovial cells, and has been shown to potentiate antiviral activity. *In vivo*, TNF is a major pyrogen and has been implicated as a mediator of cachexia and many of the clinical manifestations of gram negative sepsis [15]. The similarity in the biological properties of TNF and IL-1 has led to the speculation that TNF might also be used to specifically manipulate the immune response if delivered in conjunction with a vaccine.

Ghiara, et al, [26] demonstrated that a single dose of 1 ng/kg of human recombinant TNF-α increased the number of plaque forming cells in response to T-cell dependent sheep red blood cells, when administered subcutaneously at the same time as an intravenous injection of the antigen. Unlike IL-1β, however, rTNF-α was unable to augment the immune response to the T-cell independent pneumococcal polysaccharide antigen. Because of this, and because of its profound systemic effects, it is unlikely that TNF will be developed further as a vaccine adjuvant.

Gamma-Interferon

Gamma-interferon (γ-IFN) is a product of activated T-cells, serving to activate macrophages to produce its array of proinflammatory cytokines, while also upregulating the MHC Class II molecule expression on these antigen presenting cells [15]. These properties make α-IFN an obvious candidate for use as a vaccine adjuvant.

Playfair and DeSouzaz [27] first demonstrated the adjuvant effect of γ-IFN when it was used with a *Plasmodium yoelii* murine malaria vaccine. The administration of 5000 units of γ-IFN intraperitoneally at the same time and site on two occasions, two weeks apart, conferrred over 90% immunity to mice challenged with a lethal dose of parasitized red blood cells. Moreover, they showed that antibody, delayed type hypersensitivity (DTH), and T-helper cell responses were all increased with the use of r-IFN as an adjuvant. The increased survival was a result of the adjuvant effect of the γ-IFN rather than a direct result of γ-IFN on the parasitized cells, since no survival benefit was seen with γ-IFN alone.

The administration of rγ-IFN at the time of primary immunization with glycoprotein G of vesicular stomatitis viruse enhanced the secondary antibody response to a booster dose of the viral protein [28]. In each of these studies, γ-IFN was most effective when administered at the same time and site as the vaccine antigen. To insure γ-IFN delivery with the antigen, Heath and Playfair [29] conjugated biotinylated γ-IFN with avidin antigen and compared the DTH and antibody response to avidin in mice immunized with the conjugate or with avidin and γ-IFN. They noted a 50% increase in the DTH response and no significant difference in the antibody response in animals immunized with the conjugate. An explanation proposed to explain the increased adjuvanticity of the conjugate is that it allows specific activation of those antigen presenting cells that phagocytose the antigen, thus resulting in a more focused increase in the immune response.

In studies particularly relevant to the immunocompromised host, Heath, et al, [5] deomonstrated that γ-IFN could increase the response rate to a malaria vaccine in different strains of immunocompromised mice. They inoculated several strains of immunodeficient mice with two biweekly doses of P, yoelii vaccine mixed with γ-IFN as an adjuvant. Biozzi low responder mice, which normally produce low levels of antibody, were 100% protected against lethal challenge by the addition of the γ-IFN to the vaccine; mice administered only the vaccine were totally unprotected. Mice depleted of CD4 cells by the use of cytotoxic anti-CD4 monoclonal antibody, also showed 50–66% increased survival when γ-IFN was added to the vaccine. In contrast, IL-1 administered accoring to the same schedule as the γ-IFN did not confer any added benefit to the vaccine in these immunodeficient mice.

γ-IFN probably acts as an adjuvant by increasing MHC Class II expression on macrophages and dendritic cells. The increase in MHC Class II expression allows for increased contact between the MHC-antigen complex and the T cell receptor, causing enhanced T helper cell proliferation and augmentation of both humoral and cellular immunity. Efforts to elucidate the exact mechanism by which-γ-IFN functions as a vaccine adjuvant were greatly helped by studies in which it was shown that the administration of γ-IFN either prior to the antigen or with the antigen promotes the T_H1 response, thus augmenting a cell mediated immune response.

Granulocyte-macrophage colony stimulating factor

Granulocyte-macrophage colony stimulating factor (GM-CSF) is a cytokine produced by T-cells, endothelial cells, fibroblasts, and macrophages that is involved in the proliferation of hematopoietic progenitor cells and the activation of macrophage antimicrobial activity. For purposes of this discussion, it is particularly important that GM-CSF augments both cellular and humoral immunity by increasing the expression of MHC Class II antigens on such antigen presenting cells as the dendritic cells [15].

The ability of GM-CSF to increase MHC Class II expression on antigen presenting cells suggested that GM-CSF could be useful as a vaccine adjuvant. In a series of elegant studies, Dranoff, et al, [30] have introduced retroviruses that cause the expression of GM-CSF into irradiated murine tumor cells. When these were injected into mice, those irradiated tumor cells that express GM-CSF were far more effective as anti-tumor vaccines than cells expressing IL-2, IL-4, IL-5, IL-6, γ-IFN, or TNF (although cells expressing IL-4 and IL-6 did induce some enhanced anti-tumor activity). Neither GM-CSF itself nor irradiated, non-transduced tumor cells were able to confer tumor immunity. Moreover, the tumor cell-GM-CSF constructs conferred immunity only to the specific tumor used, not to a different murine tumor. Selective depletion of CD4, CD8, and NK cells in the experimental animals demonstrated that both CD4 and CD8 T-cells are required for the adjuvant activity of GM-CSF. These observations are consistent with the hypothesis that GM-CSF promotes antigen presentation of the irradiated tumor cells to the CD4 cells, and these in turn activate specific anti-tumor cytotoxic CD8 cells.

The administration of GM-CSF is not without side effects, however. Phase I and II clinical trials using GM-CSF to increase the number of leukocytes in patients who were neutropenic from recent chemotherapy showed that the use of GM-CSF was associated with significant side effects [31,32]. At low doses (3–15 mg/kg), the common adverse effects included fever, rigors, bone pain, and rashes. Higher doses (20–30 mg/kg) were associated with pericarditis and liver function abnormalities. The problem, then, is one of drug delivery- the systemic administration of sufficient GM-CSF to effect adjuvant function causes unacceptable side effects. Either novel methods of drug delivery or the identification of peptide fragments that have adjuvant activity without the systemic effects will be necessary if the promising adjuvant effects of this cytokine are to be translated into an effective immunization strategy.

The use of cytokines as vaccine adjuvants in humans

Thus far, there is limited information available as to the potential utility of cytokines as vaccine adjuvants in humans. In uremic patients (whose response rate to hepatitis B vaccine without adjuvant varies from 44–74%)[1] the administration of IL-2 to individuals who had previously failed to respond to three or more doses of hepatitis B vaccine appeared quite promising. Six out of ten of these patients who received hepatitis B vaccine followed by 2.5×10^5 units of IL-2 one hour later at the same site, showed protective anti-H BsAg titers for up to 15 weeks after immunization as opposed to no response in the untreated patients. Moreover, the antibody response was specific in that preexisting antibodies to cytomegalovirus did not increase in titer. One mechanism proposed to explain the action of IL-2 in this instance is that IL-2 circumvented the need for macrophage cytokines for T-cell activation (macrophage dysfunction being hypothesized as the defect in these uremic individuals), thus accentuating a vaccine response to this T-cell dependent antigen [33].

In another study involving uremic patients, Quiroga, et al, [34] immunized a group of hemodialysis patients with either recombinant hepatitis B virus vaccine alone or together with 2 million units/m^2 or rγ-IFN at 0, 1, and 6 months. There was no difference in the rate of seroconversion after the full course of treatment, but the group receiving the rγ-IFN seroconverted at an earlier time (4 months rather than 7 months after the initial immunization), and achieved significantly higher titers of antibody than those receiving the vaccine alone. Since the height of titer achieved after the course of immunization is a good predictor of the duration of immunity, this finding could :be clinically significant.

In sum, these results are consistent with the hypothesis that cytokines could have similar effects as vaccine adjuvants in humans as in experimental animals.

Future considerations and challenges

Although the study of cytokines as potential vaccine adjuvants is clearly in its infancy, certain conclusions appear to be warranted at the present time: (i) Cytokines clearly have potentially beneficial adjuvant effects, even in circumstances of immunocompromise, both in terms of inducing an increased response to a given vaccine and in terms of favoring a particular form of response; i.e., a T_H1 response over a T_H2 response; (ii) Particularly encouraging are observations that the adjuvant effects of cytokines do not, in most cases, require administration of the cytokine at the same anatomical site as the vaccine, the notable exception to this being γ-IFN; (iii) The biggest challenge to the success of cytokines as vaccine adjuvants have to do with classical clinical pharmacologic issues of drug delivery and dosimetry. The solution of these problems will be the ultimate determinant of whether or not cytokines will be useful medically for the purpose of optimizing vaccine responses.

In general, cytokines are peptides with short half-lives whose primary physiologic function is to facilitate cell-to-cell communication and interaction due to their autocrine and paracrine effects. With many cytokines, the endocrine effects of these peptides, when they reach the general circulation, are extensive and may be quite injurious to the individual. There are two issues, then, of drug delivery that come from these observations: Is the short biologic half-life of most cytokines compatible with a useful vaccine adjuvant effect; and how does one optimize local delivery and minimize the systemic effects of the cytokine being administered? The available animal data suggests that continuing plasma levels may be important in terms of mediating their adjuvant effect. Thus, IL-1, IL-2, and GM-CSF must be administered not only on the day of antigen administration but repeatedly over several days to obtain optimal adjuvant effects [10,13,19–21,30]. Thus far, γ-IFN has been the only cytokine that has been shown to offer a signficant adjuvant effect with a single dose given at the same time as the antigen [27–29].

Several strategies have been investigated in order to prolong the half-life of particular cytokines following single injections: Nunberg, et al, [21] conjugated IL-2 to polyethylene glycol. This molecule was found to be as effective as twice daily IL-2 administered for 5 days after rabies vaccine administration, when it was given once daily for the same number of days at half the IL-2 dosage. These investigators also attempted to deliver IL-2 as an oil-water emulsion with the rabies vaccine as two single doses at days 0 and 7. Unfortunately, no increased protective vaccine effect was observed with this regimen. An oil/water emulsion of IL-2 and vaccine was observed to induce an increased antibody response to myoglobin in mice that are genetically low responders to this antigen [35], as well as to a *Plasmodium falciparum* circumsporozoite protein antigen [36]. It would seem likely, then, that different antigen-cytokine combinations will require different formulations to optimize their interaction in achieving optimal immunization.

An entirely different approach involves the use of fusion proteins expressing an immunogen and the cytokine in the same molecule. This stratey increases the half-life of the cytokine *in vivo* and presumably allows the use of fewer doses by a more focused accentuation of the immune response. Hazama, et al [37], used a truncated HSV-1 glycoprotein D and human IL-2 fusion protein as a vaccine against HSV-1 infection in BALB/c mice. A single injection with 1 mg of this fusion protein resulted in complete protection from HSV-1 challenge, a result also achieved with the administration of the antigen with Freund's complete adjuvant (a strategy unacceptable for human use) but not achieved with a single dose of antigen and rIL-2. This fusion protein does not act as a haptene carrier, but rather is acting as an antigen plus adjuvant, as the antibody titer was increased to the HSV-1 glycoprotein but not to IL-2. The *in vivo* half life of IL-2 administered in this fashion is increased four-fold. It has been proposed that the mechanism of the adjuvant effect in this circumstance is that the IL-2 component of the fusion protein binds to IL-2 receptors on NK cells and thus stimulates the secretion of GM-CSF which induces IL-2 receptor expression on dendritic antigen presenting cells. The fusion protein then binds these cells via the IL-2 moiety and promotes antigen presentation of the vaccine antigen, thus accentuating the specific immune response. Thus, both the half-life of the cytokine is prolonged, and its delivery to relevant sites is accentuated, possibly limiting systemic toxicity while increasing the immune response.

In analogous fashion, the administration of a fusion protein consisting of a B-cell lymphoma idiotype and GM-CSF resulted in 40–60% long term survival following tumor challenge in animals. This survival rate was significantly better than that achieved in animals immunized with the combination of idiotype and keyhole limpet hemocyanin or idiotype plus rGM-CSF [38].

An interesting approach that combines elements of both of the previously discussed delivery systems involves the incorporation of cytokines in liposomes or in polymeric microspheres. This not only increases the half-life of the cytokine, but it also targets its delivery to such cells as macrophages. Mbawuike, et al [39], demonstrated that the administration of IL-2 containing liposomes mixed with low dose influenza vaccine provided as much immunity as high dose vaccine alone. In this study, there was an increase in the level of neutralizing antibodies but not in the level of virus-specific cytotoxic T-cells. Liposomal incorporation of antigen also increases its immunogenicity [40]. This effect was further enhanced when IL-6 containing liposomes were administered at the same time as the antigen containing liposomes. Mixture of the antigen and the IL-6 in the same liposome, however, for reasons that are currently unclear, resulted in decreased antibody levels. Finally, Singh-Hora, et al [41], have encapsulated polyethylene glycol conjugated IL-2 in biodegradable poly-lactic/glycolic acid microspheres that allow the sustained release of a small amount of IL-2 for periods of weeks to months. It would be hoped that such a strategy would optimize adjuvant function and minimize systemic side effects associated with high pulse doses of the cytokine.

In sum, then, strategies are emerging for improving the pharmacokinetic properties and side effect profiles of cytokines for use as vaccine adjuvants. The strategies available range from the injection of single doses of r-IFN simultaneously at the same site with the antigen, to peptide fragments that maintain adjuvant effect without the systemic effects, to fusion proteins that simultaneously present antigen and adjuvant to the immune system, and novel delivery systems that provide low level, sustained cytokine +/- antigen delivery after a single immunization. At present, it would appear that the last two strategies are the most promising, but clearly much work remains to be carried out in this most promising area of scientific and clinical research [11, 13, 14, 35–43].

References

1. Hibberd PL, Rubin RH. Approach to immunization in the immunosuppressed host. Infectious Disease Clinics of North America 1990; 4: 123–142.
2. Fauci AS, Rosenberg SA, Sherwin SA, *et al.* Immunomodulators in clinical medicine. Ann Intern Med 1987; 106: 421–433.
3. Warren HS, Chedid LA. Future prospects for vaccine adjuvants. CRC Crit Rev Immunol 1988; 8: 83–101
4. Afonso LCC, Scharton JM, Vierira LQ, et al. The adjuvant effect of interleukin-12 in a vaccine against Leishmania major. Science 1994; 263: 235–237.
5. Heath AW, Devey ME, Brown IN, et al. Interferon-gamma as an adjuvant in immunocompromised mice. Immunology 1989; 67: 520–524.
6. Wood DD, Cameron PM. Relationship between bacterial endotoxin and human B-cell activating factor. J Immunol 1978; 121: 53–60.
7. Oppenheim JJ, Togawa A, Chedid L, et al. Components of mycobacteria and muramyl dipeptide with adjuvant activity induce lymphocyte factor. Cell Immunol 1980; 50: 71–81.
8. Skopinska E. Some effects of E. coli endotoxin on the graft-versus-host-reaction in ice. Transplant 1972; 14: 432–437.
9. Lowy I, Bona C, Chedid L. Target cells for the activity of the synthetic adjuvant: Muramyl dipeptide. Cell Immunol 1977; 29: 195–199.
10. Staruch MJ, Wood DD. The adjuventicity of interleukin 1 in vivo. J Immunol 1983; 130: 2191–2194.
11. Nencioni L, Villa L, Tagliabue A, et al. In vivo immunostimulatory activity of the 163–171 peptide of human IL-lb. J Immunol 1987; 139: 800–804.
12. Rao KVS, Nayak AR. Enhanced immunogenicity of a sequence derived from hepatitis B virus surface antigen in a composite peptide that includes the immunostimulatory region from interleukin 1. Proc Natl Acad Sci U S A 1990; 87: 5519–5522.
13. McCune CS, Marquis MM. Interleukin 1 as an adjuvant for active specific immunotherapy in a murine tumor model Cancer Res 1990; 50: 1212–1215.

14. Piera M, De Bolos C, Castro R, et al. Cytokines as adjuvants: Effect on the immunogenicity of NeuAca2-6GalNAca-O-Ser/Thr(SIALYL-Tn). Int J Cancer 1993; 55: 148–152.
15. van der Meer JWM. Defect in host defense mechanisms. In: Rubin RH, Young LS (ed.): Clinical Approach for Infection in the Compromised Host, New York, Plenum Medical Book Co, Third Edition, 1994.
16. Tagliabue A, Boraschi D. Cytokines as vaccine adjuvants: Interleukin 1 and its synthetic peptide 163–171. Vaccine 1993; 11: 594–595.
17. Dinarello CA. Interleukin-1. FASEB J 1988; 2: 108–115.
18. Kuziel WA, Green WC. Interleukin-2. In: Thomson A (ed.): The Cytokine Handbook, Academic Press, London, 1991, 83–102.
19. Anderson G, Urbano O, Fedorka-Cray P, et al. Interleukin 2 and protective immunity in Hemophilus pleuropneumoniae. Preliminary studies. In: Vaccines, Cold Spring Harbor Press, 1987, 22–25.
20. Weinberg A, Merigan TC. Recombinant interleukin 2 as an adjuvant for vaccine-induced protection: Immunization of guinea pigs with herpes simplex virus subunit vaccines. J Immunol 1988; 140: 294–299.
21. Numberg JH, Doyle MV, York SM, et al. Interleukin 2 acts as an adjuvant to increase the potency of inactivated rabies virus vaccine. Proc Natl Acad Sci U S A 1989; 86: 4240–4243.
22. Kimoto M, Kindler V, Higaki M, et al. Recombinant murine IL-3 fails to stimulate T or B lymphopoiesis in vivo, but enhances immune immune responses to T cell-dependent antigens. J Immunol 1988; 140: 1889–1894.
23. Takatsuki F, Okano A, Suzuki C, et al. Human recombinant IL6/B cell stimulatory factor 2 augments murine antigen-specific antibody responses in vitro and in vivo. J Immunol 1988; 141: 3072–3077.
24. Hsieh CS, Macatonia SE, Tripp CS et al. Development of TH1 CD4+ cells through IL-12 produced by Listeria-induced macrophages. Science 1993; 260: 547–549.
25. D'Andrea A, Rengaraju M, Valiante NM, et al. Production of natural killer cell stimulatory factor (interleukin 12) by peripheral blood mononuclear cells. J Exp Med 1992; 176: 1387–98.
26. Ghiara P, Boraschi D, Nencioni L, et al. Enhancement of in vivo immune response by tumor necrosis factor. J Immunol 1987; 139: 3676–3679.
27. Playfair JHL, DeSouza JB. Recombinant gamma interferon is a potent adjuvant for a malaria vaccine in mice. Clin Exp Immunol 1987; 6: 5–10.
28. Anderson KP, Fennie EH, Yilma T. Enhancement of a secondary antibody response to a vescicular stomatitis virus "G" protein by IFN-g treatment at primary immunization. J Immunol 1988; 140: 3500–3604.
29. Heath AW, Playfair JHL. Conjugation of interferon-gamma to antigen enhances its adjuvanticity. Immunology 1990; 71: 454–456.
30. Dranoff G, Jaffee E, Lazenby A, et al. Vaccination with irradiated tumor cells engineered to secrete murine granulocyte-macrophage colony-stimulating factor stimulates potent, specific, and long-lasting anti-tumor immunity. Proc Natl Acad Sci U S A 1993; 90: 3539–3543.
31. Leieschke GJ, Maher D, Cebon J, et al. Effects of bacterially synthesized recombinant human granulocyte-macrophage colony-stimulating factor in patients with advanced malignancy. Ann Intern Med 1989; 110: 357–364.
32. Gerhartz HH, Stern AC, Wolf-Hornung B, et al. Intervention treatment of established neutropenia with human recombinant granulocyte-macrophage colony-stimulating factor (rhGM-CSF) in patients undergoing cancer chemotheraphy. Leuk Res 1993; 17: 175–185.
33. Meuer SC, Dumann H, Meyer Zum Buschenfelde KH, et al. Low-dose interleukin-2 induces systemic immune responses against HBsAg in immunodeficient non-responders to hepatitis B vaccination. Lancet 1989; 1: 15–18.
34. Quiroga JA, Castillo I, Porres JC, et al. Rocombinant g-interferon as adjuvant to hepatitis B vaccine in hemodialysis patients. Hepatology 1990; 12: 661–663.
35. Kawamura H, Berzofsky JA, Rosenberg SA. Immunization with antigen and interleukin-2 in vivo overcomes IR gene low responsiveness. J Exp Med 1985; 162: 381–386.
36. Good MF, Pombo D, Lunde MN, et al. Recombinant human IL-2 overcomes genetic nonresponsiveness to malaria sporozoite peptides - correlation of effect with biological activity of IL-2. J Immunol 1988; 141: 972–977.
37. Hazama M, Mayumi-Aono A, Asakawa N, et al. Adjuvant-independent enhanced immune responses to recombinant herpes simplex virus type 1 glycoprotein D by fusion with biologically active interleukin-2. Vaccine 1993; 11: 629–636//
38. Tao M, Levy R. Idiotype/granulocyte-macrophage colony-stimulating factor fusion protein as a vaccine for B-cell lymphoma. Nature 1993; 362: 755–758.
39. Mbawuike IN, Wyde PR, Anderson PM, Enhancement of the protective efficacy of inactivated influenza A virus vaccine in aged mice by IL-2 liposomes. Vaccine 1990; 8: 347–352.
40. Duits AJ, van Puijenbroek A, Vermeulen H, et al. Immunoadjuvant activity of a liposomal IL-6 formulation. Vaccine 1993; 11: 777–781.
41. Sing-Hora M, Rana RK, Nunberg JH, et al. Controlled release of interleukin-2 from biodergradable microspheres. Biotechnology 1990; 8: 755–758.
42. Heath AW, Playfair JHL. Early administration of interferon-gamma as an adjuvant: an effect on a T-helper subpopulation ? Vaccine 1991; 91: 351–354.
43. Heath AW, Playfair JHL. Cytokines as immunological adjuvants. Vaccine 1992; 10: 427–434.

www.ingramcontent.com/pod-product-compliance
Ingram Content Group UK Ltd.
Pitfield, Milton Keynes, MK11 3LW, UK
UKHW050944290926
15470UKWH00005B/1631

* 9 7 8 0 7 9 2 3 3 2 6 7 1 *